Toxicokinetics and New Drug Development

Pergamon Titles of Related Interest

Dunn PARTITION COEFFICIENT
Roche BIOREVERSIBLE CARRIERS IN DRUG DESIGN
Yacobi/Halperin-Walega ORAL SUSTAINED RELEASE FORMULATIONS

Related Journals

(Free sample copies available on request)

PHARMACOLOGY & THERAPEUTICS
BIOCHEMICAL PHARMACOLOGY
CURRENT ADVANCES IN PHARMACOLOGY & TOXICOLOGY
GENERAL PHARMACOLOGY
JOURNAL OF PHARMACEUTICAL AND BIOMEDICAL ANALYSIS
LIFE SCIENCES
TOXICOLOGY IN VITRO

Toxicokinetics and New Drug Development

Edited by
Avraham Yacobi, Ph.D.
American Cyanamid Company, Lederle Laboratories
Pearl River, New York
Jerome P. Skelly, Ph.D.
The Food and Drug Administration
Rockville, MD
Vijay K. Batra, Ph.D.
American Cyanamid Company, Lederle Laboratories
Pearl River, New York

Cosponsored by
the American Association of
Pharmaceutical Scientists

PERGAMON PRESS
New York • Oxford • Beijing • Frankfurt
São Paulo • Sydney • Tokyo • Toronto

Pergamon Press Offices:

U.S.A.	Pergamon Press, Inc., Maxwell House, Fairview Park, Elmsford, New York 10523, U.S.A.
U.K.	Pergamon Press plc, Headington Hill Hall, Oxford OX3 0BW, England
PEOPLE'S REPUBLIC OF CHINA	Pergamon Press, Qianmen Hotel, Beijing, People's Republic of China
FEDERAL REPUBLIC OF GERMANY	Pergamon Press GmbH, Hammerweg 6, D-6242 Kronberg, Federal Republic of Germany
BRAZIL	Pergamon Editora Ltda, Rua Eça de Queiros, 346, CEP 04011, São Paulo, Brazil
AUSTRALIA	Pergamon Press Australia Pty Ltd., P.O. Box 544, Potts Point, NSW 2011, Australia
JAPAN	Pergamon Press, 8th Floor, Matsuoka Central Building, 1-7-1 Nishishinjuku, Shinjuku-ku, Tokyo 160, Japan
CANADA	Pergamon Press Canada Ltd., Suite 271, 253 College Street, Toronto, Ontario M5T 1R5, Canada

---

First edition 1989

Library of Congress Cataloging in Publication Data

Toxicokinetics and new drug development / edited by Avraham Yacobi, Jerome P. Skelly, Vijay K. Batra.
p. cm.
Includes index.
ISBN 0-08-036084-X
1. Pharmacokinetics. 2. Drugs--Toxicology. 3. Drugs--Testing. I. Yacobi, Avraham. II. Skelly, Jerome P. III. Batra, Vijay K., 1947- .
[DNLM: 1 Drug Evaluation. 2. Drugs--pharmacokinetics. 3. Drugs--toxicity. QV 771 T755]
RM301.5.T69 1989
615'.7--dc19
DNLM/DLC
for Library of Congress 88-28939
CIP

Printed in the United States of America

The paper used in this publication meets the minumum requirements of American National Standard for Information Sciences -- Permanence of Paper for Printed Library Materials, ANSI Z39.48-1984

Contents

Contributors

Vijay K. Batra

Pharmacodynamic Research, Medical Research Division, American Cyanamid Company, Pearl River, NY 10965

Harold Bernhard

Clinical Pharmacokinetics Laboratory, Millard Filmore Hospital, Gates Circle, Buffalo, NY 14209

John F. Brady

Department of Pharmacology, UCLA School of Medicine, Center for the Health Sciences, Los Angeles, CA 90024

Judith N. Burstyn

Department of Pharmacology, UCLA School of Medicine, Center for the Health Sciences, Los Angeles, CA 90024

Cheong C. Chah

Office of Drug Evaluation I, Center for Drug Evaluation and Research, Food and Drug Administration, Rockville, MD 20857

Willard Chappell

Center for Environmental Sciences and Department of Physics, University of Colorado at Denver 1200 Larimer St., Denver, CO 80204

Arthur K. Cho

Department of Pharmacology, UCLA School of Medicine, Center for the Health Sciences, Los Angeles, CA 90024

William E. Evans and John H. Rodman

Pharmacokinetics/Pharmacodynamics Section, Pharmaceutical Division, St. Jude Children's Research Hospital and Center for Pediatric Pharmacokinetics and Therapeutics, University of Tennessee, Memphis, TN 38105

Patricia L. Ebbeling

The Clinical Pharmacokinetics Laboratory, Millard Fillmore Hospital, 3 Gates Circle, Buffalo, NY 14209

Vera C. Glocklin

Office of Drug Evaluation I, Center for Drug Evaluation and Research, Food and Drug Administration, Rockville, MD 20857.

Peter Greaves

Park-Davis Research Institute, Sheridan Park, Mississauga, Ontario, Canada

Michael J. Iatropoulos

American Health Foundation, American Standard Testing Bureau, 6 Bruce Court, Suffern, NY 10901

Felix A. de la Iglesia

Department of Pathology and Experimental Toxicology, Parke-Davis Pharmaceutical Research, Warner Lambert Company, Ann Arbor, MI 48105

Gerhard Levy

Department of Pharmaceutics, School of Pharmacy, State University of New York at Buffalo 14260

Louis Lemberger

Eli Lilly and Company, Lilly Laboratory for Clinical Research, Wishard Memorial Hospital and the Department of Pharmacology, Medicine and Psychiatry, Indiana University School of Medicine, Indianapolis, IN 46202

Joyce Mordenti

Department of Pharmacological Sciences, Genentech Inc., 460 Point San Bruno Blvd., South San Francisco, CA 94080

John A. Morrison

Research and Development, Medical Research Division, American Cyanamid Company, Pearl River, NY 10965

Gabriela Nicolau

Pharmacodynamic Research, Medical Research Division, American Cyanamid Company, Pearl River, NY 10965

John H. Rodman

Pharmacokinetics/Pharmacodynamics Section, Pharmaceutical Division, St. Jude Children's Research Hospital and Center for Pediatric Pharmacokinetics and Therapeutics, University of Tennessee, Memphis, TN

K. Rozman

Department of Pharmacology, Toxicology and Therapeutics, University of Kansas Medical Center, Kansas City, KS 66103
and Institut fur Toxikologie der Gesellschaft fur Strahlen-und Umweltforschung Munchen mbH, D-8042 Neuherberg, Federal Republic of Germany

Jerome J. Schentag

The State University of New York at Buffalo, School of Pharmacy and Clinical Pharmacokinetics Laboratory, Millard Filmore Hospital, Buffalo, NY 14209

Robert Temple

Office of Drug Evaluation I, Center for Drugs and Biologics, Food and Drug Administration, Rockville, MD 20857

Alfred P. Tonelli

Pharmacodynamic Research, Medical Research Division, American Cyanamid Company, Pearl River, NY 10965

Grant R. Wilkinson

Department of Pharmacology, Vanderbilt University, School of Medicine, Nashville, TN 37232

Lynda L. Welage

The Clinical Pharmacokinetics Laboratory, Millard Filmore Hospital, Buffalo, NY 14209

Avraham Yacobi

Pharmacodynamic Research, Medical Research Division, American Cyanamid Company, Pearl River, NY 10965

Preface

Toxicokinetics combines the words *toxicology* and *kinetics* and is the application of pharmacokinetic principles to the investigation of toxicity and other adverse effects of drugs. Toxicokinetics encompasses the kinetics of absorption, distribution, metabolism, and elimination of large doses of drugs in the body and the safety evaluation and assessment of adverse reactions caused by excessive drug dosages. If applied rationally, toxicokinetics can be advantageous in drug development and therapy.

Generally, pharmacological activity and toxicity are associated with the blood and tissue concentrations of drugs, their metabolites, or both. It is well established that drug actions are better correlated with concentrations in blood and tissues than with administered dosages. Furthermore, the advances in analytical chemistry, separation methods, and instrumentation now easily allow the direct quantitation of drugs in the body and in the excreta. This quantitation has increasingly facilitated and encouraged the application of toxicokinetics in safety evaluation and in determining the exposure of animals to drugs. It accounts for the great interest shown by scientists in recent symposia and meetings held to address toxicokinetics and related issues.

This book provides reviews of the state of toxicokinetics and its role in drug development, with emphasis on the mechanisms of toxicity and the relationships between adverse effects and plasma concentrations in both animals and human beings. The chapters are arranged to provide continuity of subject matter. We are grateful to the distinguished scientists who contributed to the book. We are also thankful to the many pharmaceutical companies that provided generous contributions to make meetings of the American Association of Pharmaceutical Scientists and the symposia on this topic so very successful.

The authors hope that *Toxicokinetics and New Drug Development* will be helpful to pharmaceutical scientists engaged in safety assessment and drug development and to graduate students interested in this discipline. The book contains topics not reviewed adequately elsewhere and topics reviewed in literature not commonly followed by most toxicologists. The principles discussed in the book, although related to drugs, also apply to environmental and agricultural compounds. The book provides a forum for covering experimental and clinical toxicokinetics and their role in drug development.

Chapter 1

An Overview of Toxicokinetics

Vijay K. Batra and Avraham Yacobi

A few years ago, little pharmacokinetic information was included in a safety evaluation study protocol. Today, as part of the validation of safety studies and proof of exposure of animals to a test compound, many pharmaceutical companies have established either full or partial toxicokinetic programs. The support provided by these programs, however, is variable and depends largely on the drug development philosophy of the company. Nonetheless, strong evidence indicates that toxicokinetics is essential in the safety evaluation of potential drug candidates (1–6).

Toxicokinetics is defined as the application of kinetics of drug absorption, distribution, and elimination to safety evaluation studies in which traditionally large but subtoxic dosages of a test compound are administered to test species (7,8). The need of such application is obviated by the objective of the safety evaluation studies of assuring safety of a potential drug candidate within a specific dose range. Safety evaluation of drugs is costly, is of utmost importance in drug development, and can determine the fate of a potentially valuable product.

Many methods used in drug safety evaluations, including autopsy, histology, and hemotology, are empirical. They are based mostly on qualitative observations and sometimes lack a sound scientific rationale (1,9). For instance, the duration of conduct of a safety evaluation study to support the long-term clinical use of a drug is a matter of opinion. In the United Kingdom, a 6-month toxicity study done in two species is considered appropriate; in Canada, an 18-month study may be required; and in the United States, 12-month studies in a rodent and in a large animal are acceptable.

Some of the notable pitfalls of traditional toxicity testing methods (9) are as follows:

Methods are empirical and qualitative.

Data interpretation assumes complete drug absorption.

Assume animals handle high and low doses of the drug similarly.

Dosing conditions are different from those intended to be used clinically.

Species differences are usually ignored.

When an unusual toxicity is observed, the compound is abandoned and further development stopped without attempts to understand the fundamental reasons for the toxicity.

To interpret safety data when pharmacokinetic information is not available, one has to assume complete absorption of the drug. One must also assume that there is pharmacokinetic linearity between the doses being evaluated. These assumptions, unless tested, are groundless, because the kinetics of absorption, distribution, and elimination of large doses as given in safety evaluation studies can be completely different from the kinetics of smaller doses given for therapeutic purposes. For instance, what is the meaning of LD_{50} value of 5,000 mg/kg of a drug given orally when the LD_{50} of the same drug given intravenously is less than 100 mg/kg? Or, how can one claim that the highest tolerated dose of a drug is 5,000 mg/kg per day when the concentrations of the drug in blood for this high dose are essentially the same as those after the administration of the 250 mg/kg per day dose given orally?

One serious disadvantage of traditional safety evaluation testing is that when an unusual toxicity is observed, further development of the compound is generally stopped, with no attempts made to understand the mechanism of its toxicity. In many instances, the toxicity is simply due to selection of a very high dose or to the formation of a toxic metabolite that may be specific to the test species, with no relation to human beings at all. The addition of a sound toxicokinetic program to safety evaluation studies can help overcome some of these shortcomings. Since toxicokinetics deals with quantitative measures of drug dosing and body exposure, it will identify unanticipated toxicity if elicited by excessive and supratoxic dosages. Similarly, it will indicate if a lack of toxicity findings is a result of a lack of drug absorption. Overall, toxicokinetics will strengthen the safety evaluation studies and the interpretation of data, which in turn assures the administration of safe dosages to human beings.

Typical toxicokinetic support activities needed to substantiate safety evaluation data and to strengthen Investigational New Drug/New Drug Applications (IND/NDA) submission packages are as follows:

Mixed function oxidase induction potential

Selection of an optimal drug delivery system

Dose range selection

Short-term toxicity testing

Maximum tolerated dose

Species differences

Carcinogenicity, chronic toxicity, reproduction, fertility, and teratology studies

Age-dependent accumulation of drug/metabolites

Retrospective studies

In this overview, instances describing the usefulness of toxicokinetics are presented.

MIXED FUNCTION OXIDATION INDUCTION/INHIBITION

The potential of drugs to induce or inhibit the hepatic mixed function oxidase (MFO) system can be determined readily in rats using standard methodologies (10–12). Such determinations may be done early during the development of the compound, preferably during the predevelopment phase. The knowledge of potential liver enzyme induction is important for two reasons. First, it alerts the study director of the possible hepatic reaction or toxicity that may result from long-term use of the drug. Second, the information helps in the interpretation of the safety data because induction of a drug can lead to either lower plasma drug concentrations or higher metabolite concentrations that in turn determine the efficacy or toxicity of the drug or metabolite. Early availability of the MFO information can lead the pathologist to closer scrutiny of the liver tissues by electron microscopy. Unless there is a specific reason for including it, the electromicroscopic examination is usually not performed in the toxicology study protocol.

Enzyme induction is usually accompanied by enlargement of the liver and proliferation of the smooth endoplasmic reticulum system. In some cases, enzyme induction is the direct cause of hepatotoxicity. Table 1-1 shows an example of an association between the MFO induction and toxicity of five drugs in rats. Coincidentally, all four compounds that were shown to induce liver enzymes also showed hepatotoxicity. The MFO findings alone should not be used to select or reject a compound, but these data do suggest that in such instances the possibility of liver toxicity should be explored.

The MFO induction potential is usually dose dependent. Significant in-

Table 1-1. Correlation Between Mixed Function Oxidase Induction and Hepatotoxicity

Compound	Class	Induction	Hepatotoxicity
A	Diuretic	Yes	Hepatocellular necrosis
B[a]	Metabolite	High	Yes
C	Diuretic	No	No
D	Antiasthma	Yes	Preneoplastic nodules, rat
E	Antiasthma	Yes	Proliferation of bile duct
F	Anticancer	No	No

[a]Metabolite of A.

duction of the liver enzymes may occur at high dosages but not at low dosages. A case in point is an example of compound D, which, when given orally to monkeys at 5 mg/kg twice daily showed no induction, as indicated by the comparison of drug levels in the body on days 30 and 1 (Fig. 1-1). Typically, a predicted drug accumulation was attained. In contrast, at 20 mg/kg, the plasma concentrations on day 30 were significantly lower than

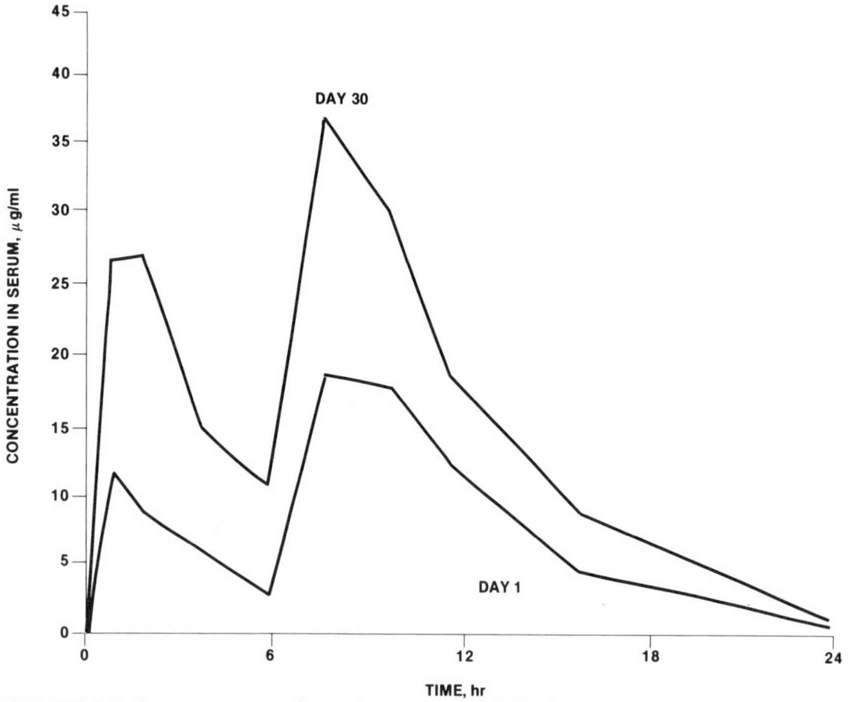

FIGURE 1-1. Serum concentrations of compound D following 5 mg/kg twice-daily administration to monkeys.

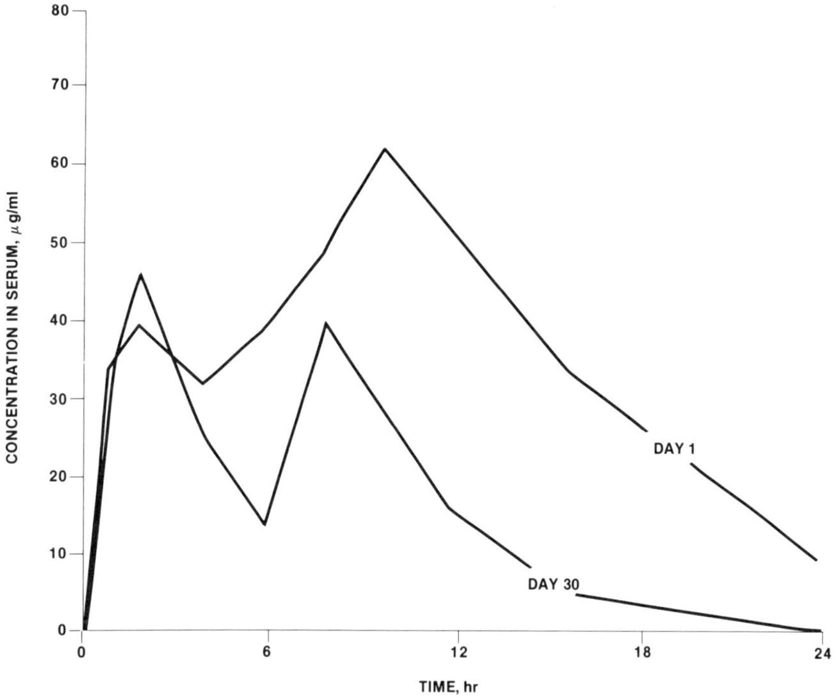

FIGURE 1-2. Serum concentrations of compound D following 20 mg/kg twice-daily administration to monkeys.

those on day 1 (Fig. 1-2). A compound with such behavior may cause more toxicity at lower doses and thus confuse the interpretation of the safety data. Occasionally, a compound might inhibit its own metabolism, thereby resulting in very high concentrations of unchanged drug in the blood, which in turn may lead to toxicity.

Repeated drug administration can influence the toxicity of the drug by changing its metabolism (MFO induction) and also by stimulating synthesis of certain proteins that can have an effect on drug activity. For example, Yacobi and colleagues (13) have shown that phenobarbital can produce a procoagulant effect on its own. The researchers showed that a 75 mg/kg intraperitoneal administration of phenobarbital for four days to Sprague-Dawley rats produces a significant increase of prothrombin complex activity (PCA) in plasma (Fig. 1-3). The rate constant for the decline of PCA after administration of a PCA synthesis-blocking dose of warfarin was not affected by treatment with phenobarbital, but the rate of synthesis of PCA was increased appreciably. It was concluded that phenobarbital increased synthesis of one or more clotting factors.

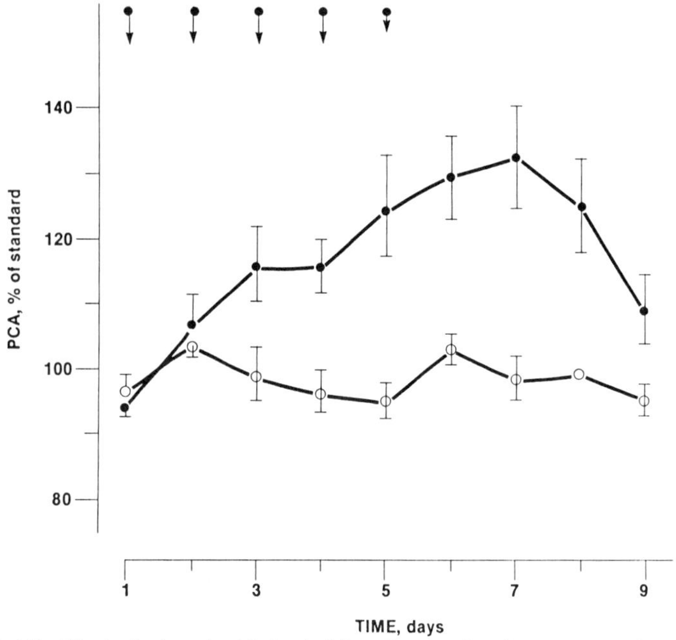

FIGURE 1-3. Effect of phenobarbital administration on the time course of prothrombin complex activity (PCA) in eight rats, determined in a crossover study. Phenobarbital injection times are indicated by long arrows (75 mg/kg) and short arrow (37.5 mg/kg). ○ = data obtained during the control phase (saline injection); ● = data obtained during and after treatment with phenobarbital. Vertical bars show standard error (13).

SELECTION OF AN OPTIMAL DRUG DELIVERY SYSTEM

In the safety evaluation studies, whenever possible the test compound is administered orally in a solution or a starch suspension to large animals, and as a drug-diet admixture to rodents. For soluble drugs, oral administration is acceptable, as exposure in most cases can be documented, but for many insoluble drugs, oral administration in suspension or drug-diet admixtures can lead to very poor drug absorption, thus leading to a lack of body exposure and consequently jeopardizing the entire safety evaluation study. A classical example is the experience with a hypolipidemic compound, CL 277,082, which is presently being tested. It is insoluble in water (<1 μg/ml) but quite soluble in various lipid solvents. In starch suspension it exhibited poor absorption (6–25%) (Table 1-2). Its absorption from various practical drug-delivery vehicles was evaluated, and the results are shown in Table 1-2. The absorption based on total radioactivity concentrations in serum was greater than 50 percent from triolein, oleic acid, and triolein

Table 1-2. Bioavailability of ^{14}C-CL 277,082 in the Monkey Following 20 mg/kg Oral Administration in Selected Drug Delivery Vehicles

Vehicle	Bioavailability[a] (%)
Starch	6–25
PEG 400	5–26
Triolein emulsion[b]	53–75
Neobee M5	14–23
Triolein	57–76
Ethyl oleate	22–29
Oleic acid	56–81
Diet	30–40

[a]Based upon comparison of the oral and intravenous serum total radioactivity data.

[b]Consisting of triolein, lecithin, and milk powder solution; 1.7 g lecithin per gram of drug.

emulsion and relatively very poor from the aqueous starch suspension. For initial safety evaluation studies, the emulsion was chosen for dosing drug to animals, but because of an unacceptable viscosity of this vehicle at high doses, it was dropped after the completion of the range-finding study. Oleic acid was chosen instead and found satisfactory in subsequent safety evaluation studies. The use of well-designed pharmacokinetic studies to select a drug-delivery vehicle proved to be extremely important in planning the safety evaluation program. In this case, had the toxicology studies proceeded in the monkey using starch suspension as a drug-delivery vehicle, the entire safety evaluation would have been compromised. In the rat, the absorption of this compound from the drug-diet admixture was close to 60 percent, and therefore this mode of administration was considered appropriate for the rat.

DOSE RANGE SELECTION

Before embarking on pivotal subchronic and chronic safety evaluation studies, range-finding studies are conducted to select a range of subtoxic doses for further evaluations. Traditionally, increasing doses of the test drug are given to animals daily for one to four weeks, and the animals are observed for signs of toxicity. The purpose is to select three or four treatment groups with tolerable doses ranging from a low to a high. The low dose is a small multiple of the intended human dose. The middle dose is selected to be one that presumably will give little or no toxic effect. And the high dose is usually selected to elicit some toxic response on chronic administration.

In the absence of data on blood drug concentrations, it is assumed that the increasing dose levels equate proportionally with a margin of safety (14). This assumption may be true in some cases in which doses administered are

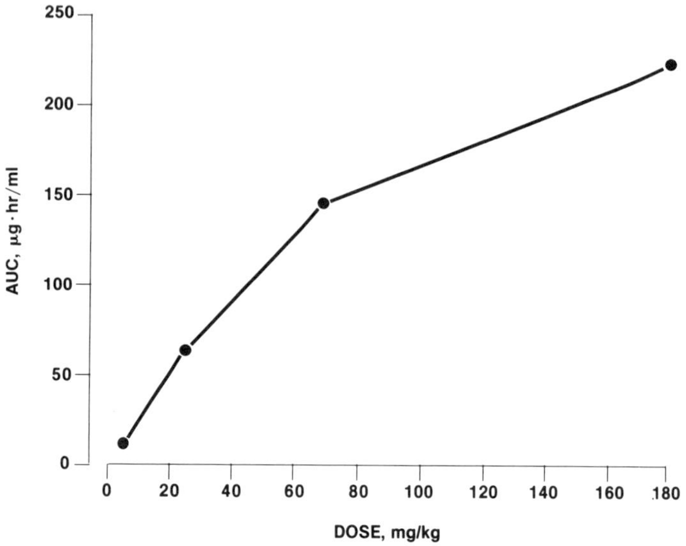

FIGURE 1-4. Correlation between the area under the serum radioactivity concentration-time curve and dose in the monkey following oral administration of 6–178 mg/kg of ^{14}C-CL 277,082 in oleic acid.

relatively small and adequate absorption occurs. But often this is an invalid assumption, because the dosages used in the safety evaluation studies are relatively high and can result in nonlinearity of absorption, distribution, metabolism, and excretion. For instance, Figure 1-4 shows the area under the serum drug concentration-time curve (AUC) as a function of dose for CL 277,082. As shown, the increase in the AUC with dose for this drug, when administered to monkeys in oleic acid, plateaus at about 200 mg/kg. In such a case, it is not meaningful to use very high doses, because no claim of tolerance beyond 200 mg/kg can be made. The plateau of the AUC with dose for CL 277,082 occurs because of saturation of absorption.

Because usually very high doses (relative to therapeutic doses) are used in the safety evaluation studies, observance of nonlinear pharmacokinetics of absorption, elimination, or both is very common; it becomes a rule rather than an exception. Toxicokinetics in the range-finding studies help in establishing a dose range in which the relationship between blood concentrations and dosage exists. These relationships introduce a quantitative measure in the study relating response to an accurate measure of the amount of drug absorbed rather than the dose administered. The knowledge can be useful in correlating toxicity with blood drug concentrations and in elucidating whether toxicity observed at any point during the short- or long-term safety evaluation is drug related.

SHORT-TERM SAFETY EVALUATION

Toxicology studies of one to three months' duration are often referred to as subchronic or short-term toxicity studies. Their purpose is to assure safety in animals over a predetermined dose range and to support the early single- and multiple-dose safety and tolerance studies in human beings involving 7- to 28-day dosing. As part of subchronic studies in animals, the toxicokinetic program will focus on providing data on assuring exposure of animals to the drug, confirming validity of the safety study, and determining the possibility of an unusual drug buildup on multiple dosing. Drug blood concentration monitoring, therefore, will serve as a quantitative measure in rationalizing the safety findings, particularly when unusual toxicity is observed in animals (3). Compound E, as shown in Table 1-3 is a good example of the usefulness of toxicokinetics in subchronic toxicity testing. The safety assessment studies with this compound were conducted in rats and dogs that received daily doses of the test compound for one month. In the rat, serum samples were obtained on days 0 and 29 of the study and analyzed for the unchanged drug. The results are shown in Table 1-3. The serum concentrations on day 29 as compared to the ones on day 0 declined significantly. During the same period, the animals exhibited liver toxicity. The data strongly indicated that the compound had resulted in the enzymatic induction of the liver enzymes and thus had produced lower serum concentrations upon multiple dosing. This induction, the formation of a possible toxic metabolite(s), or both may have been the direct cause of the toxicity.

The data in the dog were similar to those in the rat. The protocol of the one-month safety evaluation study was consequently modified to obtain a liver sample of the dog from both treated and control animals upon sacrificing on day 29 for necropsy. The liver samples were tested for indices of drug biotransformation functions. The microsomal concentrations of protein,

Table 1-3. Mean Serum Concentrations of Compound E in Male Rats Following Once-Daily Administration in Starch Suspension

Time (hr)	5 mg/kg per day[a]		60 mg/kg per day[a]	
	Day 0	Day 29	Day 0	Day 29
1	883	225	2,927	604
3	878	181	3,302	420
7	91	6	569	208
24	—[b]	—[b]	245	—[b]

[a]Concentrations expressed in ng/ml.

[b]Below assay sensitivity (5 ng/ml).

cytochrome P_{450}, and cytochrome b_5 were significantly higher in the treated dogs, thus confirming that the drug had indeed undergone MFO induction.

Another example is that of compound G, which was administered to cynomolgus monkeys at doses of 40 mg/kg per day for one month. Most of the monkeys at this dosage died by day 30 of the study. In contrast, rats were able to tolerate dosages as high as 100 mg/kg per day of the drug without any toxic symptoms. Collaborative toxicology and drug metabolism work revealed that the toxicity was probably a result of one major metabolite that was formed by both species, but that rats eliminated the metabolite faster. This information helped in interpreting the safety data and was found to be useful in the screening of other analogs of the drug by the pharmacologists.

MAXIMUM TOLERATED DOSE

It is common practice in toxicology to conduct studies in animals to determine the maximum tolerated dose, the dose that can be tolerated without signs of overt toxicity. This information is important because it helps researchers estimate the margin of safety between an effective dose and a toxic dose. As a study procedure, high doses of the drug are administered to animals until toxicity is observed. Monitoring of blood drug concentrations in such studies is extremely important, because, in most cases the pharmacokinetics of high doses of a drug can be completely different. Any of the absorption, metabolism, distribution, or excretion processes can be saturated.

A good example again is of CL 277,082, which, in the maximum tolerated dose study, was given to monkeys at 200 and 1,600 mg/kg. Serum CL 277,082 concentrations in these animals are shown in Table 1-4. No undue toxicity was observed at 1,600 mg/kg, but at the same time, the plasma drug concentrations of the unchanged drug from this dose were not any different from those obtained at 200 mg/kg. It was concluded that the amount of drug absorbed from the 200- and the 1,600-mg doses was the same. In the absence of blood drug concentration data, one would have

Table 1-4. Serum Concentrations (μg/ml) Following Oral Administration of Either 200 or 1600 mg/kg of CL 277,082 in Oleic Acid in Monkeys

Time (hr)	200 mg/kg	1,600 mg/kg
1	0.04	—[a]
2	0.36	0.09
4	0.65	0.47
8	2.27	1.18
12	1.50	1.79
24	3.94	0.38

[a]Below sensitivity limit of 0.04 μg/ml.

concluded that the monkeys had tolerated well the 1,600-mg/kg dose. The toxicokinetic information in this case served in making the true safety claims of the test compound as related to limited drug exposure at high dosages.

LONG-TERM SAFETY EVALUATION STUDIES

The objectives of long-term testing are safety evaluation of drugs for a longer duration, up to as long as 24 months of drug administration in the carcinogenicity studies (15,16). Because these drugs are usually intended for chronic use in human beings, it is essential that their long-term safety in animals be established. The purpose of toxicokinetics in long-term safety studies is to assure dose-related continuous exposure of the animals to the test compound throughout the study and to determine unusual drug accumulation and its possible association with unexpected toxicity.

A key factor to consider in long-term studies is the advancing age of the animals. It is well established that aging can affect pharmacokinetics of the drug because of age-related changes in the physiological variables. It is also known that a two-year-old rat is more reflective of an elderly person than of a young adult. In both human beings and animals, lean body mass and total body water decrease with aging. In human beings, the cardiac output decreases 1 percent per year from ages 19 to 86, and the blood flow to the kidneys appears to be reduced in a proportional manner (17). In rats, there are pronounced decreases (over 30%) in the cardiac index and in hepatic, renal, and gastrointestinal tract blood flow at 11 to 12 months of age (18). These changes can account for significant alterations in pharmacokinetics of drugs (19–23). In long-term toxicity and carcinogenicity studies in animals, which are conducted over a period of one year or more, aging may account, at least in part, for (1) diminished absorption of drugs through the gastrointestinal tract; (2) alteration in drug distribution in the body; (3) diminished rate of metabolism and renal excretion of drugs; (4) accumulation of drugs in blood and tissue; (5) changes in affinity and sensitivity of the receptor sites; and (6) increased rate of mortality.

A good example to show the effect of age on pharmacokinetics is that of *N*-acetylprocainamide (NAPA), published recently (19). In this study, a satellite group of 200 Charles River CD weanling rats were randomly taken from the same population intended for the carcinogenicity testing and were kept for a period of two years, during which feed (without any drug) and water were continuously available. Pharmacokinetic studies were performed on these rats randomly selected at ages 13, 26, and 52 weeks. At each age, the rats received 100 mg/kg NAPA.HCl by intravenous injection and by oral intubation according to a two-way crossover design (19).

Figure 1-5 depicts the time course of NAPA in plasma after administra-

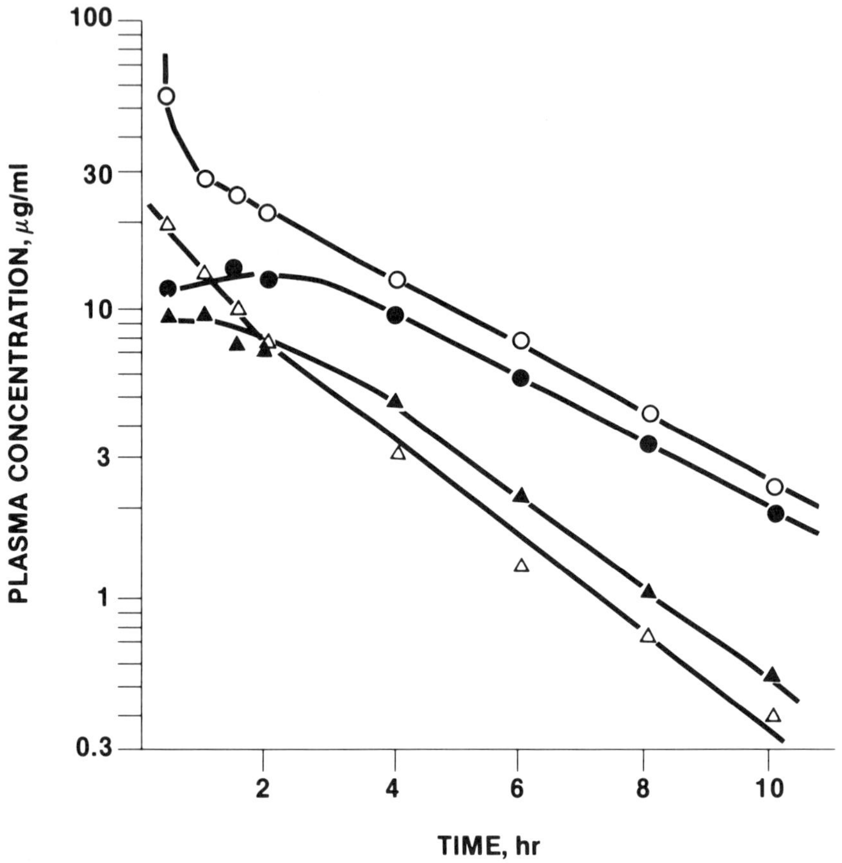

FIGURE 1-5. Time course of *N*-acetylprocainamide in plasma after administration of 100 mg of hydrochloride salt by intravenous injection (○,△) in 13-week-old rats (△,▲, *N* = 7), and in 52-week-old rats (○,●, *N* = 6) (23).

tion by intravenous injection and by oral intubation in rats at ages 13 and 52 weeks. These profiles show (1) higher plasma concentrations of the drug in 12-month-old animals after administration by either route; (2) the ratio of oral/IV plasma concentrations decreased with age, suggesting a decline in bioavailability of *N*-acetylprocainamide; and (3) the rate of decline of the postabsorption and distribution plasma concentration was slower in older rats, indicating a longer elimination half-life following administration of the drug by either route.

Table 1-5 summarizes the pharmacokinetic parameters for distribution and elimination of *N*-acetylprocainamide following intravenous administration of the drug in rats at ages 13, 26, and 52 weeks. In the 52-week-old animals compared to the 13-week-old rats, biological half-life was significantly pro-

Table 1-5. Effect of Age on Pharmacokinetics of *N*-Acetylprocainamide Hydrochloride After Intravenous Administration of 100 mg/kg in Rats (5)

	Age[b]					
Measures[a]	13 Weeks Mean	(n = 7) CV (%)	26 Weeks Mean	(n = 11) CV (%)	52 Weeks Mean	(n = 7) CV (%)
β (hr^{-1})	0.423	11.5	0.388	12.8	0.334	26.2
$t_{1/2}$ (hr)	1.66	12.1	1.82	14.2	2.29	42.3
Co_p^c (μg/ml)	19.0	12.1	27.7	21.6	46.9	21.8
AUC (μg · hr/ml)	45.3	18.2	72.6	27.0	156.0	51.4
TC (1/hr/kg)	2.01	14.8	1.29	23.5	0.664	71.4
V_d (1/kg)	4.75	11.2	3.35	22.0	1.98	24.9

[a]Determined by model independent equations.

[b]The values of β, V_d, and TC decreased significantly ($p < 0.05$, Duncan's *t*-test) and those for other parameters increased significantly after 26 weeks ($p < 0.05$, 13 vs. 52 and 26 vs. 52 weeks).

[c]Extrapolated zero-hour plasma concentration.

longed (by 38%), and the total clearance decreased significantly (67%). The extrapolated zero-hour plasma concentrations increased 2.5-fold, and the AUC values increased 3.5-fold. Consistent with these differences, the volume of distribution decreased by 58 percent. In general, the coefficient of variation (CV) of all the kinetic parameters increased from a range of 11–18 percent in the 13-week-old rats to 22–71 percent in the 52-week-old animals, indicating a much greater animal-to-animal variation with age.

The age-related changes in the pharmacokinetic parameters obtained in this study are consistent with the age-related changes in physiological characteristics in rats. Many compounds show age-dependent elimination half-life and body clearance which alter concentrations in plasma and tissues. Lack of appropriate adjustments in dosage levels can lead to accumulation of the drugs in blood and tissues in elderly human beings and in animals. In long-term safety evaluation, therefore, it becomes essential to account for the age factor. Age-dependent drug blood level monitoring in parallel to the toxicity tests can help researchers interpret the toxicological response and can provide a basis for appropriate dosage adjustment, when necessary. Yacobi and colleagues (24) have suggested that, in any long-term study, specifications for dosing, among other factors, should be established based on blood levels of the test compound.

SPECIES DIFFERENCES

Species differences must be recognized in extrapolating safety from animals to human beings. The species differences can be observed in both the absorption and the disposition characteristics of the drug. While examples showing species differences in the metabolism or disposition of the drug are well documented, very few cases exist that focus on the differences in absorption characteristics. Researchers have convincingly discussed species differences in the transdermal absorption of the drug and its impact on safety evaluation. Specifically, examples of transdermal absorption may be of interest because of advances in drug-delivery systems and their therapeutic use, which is of increased interest. The transdermal route is expected to show greater interspecies differences because of morphological and physiological differences in skin among species. In drug safety evaluation, transdermal dosage forms present a unique problem of suitability of the formulation to the test animal, the application of the formulation and its retainment, and the cost of the studies. Prior to embarking on long-term transdermal studies, it is necessary to define the most suitable transdermal dosage form that can be easily applied and will ensure the absorption of the drug from the site of application and also the presence of adequate concentrations of the test compound in blood and other biologic fluids. The choice of animal models for long-term safety evaluations is another critical issue in the development of new drugs intended for transdermal use.

The example discussed here presents data generated from drug-disposition studies conducted in support of the preclinical development and to support safety evaluation of a transdermally effective antihypertensive agent, viprostol (25–26), which is a synthetic prostaglandin effective in reduction of blood pressure after systemic and transdermal administration in animals. Its duration of action is significantly longer following topical administration than oral or intravenous administration in rats. Drug-disposition studies to support safety evaluation of viprostol were conducted in several pertinent test species; these studies are described in detail in Chapter 14.

In the rat, 95 percent of the applied drug penetrated the skin, and almost all of it was absorbed into the systemic circulation. Data in the mouse were similar. In all other species, the systemic absorption values were lower than the penetration values, indicating that not all of the penetrated dose was released for systemic absorption. The results indicated that skin acted as a natural reservoir or delivery system for viprostol. The ability to release the drug following penetration varied considerably among species, being relatively rapid in the rat and mouse, moderate in the monkey and rabbit, and poor in the dog.

From the data, it was concluded that, although the rat was appropriate for the long-term safety testing by the topical route, the dog was not because of the poor transdermal drug-release characteristics. However, the dog was considered to be a reliable and practical animal model for toxicity testing. The suitability of the subcutaneous (SC) route as a possible alternative to test long-term safety in the dog was examined (27). The results revealed that the absorption of viprostol following the SC route was complete within two to five hours after dosing, and there was a corresponding significant reduction in mean arterial blood pressure over the same time period. Like the topical route in other species, the subcutaneous route in the dog provided a hypertensive response for a duration longer than that following intravenous administration. The subcutaneous route was therefore considered a viable route for evaluating chronic toxicity studies in the dog.

The safety evaluation of drugs intended for transdermal administration should be conducted by application of the transdermal delivery system on the skin of the test species; however, several limitations might preclude the possibility of safety evaluation of such dosage forms in animals. The transdermal mode of drug administration during a chronic or subchronic safety evaluation will be limited to those species that will retain the delivery systems on the body without undue restraint and exhibit good skin-permeation characteristics. This will require screening of various animal models by pharmacokinetic procedures and, if possible, by pharmacodynamic procedures. Because transdermal application or absorption may not be feasible in some species, alternate modes of administration for conducting safety evaluation must be carefully examined and considered. For this purpose, thorough pharmacokinetic studies will be needed in gathering essential information for the design of the transdermal safety evaluation studies.

RETROSPECTIVE STUDIES

Occasionally, it is necessary to conduct studies to explain unexpected observations made during subchronic and chronic toxicity testing. For instance, it might be necessary to ascertain the impact of the changes in the route of administration or dosing vehicle that may be made in the safety evaluation program of a test compound. Retrospective studies thus can be of various types and are by nature compound specific (28). For example, for piperacillin, the proposed major clinical route of administration is intravenous. In safety evaluation studies, researchers desire that the route of administration in the test species be the same as that proposed for clinical use. However, for piperacillin it was not practical to administer the drug to rats by daily intravenous injections for a prolonged period of time. Reproduction studies with piperacillin in the rat were therefore done using the intraperitoneal route. Retrospectively, it became necessary to conduct a study to determine the effect of the route of administration on the exposure of the fetus to piperacillin.

A study was conducted in which pregnant and nonpregnant rats were given piperacillin by the intravenous and intraperitoneal routes (29). Figures 1-6 and 1-7 show the comparison of the amniotic fluid and fetal ^{14}C-piperacillin concentrations, respectively, following intravenous and intraperitoneal administration on day 18 of gestation. As compared to the intravenous

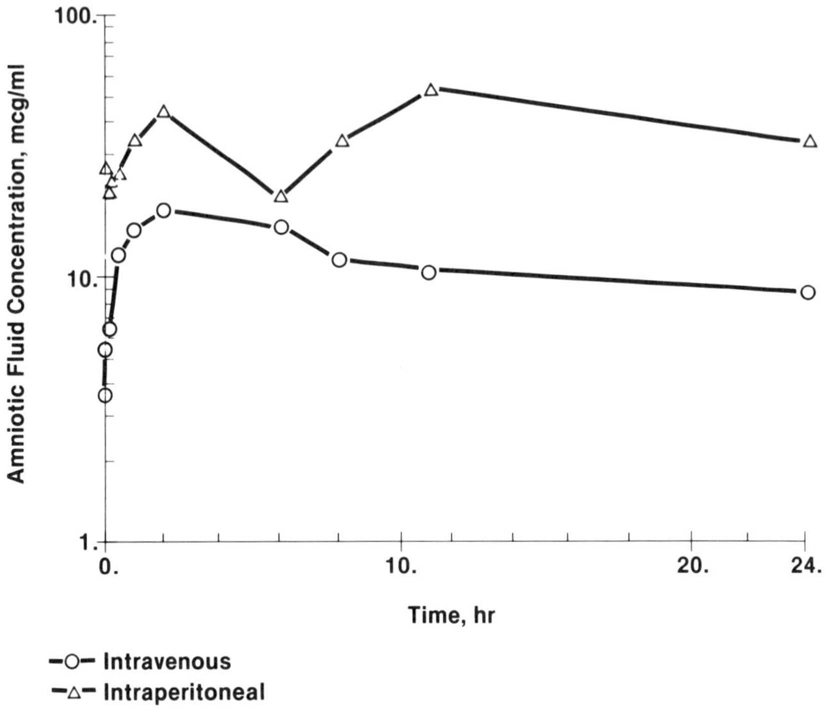

FIGURE 1-6. ^{14}C-piperacillin concentrations in the amniotic fluid in the pregnant rat following intravenous and intraperitoneal administration of 1,000 mg/kg of ^{14}C-piperacillin. ○ = Intravenous; △ = intraperitoneal.

administration, both the amniotic fluid and the fetal drug concentrations following the intraperitoneal administration were significantly higher. From the ratio of the total area under the drug concentration-time curve for the fetus and other tissues following intraperitoneal administration to that following intravenous administration, it was estimated that the fetal exposure to ^{14}C-piperacillin following intraperitoneal administration was at least twice as great. A possible explanation may be that, during pregnancy, the uterine wall is stretched and becomes more permeable; this can allow some of the drug to pass through the uterine wall directly from the peritoneal cavity and result in higher amniotic fluid and fetal drug concentrations. It should be pointed out that the results may be different on different days of gestation. These data indicate that, at least on day 18 of gestation, the fetus was exposed to a higher extent of piperacillin following intraperitoneal administration.

The results of this study clearly showed the usefulness of the data in the interpretation and evaluation of reproduction studies. Normally, it would be assumed that the fetal exposure to a drug following intravenous administration would be either equal or greater following intraperitoneal administra-

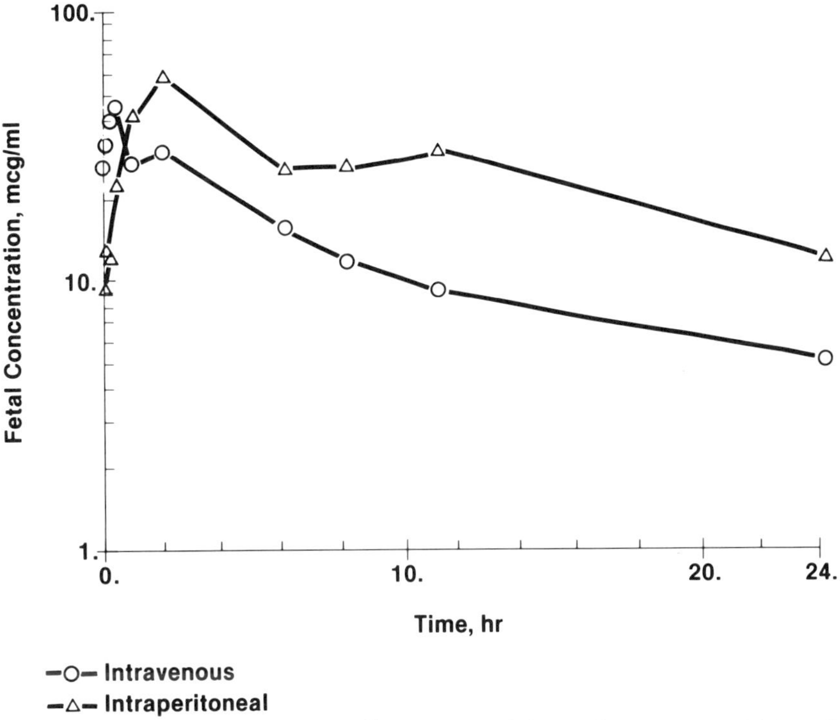

FIGURE 1-7. Fetal concentrations of ^{14}C-piperacillin following intravenous and intraperitoneal administration of 1,000 mg/kg of ^{14}C-piperacillin to pregnant rats. ○ = Intravenous; △ = intraperitoneal.

tion. Results of this piperacillin study negate such an assumption and strongly suggest that whenever safety evaluation studies are conducted using an administration route other than the proposed clinical route, tests should be done to determine the effect of route of administration on the pharmacokinetics of the drug.

IMPLEMENTATION OF THE TOXICOKINETIC SUPPORT PROGRAM

Interaction between pharmacokinetics and toxicology is continuous, occurring almost daily. A formal mechanism can facilitate the coordination and execution of activities between the two disciplines. The program is meaningful if the information obtained from the toxicokinetic studies are complementary to the results of toxicology studies. This goal is best achieved

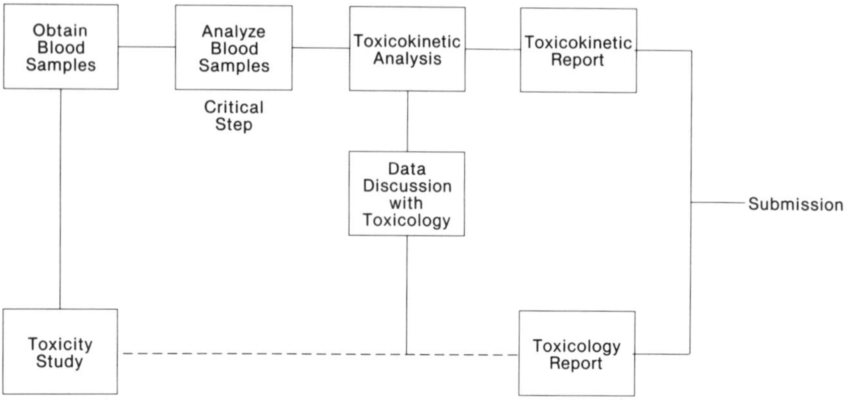

FIGURE 1-8. Flow diagram illustrating the mechanism of managing toxicokinetic data originating from the safety evaluation studies.

if blood drug concentration monitoring is built into the toxicology study protocols, and if the same animals that are undergoing toxicity testing are used for obtaining blood samples. However, this may not always be feasible because of the fear that animals may become anemic due to excessive bleeding and thus adversely affect the safety findings. In such cases, satellite groups of extra animals can be added to the toxicology study for toxicokinetic purposes. These satellite animals are handled and dosed the same way as the animals in the safety evaluation study, but they are there for the sole purpose of obtaining blood samples. In some instances, the addition of satellite animals to the safety evaluation studies may not be feasible if the addition increases the size of the study to an unmanageable level. In such cases, the toxicokinetic work will have to be done in an independent study, but under experimental and environment conditions similar to those used in the complementary safety evaluation studies.

In planning subchronic and chronic toxicity studies, the pharmacokinetic information gathered from the drug disposition studies would be used in designing toxicology protocols. Once the safety evaluation study begins, blood samples should be obtained as specified in the protocol and analyzed by a validated bioanalytical method (Fig. 1-8). Developing a sensitive bioanalytical assay before the initiation of safety studies is critical to the success of the toxicokinetic support program, because without the assay, there can be no timely toxicology support. Once the samples are analyzed, data can be discussed with the toxicology study director. In this discussion, the pharmacokinetic and toxicology information is shared and integrated, and conclusions are drawn. Preparation of the toxicology and toxicokinetic reports should take place in parallel so that the toxicokinetic report can be integrated with the toxicology report for an IND/NDA or any other submission.

CONCLUSIONS

Toxicokinetic input has become an essential part of safety evaluation studies. Several examples in this chapter were discussed to illustrate that toxicokinetic information is necessary in the interpretation of safety evaluation studies and subsequent extrapolation of data to human beings. Toxicokinetic results validate various stages of safety assessment through the measurement of blood drug concentrations, and by providing proof of exposure of the animals to the drug. Since toxicokinetics, as opposed to toxicology is a quantitative science, it tends to reduce the study variability; hence, a relevant toxicokinetic support can help in reducing the number of test animals used and the size and cost of the safety evaluation studies.

Various regulatory agencies have recognized the usefulness of a toxicokinetic program and are in strong support of substantiating the safety evaluation studies with drug-disposition studies. The type of support or input needed will depend upon the nature of the compound, the assay limitations, objectives of the safety evaluation studies, and the information to be generated. The success of the toxicokinetic program depends on the belief that the toxicity response, in addition to other factors, can be influenced by the disposition of the drug; hence, toxicokinetic input is essential to predict safety of the test drug in animals before it can be extrapolated to human beings.

REFERENCES

1. B. Clark and D. A. Smith. Pharmacokinetics and toxicity testing. CRC Critical Reviews in Toxicology *12*, 343–385 (1984).
2. R. D. Smyth and G. H. Hottendorf. Application of pharmacokinetics and biopharmaceutics in the design of toxicological studies. Toxicology and Applied Pharmacology *53*, 179–195 (1980).
3. A. Yacobi, B. L. Kamath, and C. M. Lai. Pharmacokinetics in chronic animal toxicity studies. Drug Metabolism Reviews *13* (6), 1021–1051 (1982).
4. W. J. O'Reilly. Pharmacokinetics in drug metabolism and toxicology. Canadian J. Pharm. Sci. *7*, 66–70 (1972).
5. S. Garattini. TCDD toxicology with particular reference to seveso: Introductory remarks. Drug Metabolism Reviews *13* (3), 345–353 (1982).
6. Y. Cohen. Radionuclidelabelled compounds in the approach of pharmacokinetics related to drug toxicity. Proceedings European Society Study of Drug Toxicity *14*, 20–35 (1973).
7. H. Barry, III and A. Yacobi. Preclinical toxicokinetics. In: *Experimental and Clinical Toxicokinetics*. A. Yacobi and H. Barry, III, eds. American Pharmaceutical Association, APS, Washington, DC. pp. 1–7.
8. F. J. DiCarlo. Metabolism, pharmacokinetics, and toxicokinetics defined. Drug Met. Reviews *13* (1), 1–4 (1982).
9. G. Rentsch. The use of pharmacokinetic systems for the interpretation of long-term experiments: A new approach in toxicology. Proc. Eur. Soc. Toxicol. *15*, 323–329 (1974).
10. P. Mazel. General principles and procedures for drug metabolism *in-vitro*. In: *Fundamentals of Drug Metabolism and Drug Disposition*. B. N. Ladu, H. G. Mandel, and E. L. Way. Williams and Wilkins Co., Baltimore, MD (1971) pp. 527–582.

11. Z. A. Wong, C. Wei, D. W. Rice, and D. P. H. Hsieh. Effects of phenobarbital pretreatment on the metabolism and toxicokinetics of aflatoxin B_1 in the rhesus monkey. Toxicology and Applied Pharmacology *60,* 387–397 (1981).
12. A. E. Rettie, A. W. Rettenmeier, W. N. Howland, and T. A. Baillie. Cytochrome P-450-catalyzed formation of VPA, a toxic metabolite of valproic acid. Science *235,* 890–893 (1987).
13. A. Yacobi, J. T. Slattery, and G. Levy. Procoagulant effect of phenobarbital. Life Sciences *26,* 1379–1383 (1980).
14. D. R. Hawkins and L. F. Chasseaud. Reasons for monitoring kinetics in safety evaluation studies. Arch. Toxicol., Suppl. *8,* 165–172 (1985).
15. H. G. Verschuuren and R. H. Reitz. The use of pharmacokinetics in chronic toxicity testing. Comp. Vet. Pharmacol. Toxicol. Ther. Proc. Congr. Eur. Assoc. *1,* 209–223 (1985).
16. J. M. Faccini, E. Irisarri, and A. M. Monro. A carcinogenicity study in mice of a β-adrenergic antagonist, prinidolol; increased total tumor incidence without tissue specificity. Toxicology *21,* 279–290 (1981).
17. A. D. Bender. Effects of increasing age on the distribution of peripheral blood flow in man. J. Am. Geriat. Soc. *13,* 192–198 (1965).
18. M. S. Yates and C. R. Hiley. The effect of age on cardiac output and its distribution in the rat. Experimentia *35,* 78–79 (1979).
19. A. Yacobi, B. L. Kamath, H. F. Stampfli, Z. M. Look, and C. M. Lai. Age related pharmacokinetics of *N*-acetylprocainamide in rats. Res. Commun. Chem. Pathol. Pharmacol. *24,* 197–200 (1979).
20. S. A. Friedman, A. E. Raizner, H. Rosen, N. A. Solomon, and W. Sy. Functional defects in the aging kidney. Ann. Intern. Med. *76,* 41–45 (1972).
21. T. Iga and C. D. Klaaseu. Age related pharmacokinetics of Ouabain in rats. Proc. Soc. Exptl. Brol. Med. *170,* 59–62 (1982).
22. V. Klotz, G. R. Avant, A. Hojumpa, S. Schenker, and G. R. Wilkinson. The effect of age and liver disease on the disposition and elimination of diazepam in adult man. J. Clin. Invest. *55,* 347–359 (1975).
23. L. P. Novak. Aging, total body potassium, fat free mass and cell mass in males and females between the ages of 18 and 65 years. J. Gerontal. *27,* 438–443 (1972).
24. A. Yacobi, R. W. Krasula, and C. M. Lai. Selective disposition studies in drug safety evaluation. In: *Experimental and Clinical Toxicokinetics.* A. Yacobi and H. Barry, III, eds. American Pharmaceutical Association, APS, Washington, DC. pp. 47–73.
25. P. S. Chan, P. Cervoni, M. A. Ronsberg, R. C. Accomando, G. J. Quirk, P. A. Scully, and L. M. Lipchuck. Antihypertensive activity of DL-15-deoxy-16-hydroxy-16(α/β)-vinyl prostaglandin E_2 methyl ester (CL 115,347), a new orally and transdermally long-acting hypertensive agent. Pharmacol. Exp. Ther. *226,* 726–732 (1983).
26. G. Nicoalu, V. K. Batra, S. Gordon, A. Tonelli, and W. McWilliams. Abstracts, Fifth International Conference on Prostaglandins, Florence, Italy (1982).
27. V. K. Batra, J. A. Morrison, D. B. Cosulich, W. Dougherty, N. Perkinson, M. Kohlbrenner, A. Barr, and A. Yacobi. Pharmacodynamics and pharmacokinetics of the methyl ester of 15-deoxy-16-hydroxy-16 vinyl prostaglandin E_2. J. Pharm. Sci. *74,* 1245–1246 (1985).
28. Pharmaceutical Manufacturers Association. *Strategies for Drug Disposition Studies Performed in the Context of Non-Clinical Drug Safety Evaluation (A. guide).* Washington, DC (1980) (Unpublished draft).
29. V. Batra, J. Morrison, and E. Kalerita. Comparative pharmacokinetics of ^{14}C-piperacillin following intravenous and intraperitoneal administration in pregnant and non-pregnant rats. Euro. Jour. Drug Met. and Pharmacok. *9,* 31–39 (1984).

Chapter 2

Role of Toxicokinetics in Drug Safety Evaluations*

Felix A. de la Iglesia, M.D. and Peter Greaves, M.D.**

Department of Pathology and Experimental Toxicology,
Parke-Davis Pharmaceutical Research, Warner-Lambert
Company, Ann Arbor, MI 48105

ABSTRACT

For the purposes of drug safety evaluations, toxicokinetics has been defined as the different aspects of absorption, distribution, and metabolism of therapeutic agents in the species used in toxicity trials and at dose levels extended beyond those that produce target pharmacologic responses.

The application of toxicokinetics in drug safety evaluations resides in the contribution to study design and dosing regimen, as well as in the interpretation of results. In addition, a more rationalized use of animals and technical resources is expected. The interface of toxicokinetics for drug safety evaluation is significant for the purpose of establishing rational dose levels and the differentiation between toxicity-limiting effects. The application of a systematic toxicokinetic approach in the early aspects of drug development

*Presented at the FDA-AAPS sponsored Symposium Experimental and Clinical Toxicokinetics-II, November 3, 1986 in Washington, DC.

**Dr. Greaves is Director, Parke-Davis Research Institute, Sheridan Park, Mississauga, Ontario, Canada.

is a key element for the proper selection of dose levels and validation of dose level selection and species.

The initial approach for establishing dose levels for toxicology studies is an in-depth evaluation of single- and multiple-dose pharmacokinetics in the species and strain used by the toxicology laboratory. Blood level data in acute or rising dose studies are extremely useful to correlate peak effect levels and the development of intolerance, even when overt toxic effects are not clearly delineated. The correlation of these blood level data and adverse effects in large animals or in rodents helps to determine the upper range of toxicity of the agent, without necessarily evoking mortality.

In subacute studies, the toxicokinetic analysis is of importance to determine sex differences, absorption modalities, and other differences in drug disposition. Nonspecific toxicity due to abnormal metabolism or disposition can be predicted. In longer-term studies, drug blood concentration data allow the evaluation of longer-term health effects in relation to levels achieved and in relation to intended therapeutic levels. The onset of unexpected toxicity, abnormal nonspecific responses, or long-range target effects are then viewed within a more objective framework that can indicate unsuspected pharmacokinetic behavior or extraneous sensitivities, placing a better perspective for the ultimate objective of these studies. Therefore, a more precise safety assessment for the prediction of potential adverse effects in human beings can be expected.

INTRODUCTION

The importance of metabolism and pharmacokinetics studies in the preclinical safety assessment of novel therapeutic agents has been widely appreciated for many years. Although some workers suggested that pharmacokinetic and metabolism data are frequently irrelevant for establishing proof of safety and efficacy (1), the logic of assessing the disposition of a drug in laboratory animals in study design, in understanding dose-response relationships, and in extrapolation of results of experimental studies to human beings, is inescapable (2–7).

Despite general acceptance of the importance of such information, the closeness with which pharmacokinetic and metabolism studies need to be coordinated and integrated with regulatory toxicity studies seems less widely appreciated. Indeed, poor coordination of preclinical data from toxicology and metabolism studies has been the subject of comment by a number of regulatory scientists (8–9). This situation provided the stimulus for the recent publication of regulatory guidelines for animal pharmacokinetic and metabolic studies in drug safety evaluation.

A number of reasons account for the difficulty of coordinating such studies. Zbinden (10) observed that toxicologists are liable to be torn between old loyalties to classical standardized testing procedures and the approach in which pharmacokinetic considerations play a part. Furthermore, these older traditions of standardized testing still are an integral part of regulatory requirements for toxicity testing. Thus, the inescapable dictum of a rodent and nonrodent requirement for toxicity testing leaves no choice to toxicologists, even if one or the other species included in the testing program may be totally irrelevant in terms of metabolic handling of a particular compound. Therefore, one could idealize the day in which a regulatory submission may contain in-depth studies, but only in one species! Bridges (11) cited logistical factors and poor communications between departments contributing to toxicokinetics as being further impediments to the efficient use of metabolism and pharmacokinetic studies in toxicity testing.

Undoubtedly, the logistics of developing a large body of comprehensive preclinical safety data are extremely complex. It is also difficult to achieve a balance between information gained through animal experiments and data that are more appropriately obtained in well-designed clinical studies, for this requires very effective collaboration between preclinical scientists and clinical pharmacologists.

The aim of this chapter is to address some of the factors involved in acquiring pharmacokinetics and metabolism data within the context of preclinical drug safety evaluation, to review some of the benefits to toxicologists in processing toxicokinetic information, and to update some of the concepts presented earlier at this forum (12).

DRUG TOXICOKINETICS: WHAT IS IT?

Although use of the term *toxicokinetics* in the context of drug safety evaluation has been criticized as being inappropriate (5,8), this inelegant neologism is nevertheless a convenient term to describe the study of the absorption, distribution, metabolism, and excretion of drugs in the species and at the dose levels chosen for toxicity studies. (Fig. 2-1) Thus, the term focuses on studies designed specifically to help toxicologists in safety evaluation, in the design and interpretation of animal toxicity studies, and in the extrapolation of results to human beings for safety assessment purposes. The key differences, therefore, between toxicokinetics and conventional pharmacokinetics reside in the doses employed that are beyond those that elicit pharmacological responses and significantly above those usually contemplated for use in human beings. However, it is important to add that no sharp separation between toxicokinetics and conventional pharmacokinetics is warranted, for such data are complementary.

Hawkins and Chasseaud (6) summarized the basic objectives of pharmacokinetics when applied to toxicity studies: (1) to define relationships

DRUG TOXICOKINETICS

Studies designed to establish the kinetics of absorption, distribution, metabolism and excretion in the same species and doses chosen for toxicity studies

FIGURE 2-1. The Concept of Drug Toxicokinetics.

between dose levels and the extent of absorption of the test compound; (2) to show effects of repeated doses on pharmacokinetics of the test compound; (3) to establish relationships between the age of animals employed and pharmacokinetics of the test compound; and (4) to define the relationships between dose regimens used clinically and those used in toxicity studies. (Fig. 2-2)

To this, it is important to add that because the formation of metabolites is not necessarily the same across species, knowledge of metabolic transformation and of the kinetics of metabolites is of considerable importance.

SCHEDULING AND SEQUENCE OF TOXICOKINETIC STUDIES

No program of preclinical toxicity testing is an end in itself; nor should it be regarded as a box-checking exercise to meet minimum regulatory requirements before an experimental drug is administered to a human being.

A preclinical toxicity program (Fig. 2-3) is, above all, a rational aggregate of preclinical studies designed, executed, and appropriately analyzed to support well-defined clinical objectives for the study and eventual therapeutic use of a potential new drug in human beings (13).

Clinical objectives are initially the evaluation of tolerance in small numbers of patients or volunteers, and this is followed by demonstration of activity or efficacy. As development progresses, therapeutic benefit must be demonstrated in larger numbers of patients, and this may include older people, women of childbearing age, or even children.

These patient populations may be highly variable in their metabolic handling of xenobiotics, particularly as age-dependent or genetic alterations in drug disposition may be important (14,15). To justify such extended clinical programs, it is necessary to perform extensive toxicity testing, including reproductive studies and carcinogenicity bioassays.

TOXICOKINETICS - OBJECTIVES

- *Define biovailability, dose proportionality, and sex differences*
- *Predict target organ toxicity and explain unanticipated toxic effects*
- *Establish species differences in metabolite profile and kinetics*
- *Define relationship between clinical doses and those used in toxicity studies*

FIGURE 2-2. Main objectives of toxicokinetic studies.

In the initial evaluation of certain compounds, relatively small amounts of in vivo data may be available at the time the toxicologist is required to make a preliminary assessment of the toxicity profile. In such situations, particularly if the compound under study is from well-studied chemical series, the toxicologist needs not to wait further before proceeding to preliminary studies in laboratory animals, in range finding, in rising dose, or in the screening toxicology studies suggested by Zbinden (16). Nevertheless, Monro (2) made a point on the importance of having a good assay for *parent drug in blood and body fluids before proceeding* to formal toxicity studies (Fig. 2-4). The assay should be specific with good sensitivity, and it should be reproducible. Ideally, it should also be rapid and simple to avoid the risk of error that can occur with multiple manipulations.

In the initial preclinical evaluation of more unusual compounds, a far more extensive pharmacokinetics and metabolism profile may be warranted before initiation of formal toxicity evaluations. An example of this is the neuromuscular blocking agent atracurium, in which prolonged toxicity testing

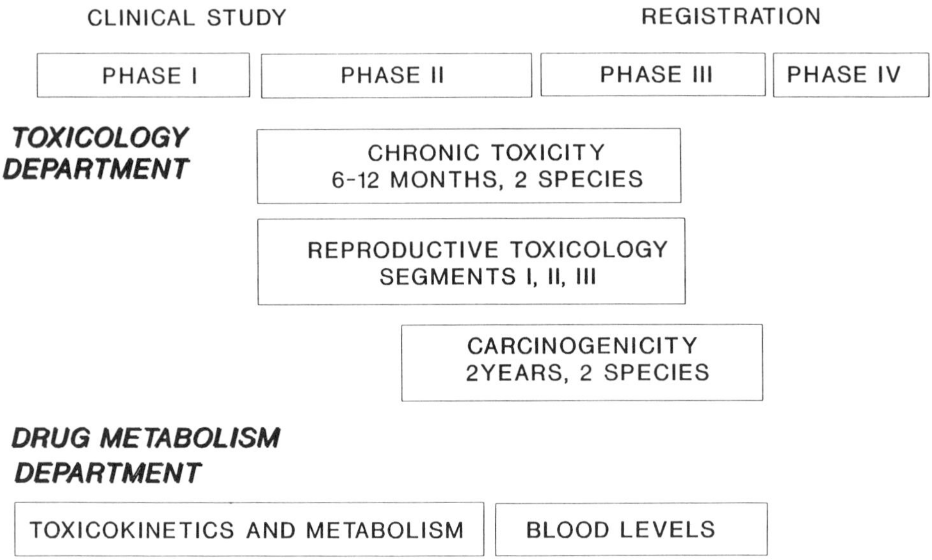

FIGURE 2-3. Development of toxicology studies during the clinical study phases of a drug, with the interrelationships with drug metabolism studies.

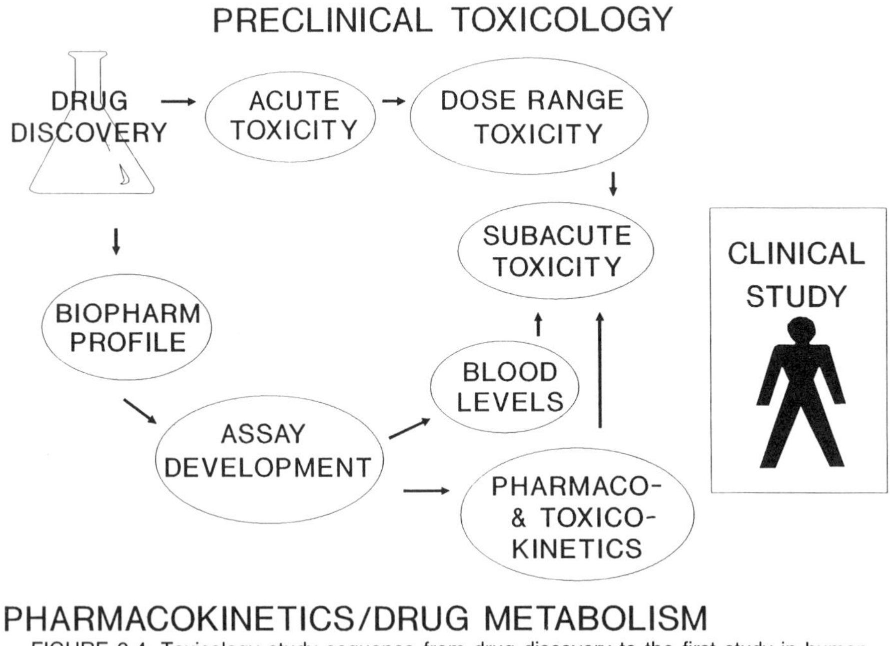

FIGURE 2-4. Toxicology study sequence from drug discovery to the first study in human beings. Corresponding pharmacokinetic studies are also shown.

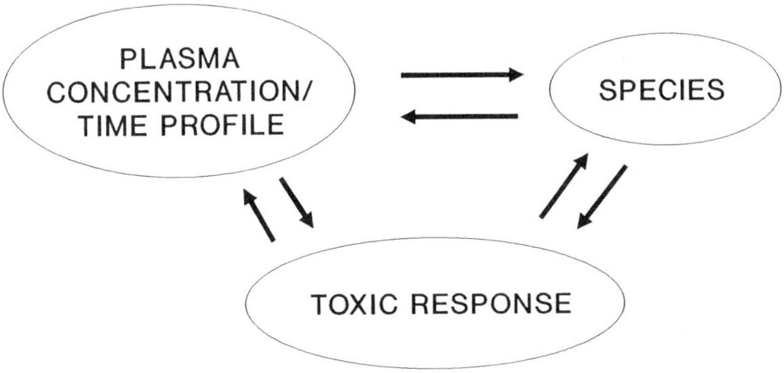

FIGURE 2-5. Relationship between species, toxic effects, and plasma levels.

by the most appropriate intravenous route in the usual test species was precluded because of resultant muscular paralysis. Here, pharmacokinetic data had an important place in early study design (17). In the toxicity testing of interferons and other biotechnology products, a clear understanding of how these agents move through body fluids is important in defining the best routes of administration and dosage schedule (18).

A key element in the whole development process is close collaboration between scientists performing the toxicologic, pharmacokinetic, and clinical work. It is highly desirable to obtain pharmacokinetic data from human beings as early as possible in development, for this allows the toxicologist to reassess toxicity studies and to consider dispositional data in the design of longer and far more expensive long-term toxicity studies. This iterative information feedback influences design of subsequent studies and has been aptly termed the "ping-pong" approach (19).

A particular issue that relates to the comparison between human beings and animals is the timing of studies with a radioactively labeled compound. Although the availability of a labeled compound may not be essential at an early stage of development, radiolabeled studies in animals and human beings may frequently provide good preliminary information about disposition and metabolic profile that far outweighs apparently excessive costs and efforts.

DOSE LEVEL SELECTION AND DESIGN OF TOXICITY STUDIES

Toxicity studies consist mainly of four groups of animals, including a control and three treated groups receiving low, intermediate, and high doses, frequently administered once daily, by gavage, or admixed in the diet. Selection of dose levels remains as the most difficult issue in the design of toxicity studies. Initially, dose selection is based on some form of rising dose or dose-finding study, although the protocols for these studies may vary significantly between laboratories. The use of drug-disposition data to justify doses that avoid the expression of high-dose toxicity has been criticized from a regulatory standpoint (8). However, this information can be helpful in providing that reasonable tissue exposure will be achieved when the high dose is limited by pharmacodynamic effects or where there are physical limitations to higher dosing levels.

Equally important in study design is defining doses that lead to the characterization of the highest no-effect level. Here, pharmacokinetic information can be extremely helpful, because it enables the no-effect level to be accurately and appropriately defined in terms of blood or tissue concentrations (5). A secondary, but no less important, point is that the no-effect level is based on relevant toxicity endpoints, since secondary effects are usually misleading. A valuable source of information in selecting doses is the pharmacodynamic profile of the drug. A careful evaluation of this process usually helps to predict exaggerated pharmacologically mediated effects.

Prior knowledge of the time at which peak plasma concentrations are attained under standard conditions and of dosage regimens is helpful for the timing of useful parameters. For example, blood pressure, ECG, and other physiological measurements or detailed clinical observations can be undertaken at the most appropriate times following dosing (Fig. 2-5).

Toxicokinetic data are also helpful in the selection of the mode or frequency of administration. Time and labor constraints usually dictate single daily dosing by gavage, capsule administration, or the parenteral route. This may or may not provide the most appropriate exposure to drug, and a clear indication of the exposure actually occurring under conditions of the study is helpful in deciding whether twice-daily or more frequent administration is necessary, or whether an effort should be made at an early stage of drug development to administer drug in diet to rodents. Toxicokinetic information can help in the justification of routes other than those intended clinically. This is important if the intended route is technically unachievable for long periods in animals (e.g., sublingual route). It may also be necessary to justify alternative routes to avoid excessive pharmacological effects such as neuromuscular blocking activity (17).

Although selection of appropriate species is often cited as an important contribution of pharmacokinetic and metabolism data, actual choices open to toxicologists are limited, being dictated by animal supply, facilities, and basic knowledge of physiology and background pathology. Even appropriateness of a nonhuman primate species for certain compounds on metabolic grounds may be largely offset by difficulties in histopathological assessment as a result of the high level of intercurrent pathology in many primate colonies. Nevertheless, disposition data may help to justify exclusion of a particular species that is highly inappropriate from a metabolic point of view.

DESIGN OF TOXICOKINETIC STUDIES

A key question usually asked is how toxicokinetic data should be generated. Samples taken at single time points are relatively simple to obtain from animals during toxicity studies, and these can be useful in monitoring drug blood concentration over the course of a chronic study. It may not be possible, however, to relate these data to those obtained from conventional pharmacokinetic studies in which different doses and vehicles may have been employed. Multiple time points in the context of toxicity studies may be difficult to obtain for a number of logistical reasons. Large volumes of blood at each time point may be required, and the sampling times may conflict with the need to obtain samples for clinical pathology and with measurement of other parameters.

In our laboratory, separate single-dose toxicokinetic studies are frequently preferable on logistical grounds at an early stage of toxicity testing. Doses can be chosen based on those proposed for toxicity studies. Dosing solutions and experimental conditions can be identical to those in toxicity studies, and blood samples can be taken over at least a 24-hour period without the constraints that occur in regulated toxicity studies. Data obtained from these studies then form a firm baseline from which to plan intervals for monitoring of blood drug levels in a more modest way in subsequent toxicity studies.

INTERPRETATION OF TOXICITY STUDIES

There are many constraints in the design of regulated toxicity studies, including the need to demonstrate overt toxicity, to establish no-effect dose levels, limited choice of species, and intended length of study. Therefore, toxicokinetic data can influence actual study design only in a relatively modest fashion. By contrast, it can have a major impact on study interpretation.

The nature of the interpretation of preclinical toxicity data is frequently misunderstood. It has more in common with the clinical methods employed in the investigation of a patient with a disease process than with a rigorous scientific experiment with an expected outcome. As in clinical practice, therefore, it is of fundamental importance that findings in toxicity studies be evaluated in the context of all salient information, including pharmacological and pharmacokinetic data to reach appropriate conclusions. A particular constellation of findings may have one or more different interpretations, depending on the circumstances in which findings developed. An obvious example is a toxicity study in which there are few or no clinical or pathological findings even when large doses are administered. The entire interpretation depends therefore on an assessment of how much drug was absorbed at the doses administered.

Prior knowledge of drug disposition and its relationship to administered dose may be particularly helpful in the assessment of dose-response relationships in group organ weight differences and associated pathological findings. Disposition data may enable the pathologist to focus the assessment using special techniques on organs that may be particularly exposed to the parent drug or to several metabolites.

In vitro studies can be helpful in the interpretation of the effects of toxicity studies and problem solving, but for their correct interpretation it is axiomatic that concentrations used in vitro need to be correlated with levels actually achieved in whole animals and with intended therapeutic use in human beings.

SAFETY ASSESSMENT AND PREDICTION OF EFFECTS IN HUMAN BEINGS

Risk assessment of novel drugs in human beings, based on animal data, has assumed far greater importance in recent years, particularly as major debilitating or life-threatening diseases have diminished. As the gain from therapy has become more marginal, side effects have become more visible (20). However, simple comparisons between results of toxicity studies in different animal species and adverse effects in human beings have shown that considerable differences occur and that only about 25 percent of adverse effects in animal studies can be expected to occur in human beings (21,22). Such findings bring into question the predictability of effects observed in animal studies and anticipated reactions in larger patient populations. However, risk assessments require critical comparisons of both animal dose-response relationships and expected human exposure data. This process requires human and animal pharmacokinetic data to express an appropriate unit of comparison between species. There is also a need for knowledge of comparative metabolism and a detailed understanding of differences in endogenous metabolic processes (7). Pharmacokinetics may be particularly helpful in the extrapolation of carcinogenicity bioassay data obtained in rodents to human beings (23).

Any attempt, therefore, to improve predictability of animal studies must include a good knowledge of species differences in absorption, distribution, metabolism, and excretion of a potential new drug, and this requires above all close cooperation between toxicologists, metabolism scientists, and clinical pharmacologists.

REFERENCES

1. P. Cuatrecasas. Contemporary drug development—Dilemmas. Reg. Toxicol. Pharmacol. *4,* 1–12 (1984).
2. A. M. Monro, The role of metabolism studies in drug safety evaluation. Drug. Dev. Comm. *2,* 377–392 (1976).
3. R. D. Smyth and G. G. Hottendorf. Application of pharmacokinetics and biopharmaceuticals in the design of toxicological studies. Toxicol. Appl. Pharmacol. *53,* 179–195 (1980).
4. A. Yacobi, B. L. Kamath, and C. M. Lai. Pharmacokinetics in chronic animal toxicity studies. Drug Metab. Rev. *13,* 1021–1051 (1982).
5. B. Clark and D. A. Smith. Pharmacokinetics and Toxicity Testing. CRC Critical Rev. Toxicol. *12,* 353–385 (1984).
6. D. R. Hawkins and L. F. Chasseaud. Reasons for monitoring kinetics in safety evaluation studies. Arch. Toxicol. *8,* 165–172 (1985).
7. S. Garattini. Toxic effects of chemicals: Difficulties in extrapolating data from animals to man. CRC Crit. Rev. Toxicol. *16,* 1–29 (1986).
8. V. C. Glocklin. General considerations for studies of the metabolism of drugs and other chemicals. Drug Metabs. Rev. *13,* 929–939 (1982).
9. D. G. Grahame-Smith. What is expected from repeated-dose studies by the regulatory authorities. In: *Long-Term Animal Studies. Their Predictive Value for Man.* S. R. Walker and A. D. Dayan, eds. MTP Press, Lancaster, PA (1986). pp. 23–27.
10. G. Zbinden. Comparative and pharmacokinetic toxicity. In: *Progress in Toxicology, Special Topics.* Springer-Verlag, Berlin (1976). pp. 244–69.
11. J. W. Bridges. Pharmacokinetic factors. In: *Long Term Animal Studies. Their Predictive Value for Man.* S. R. Walker and A. D. Daxan, eds. MTP Press, Lancaster, PA (1986). pp. 9–26.
12. G. J. Yakatan and F. A. de la Iglesia. Toxicokinetics—A role in drug discovery and development. In: *Experimental and Clinical Toxicokinetics.* A. Yacobi and H. Barry, eds. Pharmaceut. Assoc., Washington, DC (1984). pp. 615–626.
13. S. R. Walker and C. E. Lumley. Regulatory requirements for the preclinical safety testing of pharmaceuticals. In: *Development of Drugs and Modern Medicines.* Goorod, Eltorwood, eds. Chichester, England (1986). pp. 133–148.
14. D. L. Schmucker. Aging and drug disposition: An update. Pharmacol. Rev. *37,* 133–148 (1985).
15. F. J. Gonzalez, R. C. Skoda, S. Kimura, M. Umeno, U. M. Zanger, D. W. Nebert, H. V. Gelboin, J. P. Hardwick, and U. A. Meyer. Characterization of the common genetic defect in humans deficient in debrisoquine metabolism. Nature *331,* 442–446 (1988).
16. G. Zbinden, J. Elsner, and U. A. Boelsterli. Toxicological screening. Reg. Toxicol. Pharmacol. *4,* 275–286 (1984).
17. M. Skarpa, A. D. Dayan, and M. Follenfant. Toxicity testing of atracurium. Brit. J. Anaesth. *55,* 278–295 (1983).
18. V. Bocci. Distribution, catabolism and pharmacokinetics of interferons. In: *Interferon, Vol. 4: In Vivo and Clinical Studies.* N. B. Finter and R. K. Oldham, eds. Elsevier, Amsterdam (1985).
19. Council for International Organizations of Medical Sciences. Safety requirements for the first use of new drugs and diagnostic agents in man. *A review of safety issues in early clinical trials of drugs.* CIOMS, Geneva (1983).
20. A. W. Asscher. Analysis for risk assessment. In: *Long Term Animal Studies. Their Predictive Value for Man.* S. R. Walker and A. D. Dayan, eds. MTP Press, Lancaster, PA (1986). pp. 119–122.

21. A. P. Fletcher. Drug safety tests a subsequent clinical experience. J. Royal Soc. Med. *71,* 693–696, (1978).
22. J. P. Griffin. Predictive value of animals toxicity studies. In: *Long Term Animal Studies. Their Predictive Value for Man.* S. R. Walker and A. D. Dayan, eds. MTP Press, Lancaster, PA (1986). pp. 107–116.
23. A. S. Whittemore, S. C. Grosser, and A. Silvers. Pharmacokinetics in low dose extrapolation using animal cancer data. Fund. Appl. Toxicol. *7,* 183–190 (1986).

Chapter 3

Toxicokinetics in Preclinical Evaluation of Drug Safety

V. C. Glocklin and C. C. Chah

Office of Drug Research and Review
Center for Drug Evaluation and Research
Food and Drug Administration

INTRODUCTION

The U.S. Food and Drug Administration has long proposed that information about a new drug's absorption, distribution, metabolism, and excretion (ADME) should be developed to improve the predictive usefulness of its toxicology studies (1,2). Although still regarded to be pilot or research information that does not need to comply with the Good Laboratory Practices regulations (3), the importance of ADME data to drug evaluation is nevertheless recognized in current regulations for new drug investigation (IND) and marketing (NDA) applications that specify expected submission of ADME data in their preclinical sections, and comparison of animal and human ADME data in their summary sections and physicians' information (4,5). Format guidelines, recently developed to supplement the NDA regulations, include recommendations for organizing preclinical ADME data within the appli-

Based on a presentation at the First National Meeting of the American Association of Pharmaceutical Sciences (AAPS), Washington, DC, November 3, 1986.

cation to facilitate their evaluation for use as an interpretive bridge between animal toxicology and human ADME data (6,7).

The various types of ADME data identified in these format guidelines represent typical information that may be available for NDA submission, with no intention of indicating either the extent of testing that might actually be required for a particular drug or how this information should be developed during the drug's investigation. In updating our preclinical testing guidelines to incorporate the principles of toxicokinetics, we must attempt to reconcile a variety of conceptual, procedural, and interdisciplinary issues, long debated by the FDA and the pharmaceutical industry (8). These issues have since become central to discussion in the broader arena of toxicology and regulatory communities worldwide. Although the toxicologic importance of ADME data is generally acknowledged in concept and is supported by an increasing variety of notable examples, there is still little agreement about how to use ADME studies in a systematic way for best advantage in decisions about the safety of new drugs and other chemicals. Thus, a recent review on this subject noted that pharmacokinetic data are said to be important for every aspect of safety evaluation, even though the way that this information is to be used for that purpose is seldom clear (9). It has also been observed that meaningful correlations sometimes cannot be made between ADME and toxicology data because of their independent development in studies using different types of animals, different doses, and different experimental conditions (10).

Suggestions for correcting a similar lack of ADME and toxicology study coordination in drug applications have already been published (8,11), and the need for improvement in this regard was also confirmed by an examination of preclinical data in 36 INDs submitted by 18 companies in 1982–1983 (12). All of these INDs included blood level, drug metabolism, and other types of ADME data in one or more animal species. However, the doses were often inconsistent, as were the species used in these studies and in the toxicology studies. For example, one IND had ADME data in one rat strain and in dogs and subchronic toxicology studies in a different rat strain and in monkeys. Generally, however, rat strains in the ADME studies were poorly identified or not identified at all, so their correspondence to the toxicology study animals was unclear. Very few dose-ranging or repeated-dosing ADME studies were found in this survey; only two INDs (from the same sponsor) had steady-state blood level data at all doses, and in the same rodent and nonrodent species that were used in the subchronic toxicology studies. Almost all of the ADME studies in these INDs were acute-dosing, single-dose experiments, and the doses used were often lower than those in any toxicology study dose. Sometimes the doses selected were even lower than the pharmacologically active dose in that species.

To determine what further progress has been made and to gather additional background for guideline development, we expanded this preliminary survey to a more detailed examination of the preclinical ADME data in a group of more recently submitted INDs and in a group of recent NDAs.

DRUG APPLICATION SURVEY

For this survey, applications for new molecular entities were selected arbitrarily, without specific prior knowledge of their contents, to represent a broad variety of sponsors and drug categories. The survey sample consisted of 12 NDAs submitted by different companies between 1982 and 1985, and 18 INDs submitted by different companies in 1984 and 1985; four sponsors were common to both groups. The intent of this survey was to compare ADME data being submitted in early IND submissions during the 1980s with ADME data in NDAs that represent cumulative data developed since the late 1970s. It can be assumed that the ADME data in the early IND submissions for these NDA drugs would have shown the limitations and variability evident in the survey of 1982–1983 INDs described above.

ADME data, of the general types identified in the NDA format guideline (6), were submitted as shown in Table 3-1. All of the NDAs had pharmacokinetic, distribution and excretion studies in one or more species. All of the INDs also had pharmacokinetic data in at least one species, but fewer (about 80%) had distribution or excretion studies. Drug metabolism data, although present in most of the applications, were not found in one NDA and in four INDs. Only about half of the applications had information about the drug's protein binding. Half of the NDAs and fewer of the INDs had information about induction of specific enzymes.

The number of species used for pharmacokinetic studies are shown in Table 3-2. All of the NDAs had studies in two or more (usually three or four) different types of animals. Most of the INDs had pharmacokinetic data in two or three species, but two INDs had data in only one species. On the other hand, there was one IND, as well as three NDAs, with pharmacoki-

Table 3-1. Preclinical ADME Data

Type of Data Found	NDAs (n = 12)	INDs (n = 18)
Pharmacokinetics		
Acute-dosing	12	18
Repeated-dosing	3	2
Protein binding	7	9
Tissue distribution	12	14
Drug metabolism	11	14
Enzyme induction	6	3
Excretion pattern	12	15

Table 3-2. Pharmacokinetic Study Species

Number of Species Studied	NDAs (n = 12)	INDs (n = 18)
1	—	2
2	1	8
3	6	7
4	2	—
5	1	—
6	1	1
7	1	—

netic studies in four or more species, including several types of monkeys. This IND and one of these NDAs had the same sponsor.

The various species used for pharmacokinetic studies are identified in Table 3-3. All of the NDAs had pharmacokinetic data in rats and dogs, and more than half also had data in one or more monkey species. All 18 INDs had rat data, but only 13 and 3 had dog and monkey data, respectively, including 2 INDs that had data in both of these species. Fifteen of the INDs, as well as all of the NDAs, had pharmacokinetic studies in the same rodent and nonrodent species used in the subchronic or chronic toxicology studies. As in the previous survey, however, rat strain identification in the pharmacokinetic (and other ADME) studies was often vague or absent, so correspondence with the toxicology strain was not certain. Some other species that were used for pharmacokinetic studies, such as guinea pigs and baboons, are not typical candidates for chronic toxicology testing and were not used for this purpose in these applications. Rabbit pharmacokinetic studies were submitted to 6 of these NDAs and 4 of these INDs, but it is not clear whether these studies were done because of the use or intended use of this species in teratology studies, or merely because of their convenient attributes for serial blood sampling. There were relatively few mouse phar-

Table 3-3. Pharmacokinetic Studies Species

Species Used	NDAs (n = 12)	INDs (n = 18)
Rat	12	18
Dog	12	13
Monkey[a]	7	3
Rabbit	6	4
Mouse	4	3
Guinea pig	2	2
Hamster	—	1

[a]Includes one or more of rhesus, cyanomologus, squirrel, or baboon.

macokinetic studies, despite prevalence of carcinogenicity studies in this species in the NDAs and the prospect of such studies in the INDs.

As indicated in Table 3-1, all of the NDAs and INDs had acute-dosing pharmacokinetic studies in at least one species, but there were relatively few applications with repeated-dosing studies to explore steady-state pharmacokinetics. Only 3 of the 12 NDAs had repeated-dosing studies. One of these NDAs had a 5-to-10-day single-dose level study in pregnant and nonpregnant rats; another NDA had 15-day, three-dose level studies in dogs and monkeys; the third NDA had blood level measurements incorporated into a 3-month, three-dose monkey toxicology study.

Table 3-4 compares the dosing characteristics of these repeated-dosing and the acute-dosing studies in rats, dogs, and monkeys. In addition to the repeated-dosing study in pregnant and nonpregnant rats in 1 NDA, there were 2 INDs with similar acute-dosing comparisons. Acute, single-dose administration predominated in all of the rat, dog, and monkey studies, 69, 79, and 80 percent of the NDA studies in these respective species, and 60, 53, and 100 percent, respectively, in the IND studies. However, the more recently developed IND data had a greater proportion of rat and dog studies in which 2 or 3 dosage levels were used (i.e., 40% of all acute-dosing studies in the INDs as compared with less than 20% in the NDAs). The comparative use of oral and intravenous administration predominated over single-route administration in these acute-dosing studies in both groups of applications, with slightly greater proportion of oral-intravenous comparisons in the INDs (i.e., 78% vs. 71% of rat studies, 62% vs. 58% of dog studies, and 67% vs. 60% of monkey studies in the INDs and NDAs, respectively).

Table 3-4. Pharmacokinetic Study Dosing

	Rat	Dog	Monkey
Number of NDAs with Studies	12	12	7
Total number of studies	16	13	10
Acute, single dose	11	10	8
Acute, dose range	3	2	
Repeated, single dose	1[a]	—	—
Repeated, dose range	—	1	2
Number of INDs with Studies	18	13	3
Total number of studies	20	15	3
Acute, single dose	12[b]	8	3
Repeated, single dose	—	1	—
Repeated, dose range	—	—	—

[a]Includes pregnant-nonpregnant comparison in one study

[b]Includes pregnant-nonpregnant comparison in two studies.

Table 3-5. Comparison of Pharmacokinetic and Toxicology Study Doses

Pharmacokinetic Study Dose	Subchronic Toxicity Study Dose	NDAs			INDs		
		Rat	Dog	Monkey	Rat	Dog	Monkey
One-Dose Studies							
Less than	Low	1	1	1	5	3[a]	—
Same as	Low	3	1	—	3	2	—
Same as	Mid	1	1	—	2	3	1
Same as	High	2	1	—	—	—	—
Exceeds	High	2	2	—	—	—	—
Dose Range Studies							
High dose Less than	Low	1	—	—	—	—	—
High dose Same as	Low	—	—	3	1	1	—
High dose Same as	Mid	1	—	4	1	—	—
High dose Same as	High	1	—	1[b]	1	—	—
High dose Same as	High	—	2[a]	1	—	1	—

[a]Includes one repeated-dosing study.

[b]Incorporated into toxicology study.

Table 3-5 shows how the doses in the pharmacokinetic studies compared with the ones used in the corresponding species in the subchronic toxicity studies. No systematic approach was evident. As in the earlier IND survey, there were relatively few pharmacokinetic studies in these NDAs and in the more recent INDs with doses higher than the midrange of the ones used in the toxicology studies. There were pharmacokinetic studies in all three species with doses that were lower—sometimes considerably lower—than the lowest dose in corresponding toxicology studies. Only one rat, two dog, and two monkey studies were among the NDAs, and one rat and two dog studies were among the INDs that could be called toxicokinetic studies by virtue of their having acute or repeated-dosing dose range studies that encompassed or exceeded the toxicology study dose ranges.

The other types of ADME studies listed in Table 3-1 were too variable in design and reporting to compare in the above manner. In general, most appear to have been done as independent experiments, with little consistent evidence of coordination with the pharmacokinetic studies, toxicology studies, or each other with regard to dose, duration, and species use.

Plasma protein binding did not routinely accompany the preclinical pharmacokinetic studies; this type of data was submitted to only about half of these NDAs and INDs. When done, however, rat and nonrodent data were usually provided.

Tissue distribution studies were particularly variable in design and comprehensiveness. Relative tissue concentrations, usually as radioactivity, were determined quantitatively in all tissues or in selected tissues, and/or qualitatively by radioautography, at single or several sacrifice times that usually seemed to be selected arbitrarily rather than based on information derived from excretion or pharmacokinetic studies. Rats were used more frequently than other species; 2 NDAs and 2 INDs also had distribution studies in pregnant rats. There were two 15-day repeated-dose distribution studies among the NDAs, but all others were of acute-dosing design. There were no dose ranging distribution studies. The single doses used were sometimes unusually low, apparently to conserve the specific activity of the radiolabel. Drug metabolite identification was variably qualitative, quantitative, or lacking (as in 1 NDA and 4 INDs). Metabolites were identified primarily in urine and less frequently in feces, bile, and plasma of rats and, occasionally, dogs and other species. There was little information about dose- and time-related effects on drug metabolism, although a few of the pharmacokinetic studies did include quantitative plasma measurements of metabolites as well as of the parent compound. Investigation of the induction of drug-metabolizing enzymes was sporadic, without apparent link to related observations made in other studies, such as hexobarbital potentiation, evidence of tolerance, or increase in liver weight.

All of the NDAs, but fewer of the INDs, had quantitative urinary and fecal excretion studies. This suggests that this type of information was not always developed as part of the preliminary screen. Most of these excretion studies were conducted in rats; fewer were conducted in nonrodents. About one-third of these NDAs and INDs had biliary excretion data, but it was not clear whether this was a routine determination or a follow-up to fecal excretion data or other observations suggesting the need for such information.

DISCUSSION AND CONCLUSIONS

The FDA's early recommendation for drug-disposition comparison was intended to ensure, or at least improve, selection of the most humanlike animal models for chronic toxicity studies (2). Because of practical limits on species selection that make this objective unattainable, there is now greater emphasis on identification of species, dose, and duration-related similarities and differences in absorption, distribution, metabolism, and excretion to improve the interpretation of observed toxicity and, in some cases, to guide the design of chronic toxicity studies for predictive use. Technological advances have also had an enormous influence on what can be determined quantitatively as well as qualitatively, and there is an increasingly evolving interest in the ADME study aspects of toxicology testing of chemicals in general, as well as in drugs.

Greater diligence still is needed to improve interdisciplinary education and communication to ensure that ADME studies are well coordinated among themselves and with toxicology study design, so that conclusions may derive from a coherent data base rather than from individual or disconnected observations. For example, even though discussion of possible multicompartment, nonlinear toxicokinetic influences on carcinogenic or other toxicologic endpoints continues, interspecies or toxicology dose extrapolations are still often based on acute, single-dose pharmacokinetic studies that assume single-compartment linearity into the toxic range.

The preclinical ADME data submitted in the NDAs and early INDs in this survey place greater emphasis on pharmacokinetic studies than was evident in the earlier survey of INDs submitted in 1982–1983. This suggests that the development of such data for submission to these NDAs was late rather than early. However, few of these NDA or IND studies can be regarded as toxicokinetic studies by anyone's definition, because of the low doses used. Only two of the NDAs surveyed had steady-state blood level observations in dogs and monkeys. In the monkeys this was part of a three-month toxicology study. Steady-state blood level characteristics were not explored in the early IND submissions, nor in rodents in the NDAs.

In more recently submitted drug applications, we have begun to see an increasing number of rodent carcinogenicity studies that include drug blood level determinations. Although this eliminates uncertainties about animal strain, gender, and age comparability that are frequently not met by independently conducted ADME studies, the blood level determinations in these carcinogenicity studies often appear to represent add-on procedures that may be limited to parent drug blood level determinations at the time of terminal sacrifice. Apart from occasional exemplary effort, there has been little general indication of careful, collaborative planning to ensure that toxicokinetic principles, knowledge about dose- and time-dependent changes in drug metabolism, and so on are appropriately addressed in blood level monitoring.

Regardless of whether or not toxicokinetic studies are incorporated into the toxicology studies or conducted in parallel, there appears to be no disagreement between the FDA and industry about the need for a systematic approach (8,13), with particular emphasis on the following recommendations for ADME data development (13):

Use animals in the toxicology study, or parallel groups of same species, strain, weight, age, and sex.

Use doses encompassing the dose range by the same route of administration as in the toxicology studies.

Evaluate drug absorption and excretion as a function of dose level in the test species.

Determine the duration of exposure to the drug, metabolites, or both in the test species.

Determine the effects of a multiple-dose regimen on the absorption and excretion of a drug in the test species.

REFERENCES

1. A. J. Lehman, W. I. Patterson, B. Davidow, E. C. Hagan, G. Woodard, E. P. Laug, J. P. Frawley, O. Fitzhugh, A. R. Bourke, J. H. Draize, A. A. Nelson, and B. J. Vos, Procedures for Appraisal of the Toxicity of Chemicals in Foods, Drugs and Cosmetics. Food, Drug Cosmetic Law J., 679–748 (Oct. 1955).
2. E. I. Goldenthal. Current Views on Safety Evaluation of Drugs. FDA Papers, 1–8 (May 1968).
3. Good Laboratory Practices Regulations, Title 21, Sec. 58, Code of Federal Regulations; Federal Register *43,* 59986–60135 (Dec. 22, 1978); Federal Register *52,* 33768–33782 (Sept. 4, 1987).
4. New Drug, Antibiotic, and Biologic Drug Product Regulations, Title 21, Sec. 312, Code of Federal Regulations; Federal Register *50,* 8831–8846 (Mar. 19, 1987).
5. New Drug and Antibiotic Regulations, Title 21, Sec. 314, Code of Federal Regulations; Federal Register 52, 7493–7516 (Feb. 22, 1985).
6. Guideline for the Format and Content of the Nonclinical Pharmacology/Toxicology Section of an Application, U.S. Food and Drug Administration (Feb. 1987).
7. Guideline for the Format and Content of the Summary for New Drug and Antibiotic Applications, U.S. Food and Drug Administration (Feb. 1987).
8. V. C. Glocklin. General considerations for studies of the metabolism of drugs and other chemicals. Drug Metab. Rev. *13,* 929–939 (1982).
9. B. Clark and D. A. Smith. Pharmacokinetics and toxicity testing. CRC Critical Reviews Toxicol. *12,* 343–385 (1984).
10. J. R. Gillette. Solvable and unsolvable problems in extrapolating toxicological data between animal species and strains. Pages 237–260 in: *Drug Metabolism and Drug Toxicity.* J. R. Mitchell and M. G. Horning, eds. Raven Press, New York (1984).
11. V. C. Glocklin. Correlation of drug disposition and toxicity studies. Pages 75–85 in: *Experimental and Clinical Toxicokinetics.* A. Yacobi and H. Barry, III, eds. Am. Pharmaceut. Assoc., Washington, DC (1984).
12. V. C. Glocklin. Current FDA perspectives on animal selection and extrapolation. Pages 15–22 in: *Human Risk Assessment—The Role of Animals Selection and Extrapolation.* M. V. Roloff, ed. Taylor and Francis, New York (1987).
13. H. Barry, III and A. Yacobi. Preclinical toxicokinetics. Pages 1–7 in: *Experimental and Clinical Toxicokinetics.* A. Yacobi and H. Barry III, eds. Am. Pharmaceut. Assoc., Washington, DC (1984).

Chapter 4

The Use of Interspecies Scaling in Toxicokinetics

Joyce Mordenti, Ph.D.

Department of Pharmacological Sciences
Genentech Inc.

Willard Chappell, Ph.D.

Center for Environmental Sciences and
Department of Physics
University of Colorado at Denver

INTRODUCTION

The pharmaceutical research and development process depends on studies in small laboratory animals—primarily mice, rats, rabbits, monkeys, and dogs—for the selection and screening of candidate pharmaceutical compounds. In the ideal animal model, the pharmacokinetic data and toxicity response in the animal are identical to those data in humans. With the spirit of Ponce de Leon, many scientists have pursued the mythical ideal animal, yet it remains undiscovered and untamed, and animal studies continue to provide data that are qualitatively and quantitatively different from the data produced in subsequent human studies. Is the situation hopeless? Not necessarily. We can interpret pharmacokinetic and toxicologic studies in animals with more certainty with a technique called interspecies scaling.

Interspecies scaling is a method of interpolation and extrapolation based on the underlying anatomical, physiological, and biochemical similarities in mammals. It permits researchers to extrapolate animal data to human beings under many experimental conditions. When interspecies scaling concepts are incorporated into the experimental design and the data analysis of preclinical studies, we can expect (1) to produce more clinically meaningful data from animal experiments; (2) to predict the activity, efficacy, and toxicity of pharmaceutical compounds in human beings with greater accuracy; (3) to decrease the number of animals required for experimentation; and (4) to hasten the drug testing and approval process.

PHYSIOLOGIC BASIS FOR INTERSPECIES SCALING

The most obvious but commonly overlooked difference between laboratory animals and human beings is size. Once we understand how differences in animal sizes affect the size and performance of the internal organs, the methods used for pharmaceutical data extrapolation become self-evident. Figure 4-1 shows the average heartbeat rate for several mammals plotted as a function of body weight on Cartesian coordinates. As mammals increase in size, their heartbeat rate decreases. It is difficult to predict a heartbeat rate for human beings when the data are viewed in this fashion, because the exact relationship of heartbeats per minute to size is not obvious. We might conclude, in despair, that the data are insufficient for predicting the heartbeat rate for human beings, because the curve cannot be reliably extended to 70 kg. Figure 4-2 shows the same data plotted on log-log coordinates. The data for a mouse, rat, rabbit, monkey, and dog fall on a straight line; extension of this line to 70 kg predicts 83 beats per minute for humans. The equation for this straight line is

$$\log(\text{heartbeats per minute}) = -0.25 \log W + 2.38 \qquad \textbf{(1)}$$

where W is weight (kg), 2.38 is the log Y-intercept at one kg, and −0.25 is the slope. Taking the antilog of both sides produces the following power function:

$$\text{heartbeats per minute} = 240W^{-0.25}. \qquad \textbf{(2)}$$

This power function relates heartbeats per minute to species weight (1). It can be used to provide a rough estimate of the heartbeat rate in other mammals.

Empirical regression equations have been used to describe a number of physiological and anatomical properties for birds, reptiles, fish, and mammals (2–4). This type of equation arises whenever some organ or function changes in proportion to total body weight (5). Some relationships have been dramatic; for instance, a comparison of the length of an organism at the time

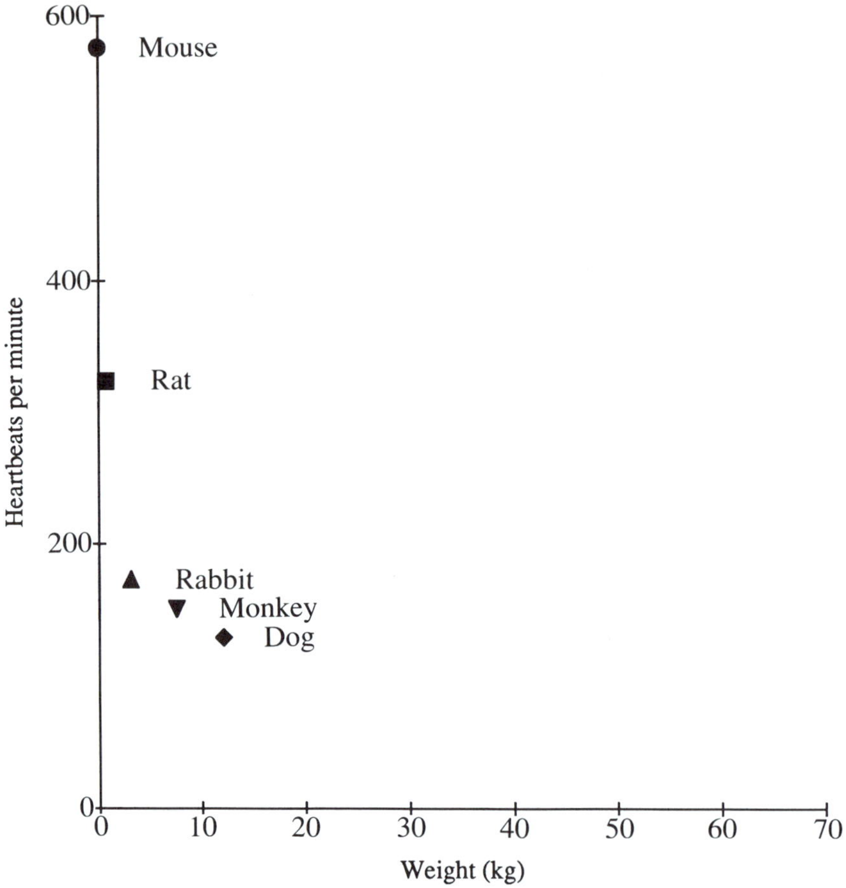

FIGURE 4-1. Cartesian plot of heartbeats per minute vs. weight.

of reproduction to the time between generations for organisms that ranged in size from bacteria to the giant Sequoia demonstrated a startling regularity on log-log coordinates (Fig. 4-3).

When the one-term power function is used in concert with body weight, it is called an allometric equation ("allometric" from the Greek word *alloios* ("different") means "by different measure") (2). The log-transformed equation is represented as follows:

$$\log \mathrm{Y} = \log a + b \log \mathrm{W} \quad \mathbf{(3)}$$

where Y is the physiological variable of interest, log a is the Y-intercept, W is weight, and b is the slope of the log-log plot. Usually, the allometric equation is represented as:

$$\mathrm{Y} = a\mathrm{W}^{b} \quad \mathbf{(4)}$$

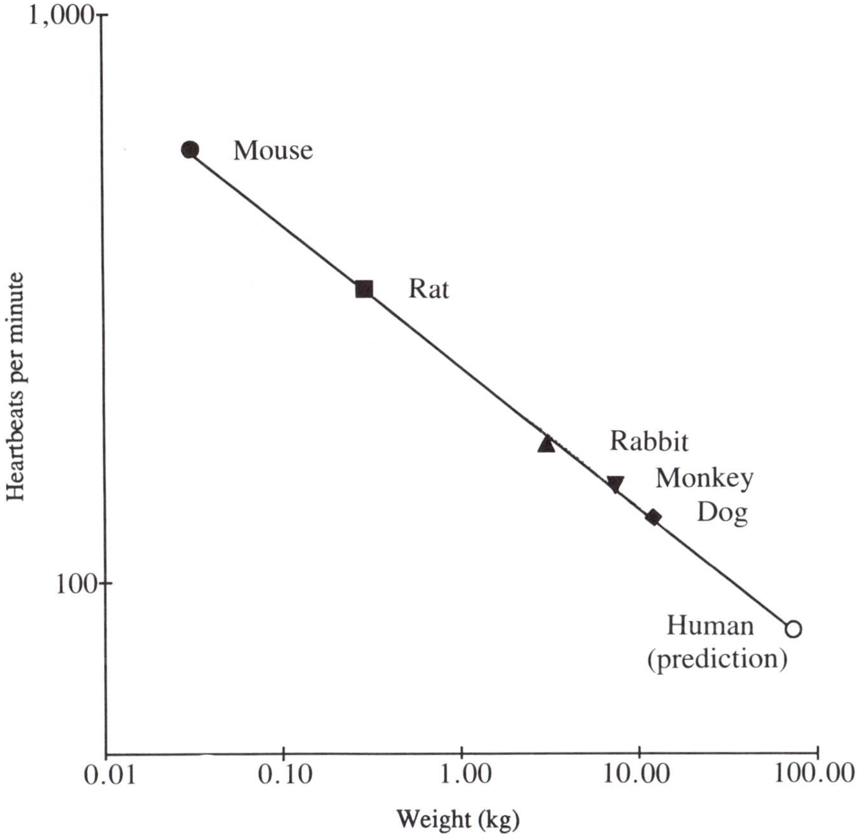

FIGURE 4-2. Log-log plot of heartbeats per minute vs. weight. Prediction for human-beings is read directly from linear regression line.

The sign and magnitude of the exponent (*b*) indicate how a physiological variable (Y) is changing as a function of weight (W). When *b* is <0, Y decreases as weight increases. In the heartbeat example (equation 2), the exponent is -0.25; as species get larger, they have fewer heartbeats per minute. When $b = 0$, Y is independent of weight; for example, the body core temperature of mammals is independent of size, with most mammals at 36–38°C.

When $0 < b < 1$, Y increases as species get larger, but Y does not increase as rapidly as weight. The allometric equation for the blood volume circulation time (seconds) as a function of body weight (kg) is $21W^{0.21}$ (1). The blood volume circulation time is 10 seconds in a 0.03-kg mouse and 51 seconds in a 70-kg person; therefore, a 2,000-fold increase in weight results in only a fivefold increase in circulation time. The allometric equa-

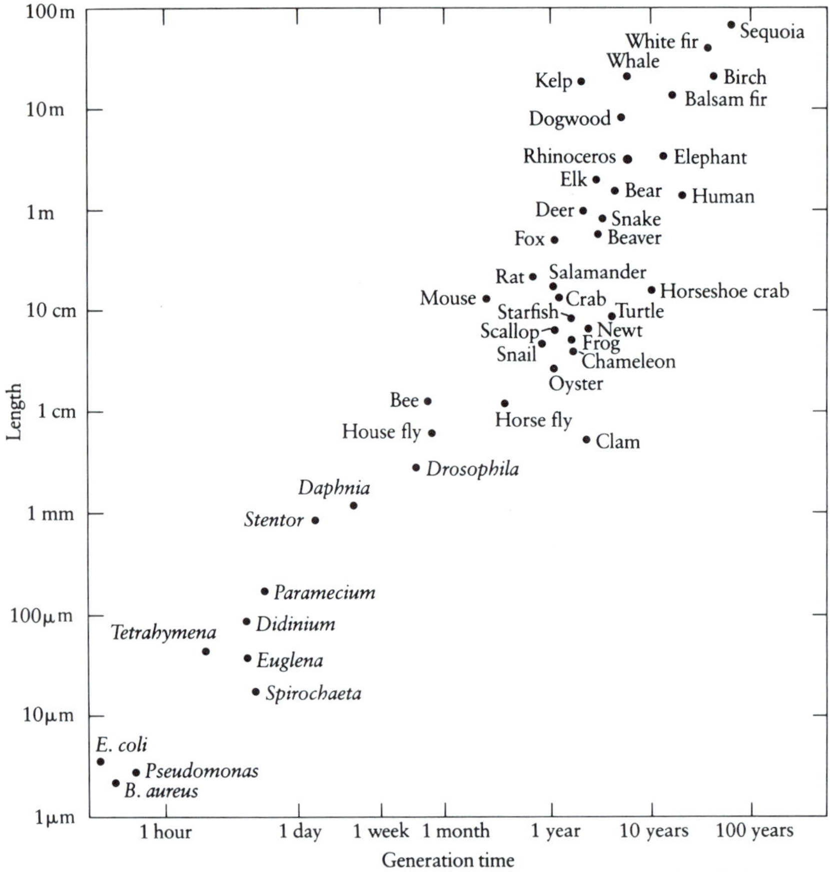

FIGURE 4-3. The length of an organism at the time of reproduction in relation to the generation time is plotted on a logarithmic scale. The first four organisms at the bottom are bacteria. The next five, going up, are protozoa. *Daphnia* is a water flea, *Drosophila* is the fruit fly made famous by experimental geneticists, and all other organisms are easily recognized by their common names. (From *On size and life,* by Thomas A. McMahon and John Tyler Bonner. Copyright © 1983. Reprinted with Permission of Scientific American Books, Inc. and the authors.)

tion for kidney weight (g) as a function of body weight (g) is $0.0212W^{0.85}$ (6). The kidneys are 1.3 percent of total body weight in a 30-g mouse, yet only 0.4 percent of total body weight in a 70,000-g person, resulting in proportionately larger kidneys in the mouse.

When $b = 1$, Y increases in direct proportion to increases in size; in this special case, the allometric equation is referred to as an isometric equation ("by the same measure") (2). Estimates for total blood volume (ml) as a function of body weight (kg) range from $65.6W^{1.02}$ (1) to $77W^{1.0}$ (7); in other words, the blood volume is a constant proportion of total body weight (approximately 6.5–8%) for all mammals.

When $b > 1$, the physiological property (Y) increases faster than increases in total body weight. The allometric equation for the weight of the skeleton of mammals (kg) in relation to body weight (kg) is $0.0608W^{1.083}$ (4, p. 47).

Several patterns have emerged from allometric analyses. In general, biological frequencies tend to have an exponent of −0.25, biological times tend to have an exponent of 0.25, surface area tends to have an exponent of 0.67, clearance and physiologic flow rates tend to have an exponent of 0.75, and volumes tend to have an exponent of 1.0. These values are only approximations; the exact values are still subject to debate, particularly the exponent for metabolic rate that is between 0.67 and 0.77, and most frequently cited as 0.75 (8–17).

SIMILARITY ANALYSIS

Engineers frequently employ similarity analysis and modeling theory to calculate the working characteristics of the prototype from the physical dimensions of a model. As one researcher points out, "A basic requirement for similarity analysis is that a given system exists in at least two discernible alternative forms that are considered similar to each other; preferably there should be many forms, with smooth gradations. Very commonly this means that a certain system must exist in a range of sizes, while retaining clear geometric similarity" (18). Engineering similarity analysis and modeling theory can be used to compare mammals as physical systems (18,19). Physical similarity, in the engineering sense, is defined specifically by dimensionless numbers called criterion of similarity. These numbers are obtained by forming quotients of allometric equations; for example, division of renal blood flow by cardiac output reveals that renal blood flow is approximately 25 percent of cardiac output regardless of mammalian species:

$$\frac{\text{Renal blood flow}}{\text{Cardiac output}} \times 100 = \frac{43.06W^{0.77}}{166W^{0.79}} \times 100 = 25.9\% \quad (5)$$

where renal blood flow and cardiac output are measured in milliliters per minute and weight is in kilograms (20). The residual mass, $W^{-0.02}$, is not considered significantly different from unity and is dropped from the equation.

Another criterion of similarity can be obtained by dividing the time for one breadth by the time for one heartbeat:

$$\frac{\text{Breath time}}{\text{Heartbeat time}} = \frac{4.7 \times 10^{-5}W^{0.28}}{1.2 \times 10^{-5}W^{0.27}} = 3.9 \quad (6)$$

where time is in hours and weight is in grams (6). The breath-to-heartbeat ratio is 4 for mammals; regardless of size, a mammal usually breathes once for every four heartbeats (19). As before, the residual mass, $W^{0.01}$, is not considered significantly different from unity and is dropped from the equation.

Additionally, in many mammalian species, the number of heartbeats per maximum life span is a constant:

$$\frac{\text{Lifetime}}{\text{Heartbeat time}} = \frac{6.6 \times 10^4 W^{0.29}}{7.7 \times 10^{-5} W^{0.27}} = 8.6 \times 10^8 \quad \textbf{(7)}$$

where weight is in kilograms and time is in hours (19,21). In other words, most mammals have 800 to 900 million heartbeats in their lifetime. Small mammals have a short life span, but, at the time of their death, they have performed an equivalent number of physiological functions. Measured by the sensible internal clocks of their own hearts or the rhythm of their breathing, virtually all mammals live for an equivalent amount of time (22). This relationship does not hold for the longer-living *Homo sapiens,* who live approximately three times longer than other mammals of similar weight. Human beings have three times as many breaths and three times as many heartbeats in a lifetime as predicted by the criteria of similarity, but the ratio of four heartbeats per breath remains constant (22). Additional criteria of similarity can be found elsewhere (18,21,23).

Stahl offered these words of caution regarding criterion of similarity (18): "As is generally true in engineering, the numerical value of the criteria should not be considered as always fixed or precise. A possible deviation of 100% is entirely possible in certain cases and may be higher if animals are not similar in overall habitus. It should be noted that a residual mass exponent of more than 0.05 may introduce considerable error with larger animals."

The concept of equivalent time emerges in similarity analysis: Smaller mammals are performing the same physiological functions in the correct relative quantities but at a much quicker pace than larger mammals. Understanding this concept is paramount to understanding pharmacokinetic scaling.

INTERSPECIES SCALING IN PHARMACOKINETIC ANALYSIS

Based on comparative physiology, we can expect small animals to eliminate drugs more rapidly than human beings; small animals have proportionately larger organs and shorter blood circulation times. Based on the inseparable dependence of drug disposition on physiology, we expect that (1) pharmacokinetic scaling will be accomplished in a fashion analogous to biological scaling, and (2) the allometric equations for the pharmacokinetic parameters will be similar to corresponding physiologic variables, i.e., half-life (or time) $\sim W^{0.25}$, clearance $\sim W^{0.75}$, and the volume of distribution $\sim W^{1.0}$. Two decades of experience with interspecies pharmacokinetic scaling has proven these generalities to be true, particularly for drugs that are eliminated solely by physical processes (biliary, renal, or pulmonary excretion). As we embark on our journey of interspecies scaling, we must remember that "allometric regressions are empirically determined and apply only to size ranges represented by actual data" (24). We must be ever wary that we are stepping outside the bounds of our data when we extrapolate from small laboratory animals to human beings.

The Allometric Approach

The allometric approach to interspecies pharmacokinetic scaling is based on methods adapted from comparative physiology. In 1970, Dedrick and colleagues (25) introduced the term *equivalent time* (now called *pharmacokinetic time*). This concept is essentially the same as the ideas of physiologic time (26) and biological time (19) and acknowledges the fact that small animals are performing the same physiological functions as large animals, only at a much faster rate. These functions include heartbeats, gut beats, energy metabolism, chemical metabolism, and chemical excretion. The fact that biological half-lives are usually longer for larger animals than for smaller animals is to be expected.

The use of equivalent time in pharmacokinetic data analysis enabled Dedrick, Bischoff, and Zaharko (25) to further advance the field of comparative pharmacokinetics. They compiled data from experiments in which methotrexate was administered intravascularly or intraperitoneally to mice, rats, dogs, monkeys, and human beings. The doses ranged from 0.1 to 450 mg/kg; the body weights ranged from 22 to 70,000 grams; and the plasma (or serum) concentrations ranged from 0.0077 to 130 μg/ml. Because clearance varied considerably from one species to another, it was not surprising that the concentration-time curves for the five species studied were very different from one another in shape and magnitude. For a single species, the curves for different doses were similar in shape but transposed more or less vertically from one another. Figure 4-4 shows the curves for all species and doses, covering a range in concentration of more than four orders of magnitude over a period of nearly seven hours.

Taking the ordinate as concentration, $C(t)$ and the abscissa as time, t, Dedrick and coworkers (25) normalized the ordinate by dividing the observed plasma (or serum) concentration by dose per unit body weight. They normalized the abscissa by defining equivalent time; that is, since the biological half-life for methotrexate for a mouse was about one-tenth the half-

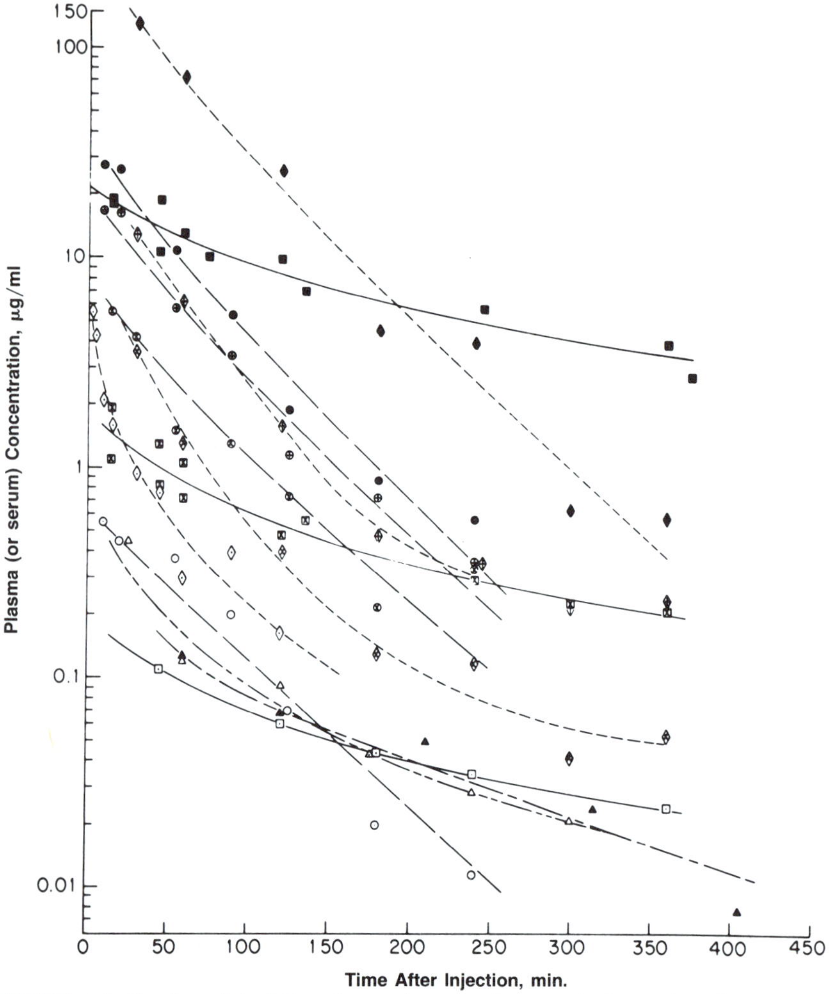

FIGURE 4-4. Semilog plot of the plasma (or serum) concentrations of methotrexate in the mouse (------), rat (———), monkey (—-—), dog (—--—), and human being (——) following IV or IP Injection (symbols refer to different dose levels and routes of administration). Reproduced from Dedrick et al. (25).

life for a human, they noted that "methotrexate pharmacokinetics occur about an order of magnitude faster in mouse than man and that an equivalent time might thus be defined." It could be said that 1 minute to a mouse is equivalent to 10 minutes for a person in terms of the amount of methotrexate eliminated. The scaling factor for the abscissa, $W^{0.25}$, was chosen empirically, based on the concept that equivalent time between species correlates with weight to the 0.25 power; however, they noted that the scaling factor could be based on any intrinsic biological property, such as creatinine clearance, blood circulation velocity, or the mean residence time of blood components in the vascular system. Thus, they normalized the abscissa by dividing time for each species by $W^{0.25}$, which means that 0.13 minutes for a 0.022-kg mouse is equivalent to 1 minute for a 70-kg person.

When they plotted the data from each species as C(t)/(D/W) vs. (time/$W^{0.25}$), they found that the data fit a single curve (Figure 4-5). Equating biological time, $W^{0.25}$, to half-life ($t_{1/2}$) was a good approximation for methotrexate; the actual value was $W^{0.2}$ (Fig. 4-6).

The methotrexate example took plasma (or serum) concentration and bi-

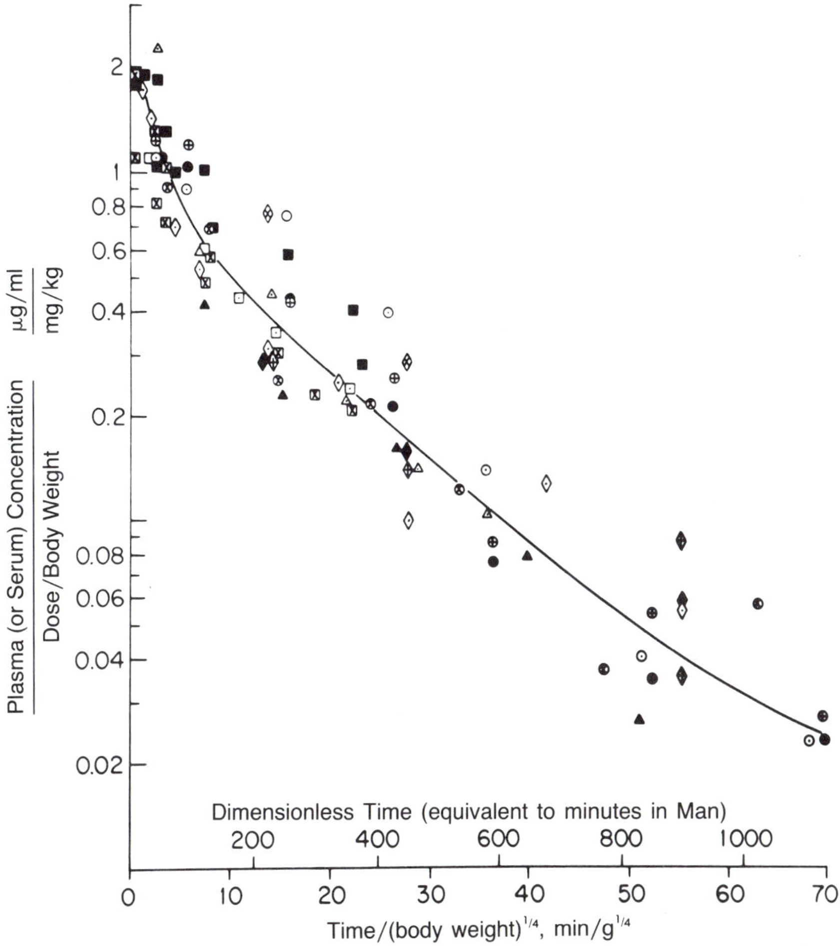

FIGURE 4-5. Semilog plot of the plasma (or serum) methotrexate concentrations from Figure 4-4 after normalization of the axes (symbols refer to different dose levels and routes of administration). Reproduced from Dedrick et al. (25).

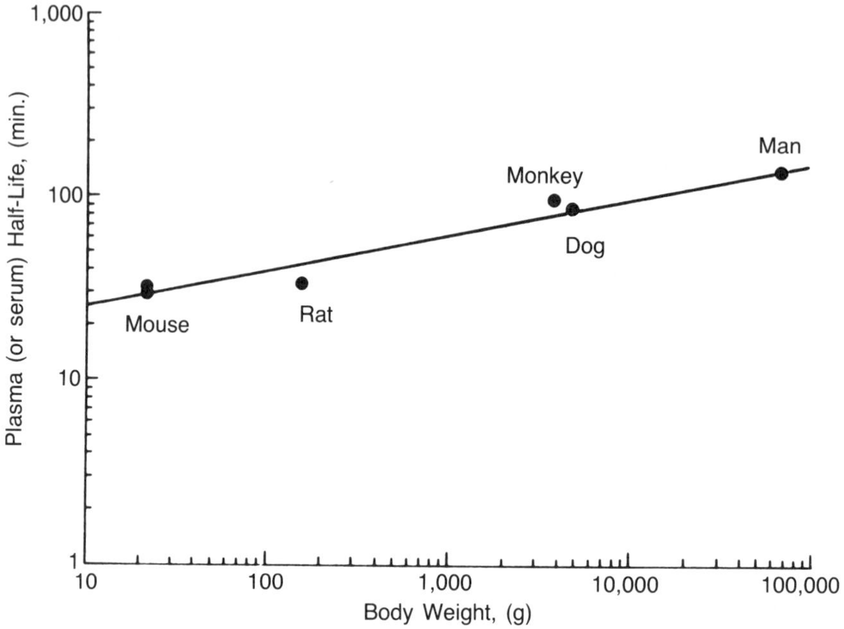

FIGURE 4-6. Reported and calculated half-lives of methotrexate in plasma (or serum) of mouse, rat, monkey, dog, and human being. Reproduced from Dedrick et al. (25).

ological half-life into account and produced superimposable concentration vs. time profiles. The fact that all the data for five species with a range of mass over three orders of magnitude fits the same curve is evidence of the applicability of allometric equations for interspecies pharmacokinetic scaling.

Boxenbaum (27) used data from the same sources as Dedrick and colleagues (25) to calculate the methotrexate plasma clearance (CL_{MTX}) and the volume of distribution (V_{β}) in five species. When these pharmacokinetic parameters were plotted as a function of species body weight on log-log coordinates, both were linearly related to body weight (Figs. 4-7 and 4-8). Boxenbaum demonstrated the use of engineering dimensional analysis by forming a quotient between the allometric equation for methotrexate clearance (CL_{MTX}) and the allometric equation for creatinine clearance (CL_{Cr}) as follows:

$$\frac{CL_{MTX}}{CL_{Cr}} = \frac{10.9W^{0.69}}{8.2W^{0.69}} = 1.33 \quad \textbf{(8)}$$

where clearance is in milliliters per minute and weight is in kilograms. Thus, CL_{MTX} is 1.33 CL_{Cr}, and this relationship is independent of species and size.

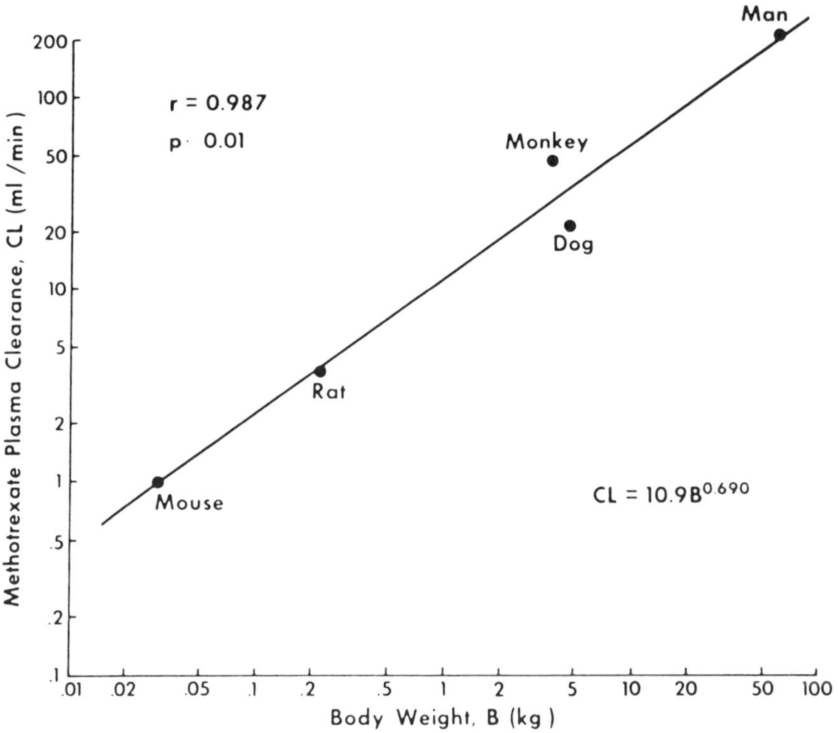

FIGURE 4-7. Interspecies correlation between methotrexate plasma clearance (CL) and body weight (B). Linear regression analysis was performed on logarithmically transformed data. Reprinted from Boxenbaum (27) with permission of the author. Copyright 1982 Plenum Publishing Co.

In a sense, all species are alike, excreting methotrexate from their bodies at a rate that correlates with their physiology.

Similar analysis was performed for methotrexate volume of distribution (V_β) and total body water (TBW) as follows:

$$\frac{V_\beta}{TBW} = \frac{0.859W^{0.918}}{0.703W^{0.963}} = 1.22W^{-0.045} \sim 1.22 \qquad \textbf{(9)}$$

where V_β and TBW are in liters and weight is in kilograms. This analysis suggests that methotrexate V_β is 1.22 times larger than total body water in all species. The residual mass exponent in this calculation (−0.045) is considered to have a modest effect on this ratio. A critical tacit assumption made by Dedrick and co-workers (25), was that the distribution volume was proportional to body mass, i.e., $W^{1.0}$. While this assumption is good as a first approximation for drugs, it is not the case for all drugs; for example, chlor-

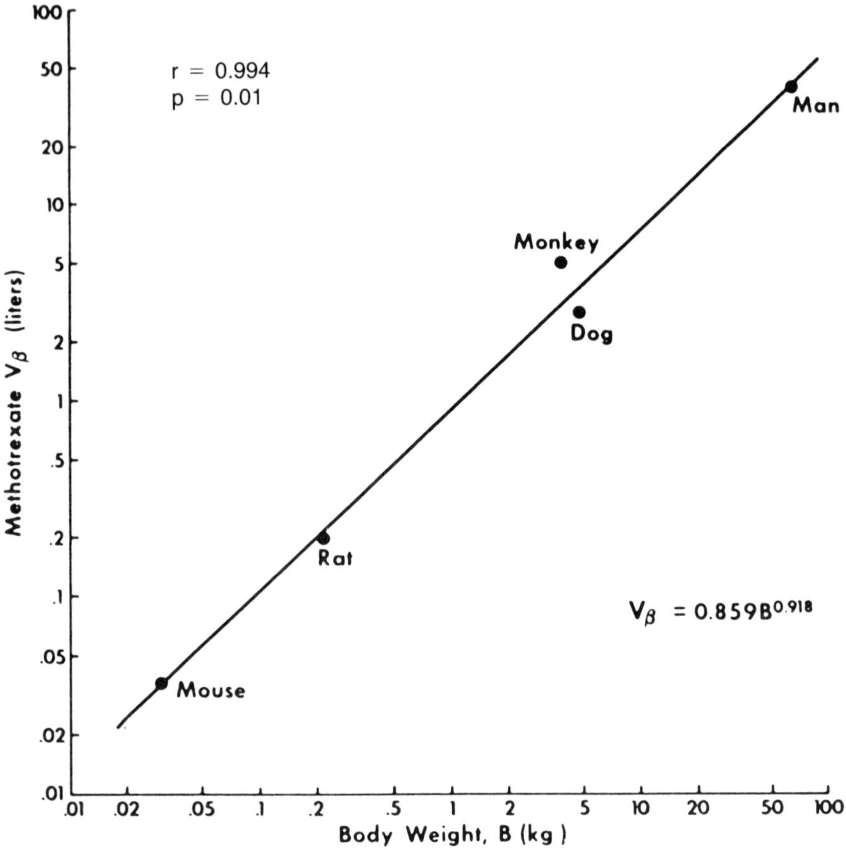

FIGURE 4-8. Interspecies correlation between methotrexate volume of distribution (V_β) and body weight (B). Linear regression analysis was performed on logarithmically transformed data. Reprinted from Boxenbaum (27) with permission of the author. Copyright 1982. Plenum Publishing Co.

diazepoxide has a volume of distribution proportional to $W^{0.58}$ (28), and ceftizoxime has a volume of distribution proportional to $W^{0.8}$ (29).

In a series of papers, Boxenbaum (27,28,30) refined the concept of physiological time first discussed by Brody (26) and the concept of pharmacokinetic scaling introduced by Dedrick and colleagues (25). He reemphasized the fact that the variation in biological half-lives with size and time scaling introduced by Dedrick and co-workers is a reflection of the faster tempo of living in small animals. When applied to pharmacokinetic events, he calls this new time scale pharmacokinetic time and notes that it is not the same for all chemicals.

Boxenbaum and Ronfeld (28) provided cross-species pharmacokinetic scaling equations for the one- and two-compartment pharmacokinetic models.

They began with one-compartment model for a single dose, D, administered at time (t) = 0:

$$C(t) = \left(\frac{D}{V}\right) \exp(-kt) \tag{10}$$

where C(t) is the concentration at time = t, V is the volume of distribution, and k is the elimination rate constant. Assuming first-order kinetics, the elimination rate constant (k) is defined by

$$k = \frac{CL}{V} \tag{11}$$

where CL = clearance. Substituting equation 11 into equation 10 produces

$$C(t) = \left(\frac{D}{V}\right) \exp(-CL/V)t \tag{12}$$

Clearance and volume of distribution can be defined by allometric functions as follows:

$$CL = aW^{x} \tag{13}$$

$$V = bW^{y} \tag{14}$$

Equations 13 and 14 can be substituted into equation 12 to produce an equation for C(t) as a function of body weight as follows:

$$C(t) = \left(\frac{D}{bW^{y}}\right) \exp(-a/b)(W^{x-y})t \tag{15}$$

A rearrangement of equation 15 produces equation 16:

$$\frac{C(t)}{\left(\frac{D}{W^{y}}\right)} = \left(\frac{1}{b}\right) \exp\left(-\frac{a}{b}\right)\left(\frac{t}{W^{y-x}}\right) \tag{16}$$

A Naperian log-linear plot of $C(t)/(D/W^{y})$ vs. (t/W^{y-x}) will produce superimposable pharmacokinetic profiles for one-compartment pharmacokinetic data from different species. The authors introduced a new unit of pharmacokinetic space-time, the apolysichron (apl), which they defined as follows:

$$apl = W^{y-x} \tag{17}$$

In this equation, an apolysichron has the same units of time as those used in the pharmacokinetic analysis, i.e., seconds, minutes, hours, or days. Referring to equation 11, Boxenbaum and Ronfeld expressed half-life ($t_{1/2}$) and mean residence time (MRT) as allometric functions and then converted them to apolysichrons as follows:

$$t_{1/2} = \frac{0.693}{k} = 0.693\left(\frac{b}{a}\right)W^{y-x} = 0.693\left(\frac{b}{a}\right)\text{apl} \quad \textbf{(18)}$$

$$\text{MRT} = \frac{1}{k} = \left(\frac{b}{a}\right)W^{y-x} = \left(\frac{b}{a}\right)\text{apl} \quad \textbf{(19)}$$

They demonstrated that half-life in one species can be related to half-life in a second species by a simple relationship:

$$t_{1/2,\text{human}} = t_{1/2,\text{dog}}\left(\frac{W_{\text{human}}}{W_{\text{dog}}}\right)^{y-x} \quad \textbf{(20)}$$

Boxenbaum and Ronfeld substituted $y = 1$ in equation 16 to solve the equation for the simplest case in which the volume of distribution is proportional to weight, i.e., $V = bW$. The equation is rearranged as follows:

$$\frac{C(t)}{\left(\frac{D}{W}\right)} = \left(\frac{1}{b}\right)\exp - \left(\frac{a}{b}\right)\left(\frac{t}{W^{1-x}}\right) \quad \textbf{(21)}$$

A Naperian log-linear plot of $C(t)/(D/W)$ vs. (t/W^{1-x}) results in superimposability of the pharmacokinetic data from the different species. When $y = 1$, the authors referred to the plot as an Elementary Dedrick Plot because it is the same data transformation introduced by Dedrick and colleagues (25). When $y \neq 1$, the authors referred to the plot as a Complex Dedrick Plot.

In the Elementary Dedrick Plot, one unit of pharmacokinetic space-time is equivalent to W^{1-x} units of chronological time. Boxenbaum and Ronfeld (28) introduced the kallynochron (kln) as a new unit of pharmacokinetic space-time and defined it as follows:

$$\text{kln} = W^{1-x} \quad \textbf{(22)}$$

In this equation, a kallynochron has the same units of time as those used in the pharmacokinetic analysis (i.e., seconds, minutes, hours, or days, etc.). Obviously, the kallynochron and the apolysichron are equivalent when the volume of distribution is directly proportional to body weight, that is, when $y = 1$.

Furthermore, since

$$\text{CL} = aW^{x}\ (\text{ml/min}) \quad \textbf{(13)}$$

or

$$\text{CL} = aW^{x-1}\ (\text{ml/min/kg}) \quad \textbf{(23)}$$

then

$$\text{CL} = a(\text{ml/kln/kg}) \quad \textbf{(24)}$$

or clearance expressed in ml/kln is directly proportional to species body weight. Area under the curve for an intravenous dose is solely a function of clearance; therefore, a plot based on kallynochrons will produce equivalent area under the curves. At one mouse kallynochron and one dog kallynochron, each species will have cleared the same volume of drug from the sampling compartment per kilogram of body weight.

The derivations presented above consider only monoexponential decay of drug in serum or plasma. Boxenbaum and Ronfeld (28) provided an equivalent derivation for the two-compartment model with input into and elimination from the central compartment. They represented the clearance and volume terms with allometric functions as follows:

$$CL = aW^x \qquad \textbf{(13)}$$

$$V_1 = cW^y \qquad \textbf{(25)}$$

$$V_\beta = dW^y \qquad \textbf{(26)}$$

$$V_{ss} = eW^y \qquad \textbf{(27)}$$

where V_1 is the volume of the central compartment, V_β is the volume of distribution during the β phase (also called V_{area}), and V_{ss} is the volume of distribution at steady state. Then, through rearrangements and substitutions, they obtained the following equation:

$$C(t) = \left(\frac{D}{W^y}\right) \frac{(cfg - af)\exp(-f)(t/W^{y-x}) - (cfg - ag)\exp(-g)(t/W^{y-x})}{ac(g - f)} \qquad \textbf{(28)}$$

where $f = a(d - c)/[c/(d - e)]$ and $g = a/d$. A limitation to this proof is the premise that V_1, V_β, and V_{ss} will all scale to body weight with the same allometric exponent, y.

A plot of $C(t)/(D/W^y)$ vs. (t/W^{y-x}) results in superimposable biexponential curves. Once again, the area under the curve is equal to $1/a$, since area is only a function of clearance. In the special case where $y = 1$, the plot reduces to $C(t)/(D/W)$ vs. (t/W^{1-x}), which is the same quantity plotted by Dedrick and colleagues (25).

To demonstrate the utility of these equations, Boxenbaum and Ronfeld used biexponential antipyrine and chlordiazepoxide data obtained from dogs and human beings. The antipyrine data are illustrated in Figure 4-9. Figure 4-10 illustrates an Elementary Dedrick Plot of these same data. Figure 4-11 illustrates chlordiazepoxide plasma concentration-time data plotted in accordance with the elementary Dedrick relationship; that is, kallynochrons are plotted on the abscissa. Superimposability is not obtained. The dog has a greater volume of distribution than the person ($y \neq 1$), making these data ill-conditioned for an Elementary Dedrick Plot. Figure 4-12 illustrates these

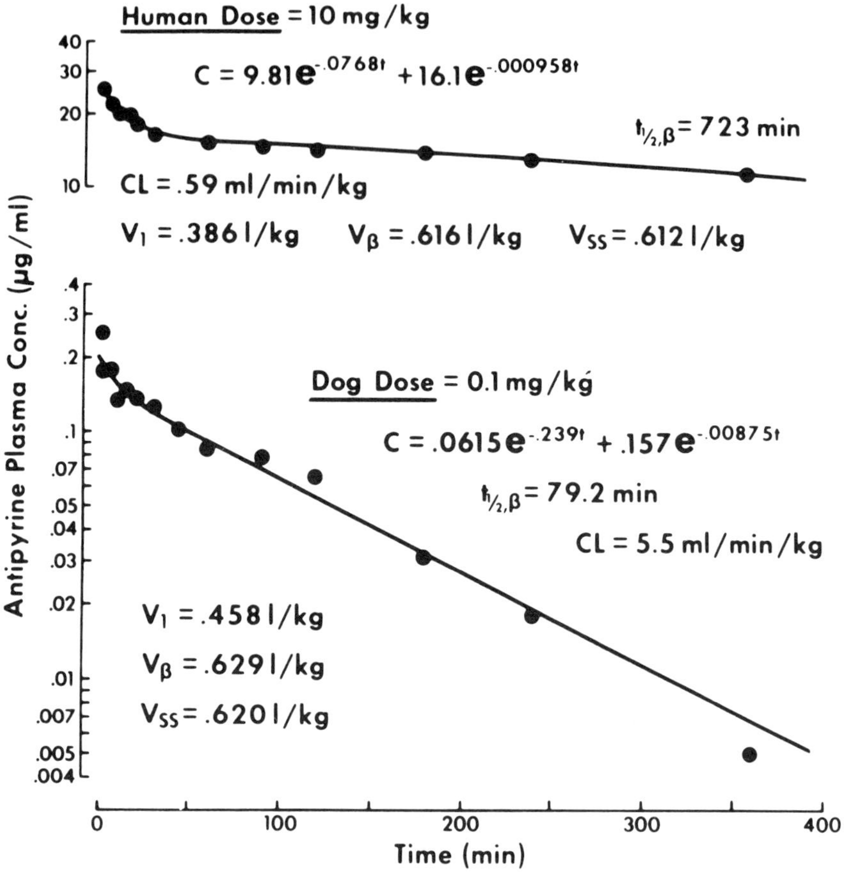

FIGURE 4-9. Antipyrine disposition in dogs and human beings after rapid intravenous injection. Reprinted from Boxenbaum and Ronfeld (28) with permission. Copyright 1983. The American Physiology Society.

same chlordiazepoxide data plotted as a complex Dedrick relationship (i.e., apolysichrons are plotted on the abscissa).

Swabb and Bonner (31), in 1983, were the first to publish a priori predictions of human serum concentration-time profiles using allometric relationships. They had pharmacokinetic data from mice, rats, rabbits, squirrel monkeys, and cynomolgus monkeys when they were confronted with the task of designing the first human clinical trials for the renally excreted antibacterial drug aztreonam. They scaled clearance and volume of distribution allometrically, assumed a one-compartment model in human begins, and predicted the serum aztreonam decay curve for humans following intravenous administration. Although aztreonam displayed two-compartment characteristics in humans, their predictions were remarkably accurate (Fig. 4-13).

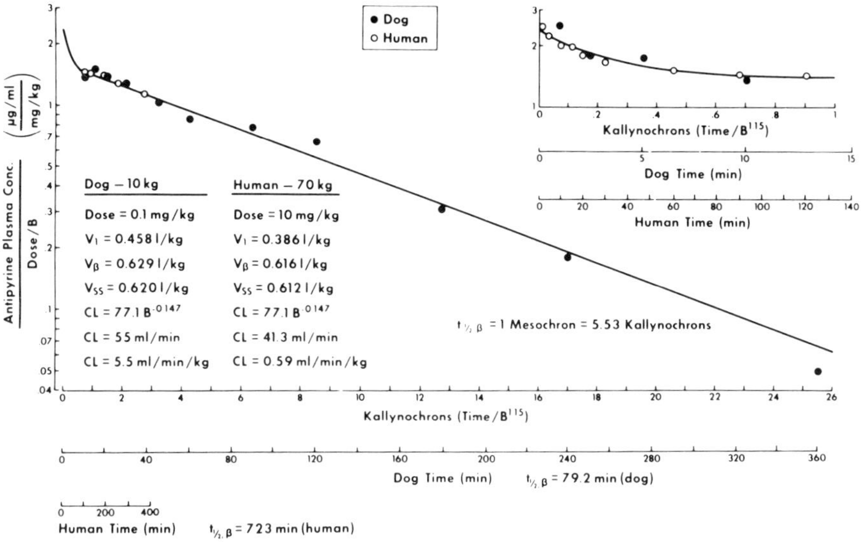

FIGURE 4-10. Elementary Dedrick Plot of antipyrine data illustrated in Figure 4-9. Reprinted from Boxenbaum and Ronfeld (28) with permission. Copyright 1983. The American Physiology Society.

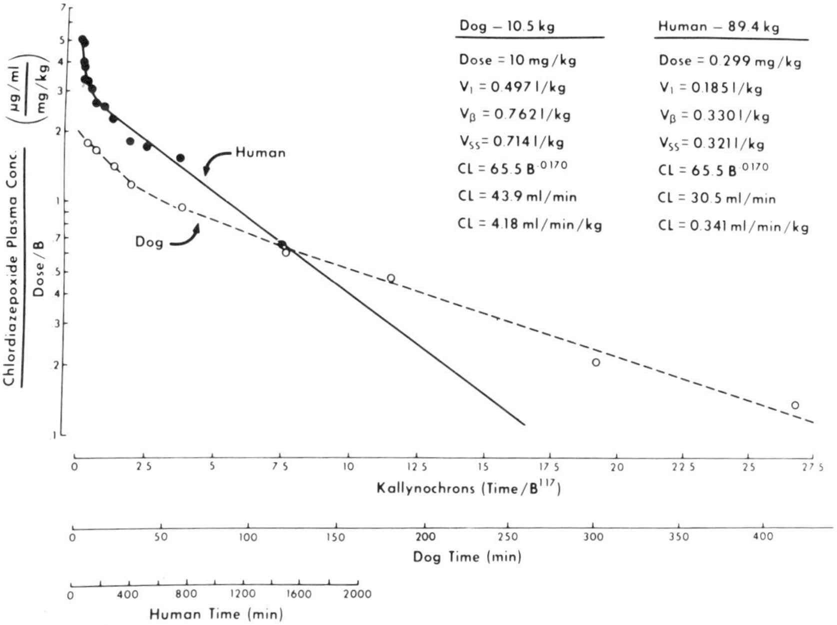

FIGURE 4-11. Elementary Dedrick Plot of chlordiazepoxide data from dogs and human beings after rapid intravenous injection. Reprinted from Boxenbaum and Ronfeld (28) with permission. Copyright 1983. The American Physiology Society.

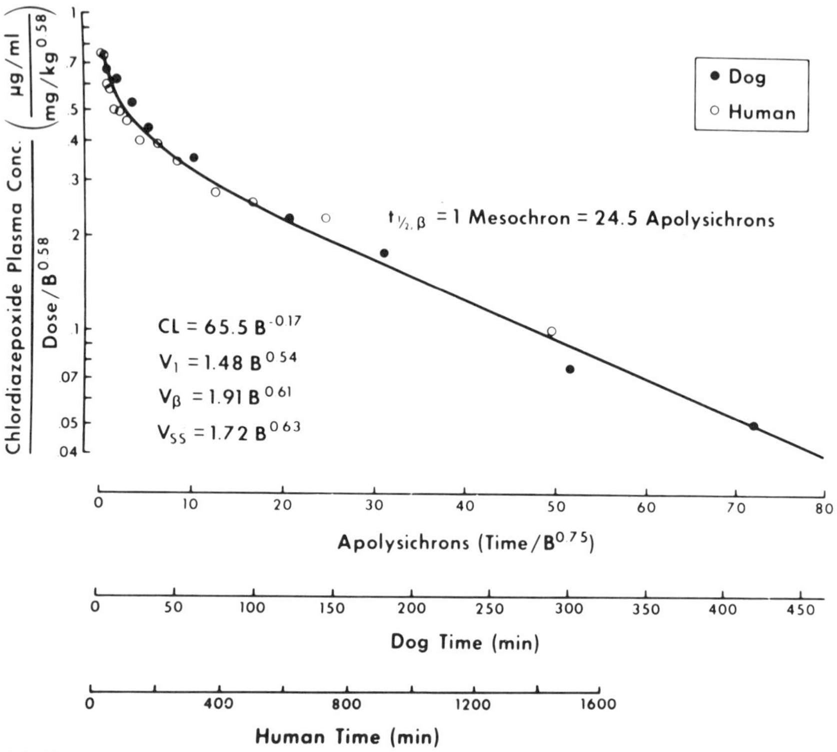

FIGURE 4-12. Complex Dedrick Plot of chlordiazepoxide data from dogs and human beings after rapid intravenous injection. Reprinted from Boxenbaum and Ronfeld (28) with permission. Copyright 1983. The American Physiology Society.

In 1985, Mordenti (29) reported the successful scale-up of biexponential pharmacokinetic data from animals to humans for the antibacterial drug ceftizoxime. This antibiotic is renally excreted and exhibits low protein binding. The pharmacokinetic parameters for ceftizoxime in mice, rats, monkeys, and dogs (32) were scaled as a function of body weight using the allometric approach. Three models were used to predict the serum concentration-time profiles for a 1-gram intravenous bolus and a four-gram, 30-minute intravenous infusion in human beings. Method I scaled the coefficients (A,B) and exponents (α, β) of the biexponential equation; Method II scaled the microconstants (k_{12}, k_{21}, k_{10}) and volume of distribution (V_1) of the two-compartment model; and Method III scaled the volumes of distribution (V_1, V_β, V_{ss}) and clearance. Irrespective of the method chosen, there was close agreement between the predicted concentrations of ceftizoxime in human serum and the concentrations reported in the literature (Fig. 4-14). Method III does not require the exponents for V_1, V_β, and V_{ss} to scale to body weight with the same allometric exponent, y, as required by equation 28.

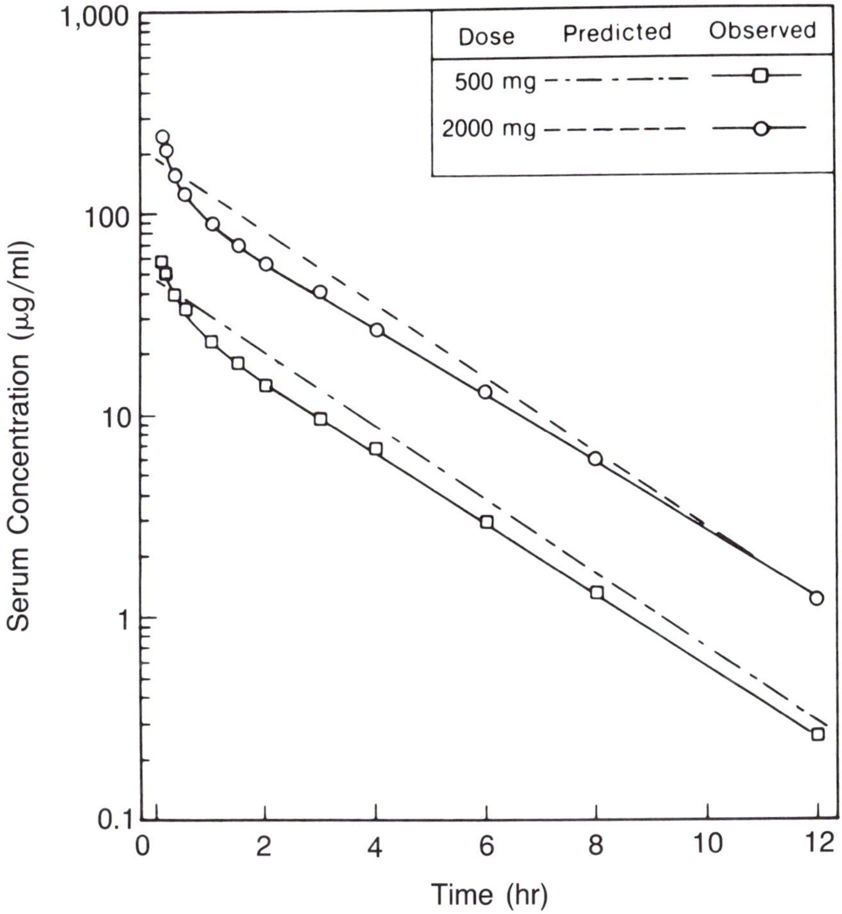

FIGURE 4-13. Comparison between predicted and observed serum concentrations for aztreonam given as 500- and 1,000-mg intravenous infusions over 3 minutes to healthy male subjects. Values are means for two groups of subjects. Reprinted with permission from Swabb and Bonner (31). Copyright 1983. Plenum Publishing Co.

Sometimes the single-term power function, i.e., $Y = aW^b$, is incapable of fully characterizing biological and pharmacokinetic processes for all mammals. Most notably, human beings live longer and have larger brains than mammals of similar size. Sacher (33) found that the maximum life-span potential (MLP) for mammals was well described by a two-term power function that contained both brain weight (BW) and body weight (W) as follows:

$$\text{MLP (years)} = 10.839\text{BW}^{0.636}\text{W}^{-0.225} \quad \textbf{(29)}$$

where brain weight and body weight are in grams. The equation can be rewritten for weight in kilograms (34) as follows:

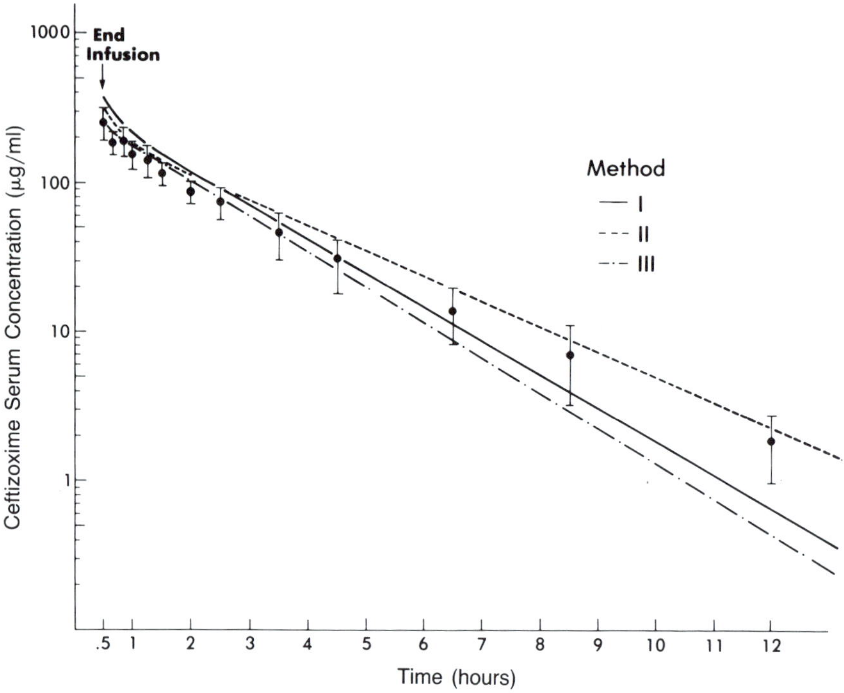

FIGURE 4-14. Comparison between predicted and observed serum concentrations for ceftizoxime given as a 4-g, 30-min intravenous infusion to healthy male subjects. The symbols represent experimental data (mean ± SD) for four healthy volunteers taken from the literature. From Mordenti (29). Copyright 1985. Reproduced with permission of the copyright owner, the American Pharmaceutical Association.

$$\text{MLP (years)} = 185.4\text{BW}^{0.636}\text{W}^{-0.225} \quad \textbf{(30)}$$

The mean values for body weight and brain weight appear in Table 4-1.

In a review of the effects of size and allometry on phylogeny and ontogeny, Gould (24), like Sacher, suggested that the one independent variable allometric equation probably needed to be replaced by a multivariable equation in some instances. He wrote: "Multivariate techniques suited for the apprehension of causal influences may soon supersede the simple allometric equation as a major quantitative technique for explanatory analysis of the phenomena of allometry" (24, p. 628).

Boxenbaum (35) reported that the intrinsic clearance of antipyrine in humans, a compound cleared solely by phase 1 hepatic oxidative metabolism, was approximately one-seventh of that which would be predicted from other species. Data on phenytoin and benzodiazepines (bromazepam, clonazepam, chlordiazepoxide) showed a similar pattern; thus, the allometric equation with one independent variable, $Y = aW^b$, and data in several mammalian species cannot adequately predict the clearance of these compounds in humans.

Table 4-1. Mean Body Weight and Mean Brain Weight for Select Mammals

Species	Body Weight (kg)	Brain Weight (kg)
Mouse	0.0288	0.000418
Rat	0.232	0.00174
Guinea pig	0.285	0.00362
Quokka	2.6	0.013
Rabbit	2.93	0.0115
Cynomolgus monkey	3.73	0.0424
Baboon	4.92	0.0312
Rhesus monkey	5.82	0.0768
Dog	14.2	0.0754
Goat	31.3	0.13
Sheep	57.6	0.11
Pig	66.5	0.0499
Human	70	1.53
Cattle	310	0.251
Horse	398	0.569

Note: Information is from Boxenbaum and Fertig (34).

Boxenbaum and Fertig (34) showed that the intrinsic clearance of unbound antipyrine (CLu_{int}) was well described by a two-term power equation based on brain weight (BW) and body weight (W):

$$CL_{u,int} = 0.387BW^{-0.619}W^{1.32} \tag{31}$$

The authors concluded: "The observation that both maximum life potential and antipyrine CLu_{int}, as well as Clu_{int} for other drugs (36), was related to the same body variables suggests that the set of genetic mechanisms regulating these constitutional characteristics has obtained increased efficiency through a harmonious integration of parts. This interconnectedness and multifactorial expression of the genome creates a design principle—the pharmacokinetic ground plan—the expression of which has rendered interspecies scaling a reality."

In a general derivation for monoexponential decay, Boxenbaum (30) used a two-term power equation for clearance (CL):

$$CL = a(BW)^{b}W^{c} \tag{32}$$

and a one-term power function for volume of distribution (V):

$$V = dW^{e} \tag{33}$$

Equations 32 and 33 were combined to produce the disposition function as follows:

$$\frac{C(t)}{\left(\dfrac{D}{W^{e}}\right)} = \left(\frac{1}{d}\right) \exp\left(-\frac{a}{d}\right)(w^{c-e})(BW^{b})t \tag{34}$$

A Naperian semilogarithmic plot of $C(t)/(D/W^e)$ vs. $[(W^{c-e})(BW^b)(t)]$ is linear with slope $-a/d$ and intercept $1/d$. This plot is illustrated for antipyrine data (terminal exponential phase) in Figure 4-15. Syndesichrons are plotted on the ordinate. Area under the curve $(0 - \infty)$ is equal to $(1/a) \times 10^{-2}$. For superimposability of biexponential data, all volume of distribution terms must scale to W^e.

Gould postulated that human beings deviate from other mammals because of neoteny, that is, the retention of formerly juvenile characteristics by adult descendants produced by the retardation of somatic development for selected organs and parts (37–39). In other words, adult humans physically resemble baby chimpanzees. Relative to other species, neoteny is associated with longer gestation periods, slower maturation (including sexual), intense parenteral care, longer learning in offspring, greater socialization, enhanced longevity, larger and more complex brains, and low reproductive effort producing few well-formed individuals with high competitive ability.

Yates and Kugler (40) elegantly tied the concept of neoteny to drug pharmacokinetics. Neoteny is a reasonable explanation for human beings appearing to have diminished oxidative drug metabolism compared to other mammals (see H. Boxenbaum and R. D'Souza for discussions on the impact of neoteny on phase 1 hepatic oxidative metabolism in humans [41,42]). It is attractive to postulate that reduced mixed function oxidase hepatic activity in human beings is linked to enhanced longevity (41). With relatively low

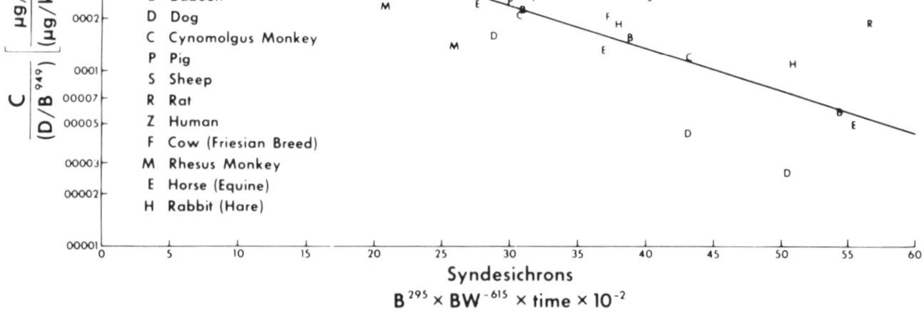

FIGURE 4-15. Semilogarithmic syndesichron plot for antipyrine disposition in 11 mammalian species. Clearance (ml/min) data were characterized by the relationship CL = $0.4063\ B^{1.244}\ BW^{-0.615}$ (B and BW in kg), and volume of distribution (V) was characterized by the relationship V = $08308W^{0.949}$ (W in kg). V and CL values used in fits were calculated from terminal exponential disposition data only. Reprinted from Boxenbaum (30), p. 91, by courtesy of Marcel Dekker, Inc. Copyright 1984.

mixed function oxidase activity, human beings possibly activate fewer procarcinogenic molecules, thereby promoting a longer life than would otherwise be possible (41).

Table 4-2 lists a summary to the equations, data requirements, uses, advantages, and limitations of the allometric approach. Additional examples of the allometric approach can be found in the literature (43–50). The allometric approach tells us how size exerts its influence, but it cannot tell us why. Although it may afford superficial characterization, it cannot generally explain in terms of constitution, events, processes, or structure (41).

The Physiologic Approach

The physiologic approach to interspecies pharmacokinetic scaling is based on methods adapted from chemical engineering. Physiologic flow models attempt to be anatomically, physiologically, thermodynamically, and biochemically realistic. The models are drawn as a flow scheme in which all the important organ and tissue compartments are connected via the circulatory system, as in the body (Fig. 4-16). Elimination can occur from any compartment. There is no simple way to decide exactly how many body regions, or compartments, are needed. One must base the initial choices upon whatever is known about the physiochemical properties (binding, lipid solubility, ionization) and the pharmacologic properties (mechanisms of transport, site(s) of action) of the drug (52).

Once the body regions have been selected, the mathematical pharmacokinetic model is obtained by writing mass balance equations for the sum of the processes occurring in each compartment. Important variables in the physiologic model include the blood flow to eliminating organs; tissue and fluid volumes; blood-to-plasma and tissue-to-plasma drug concentration ratios; drug protein binding; and enzyme kinetics.

The amount of drug in the blood of a physiologic model is written in words (52) as follows:

(the accumulation of unbound drug) + (the accumulation of bound drug)
= (flow in from organs) − (flow out from organs) + (new IV doses) **(35)**

This relationship is written mathematically (52) as follows:

$$w_B V_B \frac{dC_B}{dt} + p_B V_B \frac{dX_B}{dt} = \sum_i Q_i(w_{Bi}C_{Bi} + p_{Bi}X_{Bi}) - (Q_B)(w_B C_B + p_B X_B) + (\text{new IV doses}) \quad (36)$$

where C is the free (unbound) concentration; X, bound concentrations; V,

Table 4-2. Interspecies Pharmacokinetic Scaling at a Glance

I. Allometric Approach
   A. Equations
      1. one independent variable: $Y = aW^b$, where W = body weight
      2. two independent variables: $Y = aW^b(BW)^c$, where BW = brain weight
   B. Data Requirements
      1. Enough data are available to obtain statistical significance
      2. If protein binding is greater than 80%, it is essential that the percentage of protein binding is similar in all species and linear over the concentration range of interest. When in doubt, scale unbound drug concentrations
      3. Physical methods of elimination (renal, biliary, pulmonary) are preferred for one independent variable; oxidative metabolism scales with two independent variables
   C. Uses
      1. Estimation of pharmacokinetic parameters (clearance, volume of distribution, half-life, etc.)
      2. Estimation of entire pharmacokinetic profiles
      3. Estimation of toxicity endpoints
   D. Advantages: Easy and fast
   E. Limitations
      1. Empirical
      2. No attempt is made to give physiological meaning to the pharmacokinetic parameters
      3. May not work well for metabolized compounds, although there are data to support allometric approach for some metabolized compounds

II. Physiologic Approach
   A. Equations: Series of differential equations that are solved simultaneously
   B. Data Requirements
      1. Need anatomical, physiological, biochemical, and binding data for drug disposition, such as
         a. blood flow to eliminating organs
         b. tissue and fluid volumes
         c. blood-to-plasma and tissue-to-plasma drug concentration ratios
         d. drug protein binding
         e. enzyme kinetics
      2. Linear or nonlinear pharmacokinetic data
      3. Linear or nonlinear protein binding
   C. Uses
      1. Estimates of drug disposition in other animal species are obtained once the model is described in detail for one species
      2. Estimation of toxicity endpoints
      3. Low dose to high dose extrapolation (and vice versa)
   D. Advantages
      1. Pharmacokinetic parameters have physiological meaning
      2. Method of choice for metabolized compounds
      3. The parameters in the model can be modified to make *a priori* predictions of pharmacokinetic changes associated with various disease states, age, pregnancy, and drug-drug interactions.
   E. Limitations
      1. Requires sophisticated computer programs, mathematical prowess, lots of experimental time, and money
      2. Data in humans may not be available; therefore, may need to rely on in vitro experiments, allometric estimates, or may need to assume same value as animals

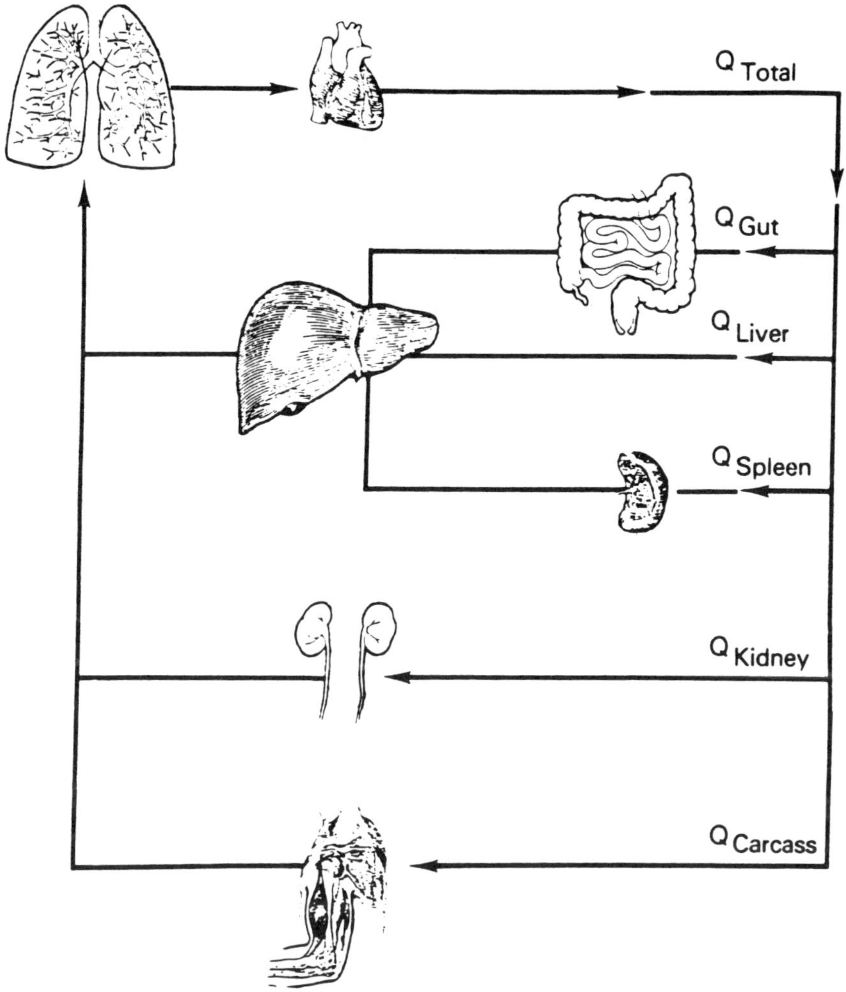

FIGURE 4-16. Physiologic flow model for IgG pharmacokinetics in mammals. Antibody is distributed to each organ according to the arterial plasma flow to that organ (Q_i). Arrows indicate the direction of arterial plasma flow. Reprinted with permission from Covell et al. (51). Copyright 1986. Cancer Research.

volume; Q, flows; w, fraction water; p, protein concentration; and the subscripts are B, blood pool; and i, the i-th tissue region.

If membrane transport is by simple diffusion (i.e., if the free concentration is the driving force), the amount of drug in equilibrium blood in a tissue includes a diffusion-mediated membrane transport term, $k_i(C_{Ti} - C_{Bi})$, where k is membrane permeability and T, tissue. If facilitated active transport is operational, the membrane transport term may have a different form. The relationship for simple diffusion is written mathematically (52) as follows:

$$w_{Bi}V_{Bi}\frac{dC_{Bi}}{dt} + p_{Bi}V_{Bi}\frac{dX_{Bi}}{dt} \tag{37}$$
$$= Q_i(w_B C_B + p_B X_B - w_{Bi}C_{Bi} - p_{Bi}X_{Bi}) + k_i(C_{Ti} - C_{Bi})$$

The amount of drug in a tissue includes a term for reaction, secretion, reabsorption, and so on, $r_i(C_{Ti},X_{Ti})$, where r is a rate constant and T, tissue. This term can have a positive or negative sign, depending on the net effect of the process. This relationship is written mathematically (52) as follows:

$$w_{Ti}V_{Ti}\frac{dC_{Ti}}{dt} + p_{Ti}V_{Ti}\frac{dX_{Ti}}{dt} = k_i(C_{Bi} - C_{Ti}) + r_i(C_{Ti},X_{Ti}) \tag{38}$$

It should be noted that each compartment can be divided into three subcompartments consisting of a vascular space, an interstitial space, and an intracellular space (53), and equations have been presented to describe the mass balance in these compartments (54).

The formal procedure for solving flow limited models is to let k approach infinity, making $C_{Ti} \sim C_{Bi} \equiv C_i$ (the free concentrations) (52). This assumption is based on the simple form of equation 37, with diffusion-mediated membrane transport, and permits combining equations 37 and 38 into the following equation:

$$(w_{Bi}V_{Bi} + w_{Ti}V_{Ti})\frac{dC_i}{dt} + p_{Bi}V_{Bi}\frac{dX_{Bi}}{dt} + p_{Ti}V_{Ti}\frac{dX_{Ti}}{dt} \tag{39}$$
$$= \quad Q_i(w_B C_B + p_B X_B - w_{Bi}C_i - p_{Bi}X_{Bi}) + r_i(C_i,X_{Ti})$$

Sets of tissue equations (equation 39) are solved together with equation 36.

When detailed binding information is available, the relationship between bound and free drug can often be represented by a Langmuir isotherm. Detailed binding information is not always available, and a further useful simplification is that of linear binding, either exactly or approximately. Then the basic mass balance equations are further condensed and written in terms of total drug concentrations, C^*, which is equal to $C_{free} + C_{bound}$ as follows (52):

$$V_B\frac{dC_B^*}{dt} = \sum_i Q_i\frac{C_i^*}{R_i} - \left(\sum_i Q_i\right)C_B^* + \text{(new IV doses)} \tag{40}$$

$$V_{Bi} + V_{Ti}\frac{dC_i^*}{dt} = Q_i\left(C_B - \frac{C_i^*}{R_i}\right) + r_i(C_i^*) \tag{41}$$

where R_i is the tissue-to-blood distribution ratio constant. It is tacitly assumed that the free concentration is the driving force in equation 41.

Once the pharmacokinetics of the drug are defined in one animal species, predictions for humans are obtained by replacing the physiological, anatomical, biochemical, and thermodynamic variables used for the experimental animal species with the values for the corresponding parameters from human beings. These values can be obtained from the literature, determined from in vitro experiments, or estimated via interspecies allometric extrapolations. Some data, such as tissue-to-plasma drug concentration ratios, are not readily available for human beings, and one sometimes assumes that the values in human beings are the same as the values in the experimental animal species. But this may not always be true. Membrane permeabilities are sometimes assumed to be less important than the amount of drug presented to a region—the so-called flow-limited approximation (52); however, models utilizing actual values of membrane permeabilities are sometimes required (55,56). Bischoff (54,56) present detailed mass balance equations for blood and tissues.

Many reviews and literature references now exist (53–63), so only a brief set of examples will be presented here. Related reviews and articles on plasma and tissue protein binding (64), hemodynamic considerations (65), in vitro estimates of drug distribution and metabolism rates (66,67), estimations of regional drug distribution and elimination (68), and estimation of partition coefficients (69) provide additional useful information.

The anticancer drug methotrexate has been the most extensively studied drug. The pharmacokinetics of methotrexate in the mouse were described by using a physiological model that included linear protein binding, strong saturable protein binding, and enterohepatic circulation (70). Scale-up of the mouse model to rats, dogs, and human beings produced predictions of methotrexate that correlated well with experimental data (71). The same mouse model, without intestinal reabsorption and with estimated parameters for the sting ray, was used to predict the disposition of methotrexate in sting rays, demonstrating the versatility of physiologic models (72).

For drugs that are metabolized, physiological models can be combined with in vitro estimates of intrinsic clearance or in vitro estimates of enzyme activity ($V_{\max}$ and K_m) to obtain reasonable estimates of drug disposition in different species. The anticancer drug cytarabine hydrochloride (Ara-C) is converted to uracil arabinoside (Ara-U) by pyrimidine nucleoside deaminase. This enzyme is distributed differently in each species, and it is highly variable in kinetic characteristics ($V_{\max}$ and K_m). A seven-compartment physiological model for Ara-C disposition was developed for human beings by using in vitro values for enzyme activity and Michaelis constants (73). The model predicted the plasma concentrations of Ara-C and Ara-U in humans after a single intravenous dose of the parent compound. Using enzyme kinetics determined in vitro, this model was extended to mice, monkeys, and dogs to produce accurate pharmacokinetic profiles for each species (74). The model was then expanded for the mouse to include the intracellular metabolism of the drug to the active metabolite, arabinoside cytosine triphosphate

(75). The variable distribution and kinetic activities of the deaminase enzymes make direct scale-up of Ara-C among species difficult unless in vitro data are available for each tissue.

An outstanding feature of the physiologically based pharmacokinetic model is the ability to predict the influence of disease, concommitant medications, age, or pregnancy on drug disposition. The drug digoxin was used to test the ability of a physiologic model to predict changes in renal function. An eight-compartment physiological model for digoxin disposition was developed in the rat (76). The model was modified to account for the interspecies differences in tissue-to-plasma digoxin concentration ratios and applied to the dog. The model provided a quantitative assessment of the time course of digoxin concentrations in dog plasma, various tissues, and urine. Also, it predicted the effect of renal failure on digoxin pharmacokinetics in the dog. The dog model was scaled up to human beings by considering differences in organ volumes, organ flow rates, and digoxin clearances. Good predictions were obtained for plasma digoxin concentrations and urinary digoxin excretion following a single dose and for plasma, heart, and skeletal muscle concentrations at steady state; however, the model predicted considerably higher kidney digoxin concentrations than were actually found. As can be seen in Figure 4-17, the model adequately characterized the time course of digoxin concentration in patients with normal renal function and moderate renal impairment.

Drug interactions have been studied in physiological pharmacokinetic models to elucidate the physiological basis of the interactions. Phenolsulfonphthalein is an indicator dye that is actively secreted by the proximal tubules of the kidney; it is a model substrate for the renal organic anion transport system. The interaction of phenolsulfonphthalein with probenecid or salicyluric acid was studied in a physiologically based kidney model (77). The five-compartment model incorporated the functional characteristics of the kidney that determine the excretion of phenolsulfonphthalein, namely, renal plasma flow, urine flow, nonlinear protein binding, glomerular filtration, tubular secretion, and tubular accumulation (Figure 4-18). The model enabled an accurate description and analysis of the measured plasma concentrations and renal excretion rates in dogs (Figure 4-19) and helped distinguish the different mechanisms of inhibitory action for probenecid and salicyluric acid.

An 11-compartment physiologically based pharmacokinetic model was developed in rats to study the drug interaction of tolbutamide, a sulfonylurea derivative, with three sulfonamides: sulfaphenazole, sulfadimethoxine, and sulfamethoxazole (78). The concentrations of tolbutamide in several tissues and plasma were predicted using in vitro estimates of the plasma binding and metabolic parameters and in vivo determinations of plasma-to-blood concentration ratios and tissue-to-plasma unbound concentration ratios. The predicted concentration curves of tolbutamide in plasma and in each tissue

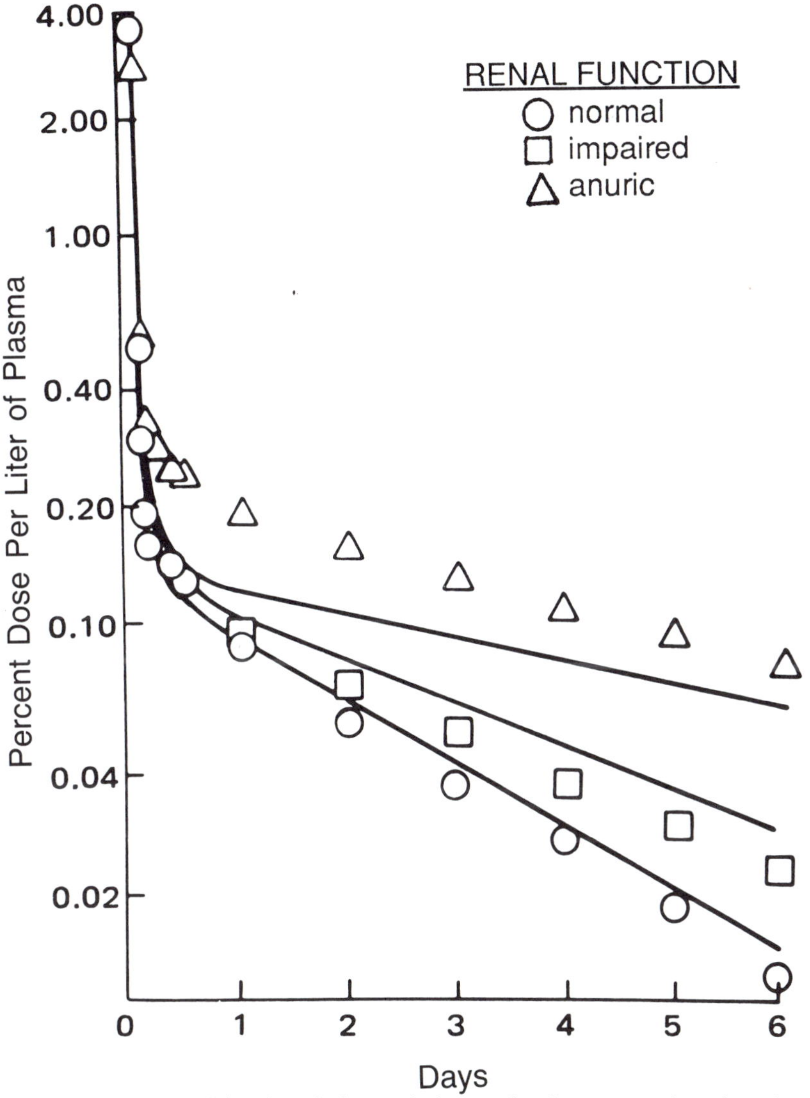

FIGURE 4-17. Predicted (——) and observed plasma digoxin concentrations in patients with normal renal function, in patients with moderate renal impairment, and in patients with severe renal failure. From Harrison and Gibaldi (76). Copyright 1977. Reproduced with permission of the copyright owner, the American Pharmaceutical Association.

showed good agreement with the observed values except for the brain, for which the predicted concentrations were lower than the observed values in the early time period (Figs. 4-20 and 4-21).

Table 4-2 lists a summary of the equations, data requirements, uses, advantages, and limitations of the physiologic approach to interspecies scaling.

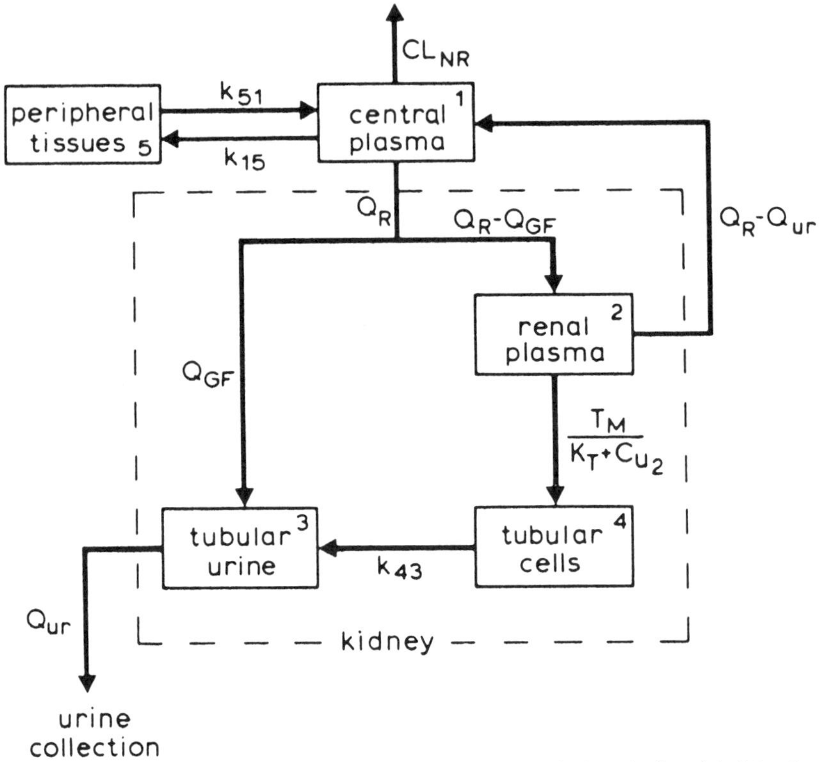

FIGURE 4-18. Physiological model for the renal clearance of phenolsulfonphthalein. Symbols: CL_{NR}, nonrenal plasma clearance; Q_R, renal plasma flow; Q_{ur}, urine flow; Q_{GF}, glomerular filtration rate; k_{ij}, first-order rate constant associated with movement of drug from compartment i to compartment j; T_M, maximum transport capacity of the tubular secretion mechanisms; K_T, Michaelis-Menten constant of the tubular secretion mechanism; and C_{ui}, unbound drug concentration in compartment i. Reprinted with permission from Russel et al. (77). Copyright 1987. Plenum Publishing Co.

INTERSPECIES SCALING IN TOXICOLOGIC ANALYSIS AND RISK ASSESSMENT

The interpretation of toxicological findings is a complex exercise requiring a large volume of kinetic, metabolic, biochemical, and pharmacological information in addition to improved knowledge of the characteristics of specific animal species and strains used for toxicological testing (79). The difficulty of designing manageable studies to detect subtle effects (80) cannot be overemphasized when reviewing the numerous examples of false-positive and false-negative findings generated by toxicology studies (81,82). One encounters many problems when predicting drug effects across species (83).

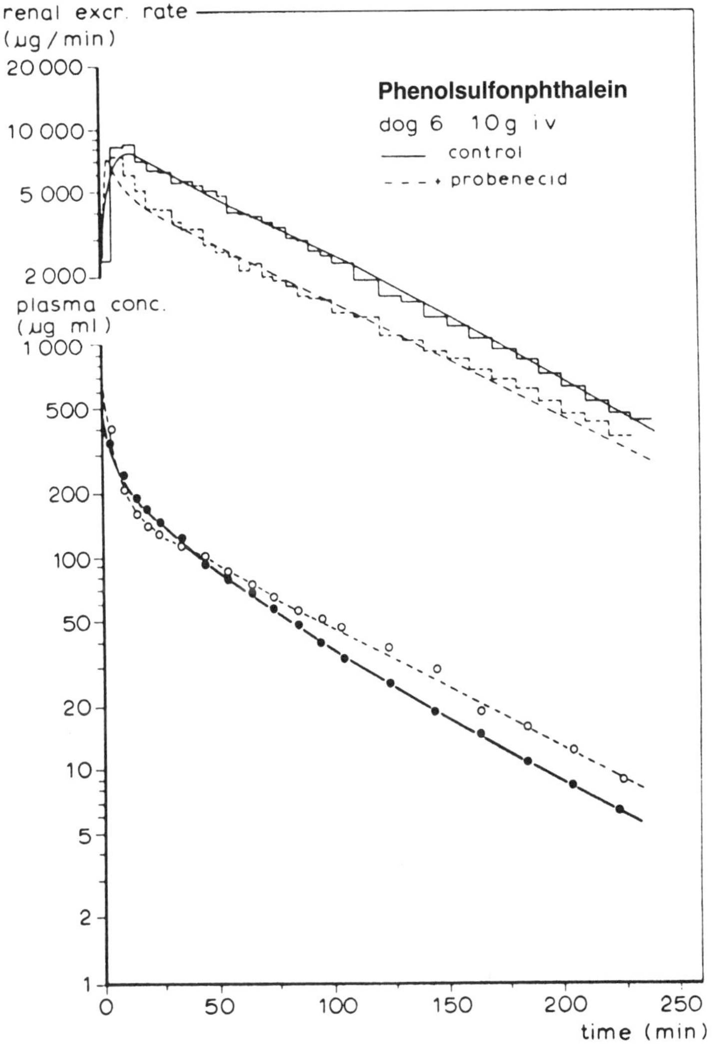

FIGURE 4-19. Renal excretion rate (top half of panel) and plasma concentration (bottom half of panel) as a function after rapid intravenous administration of 1.0 g phenolsulfonphthalein with or without concomitant infusion of probenecid (panel A) or salicyluric acid (panel B) in dogs. The solid and broken lines in the figures represent the results of data analysis according to the kidney model. The symbols and stepped line represent experimental data. Reprinted with permission from Russel et al. (77). Copyright 1987. Plenum Publishing Co.

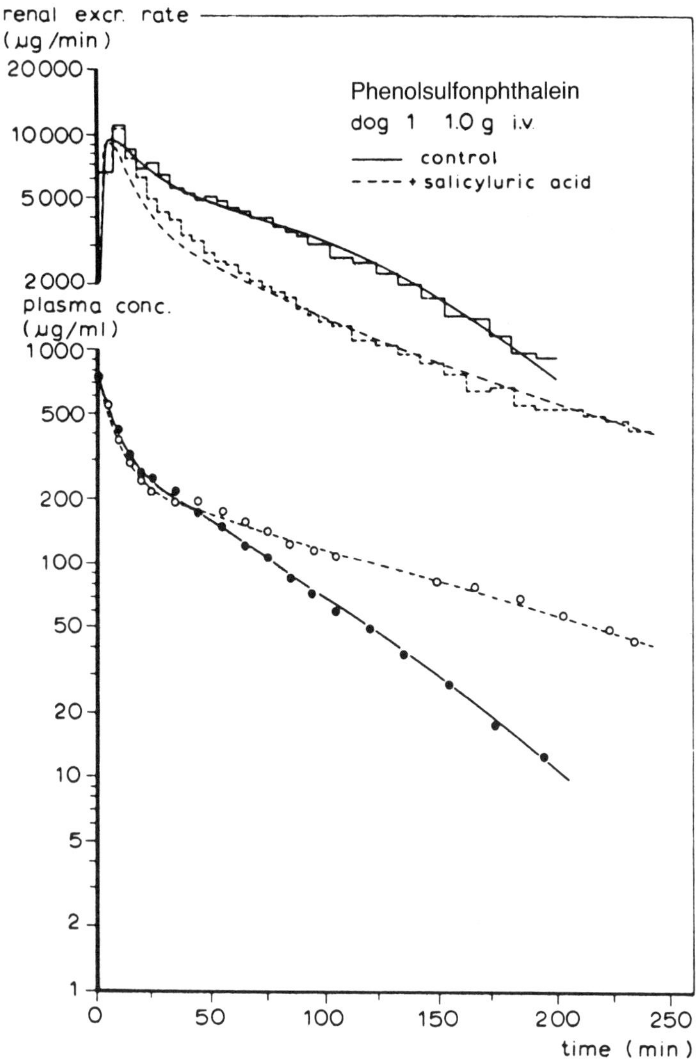

FIGURE 4-19. (*Continued*)

Pharmacokinetic drug modeling plays an important role in understanding and interpreting the results of toxicology studies. Many reviews have emphasized the role of pharmacokinetics in risk assessment (84–95). Three books on this topic are highly recommended (96–98). The pharmacokinetic parameters that are pertinent to an understanding of toxicological properties of drugs are listed in Table 4-3.

Nature has raised an enormous barrier to drug development by assigning the drug-metabolizing enzymes to various species in astonishingly diverse

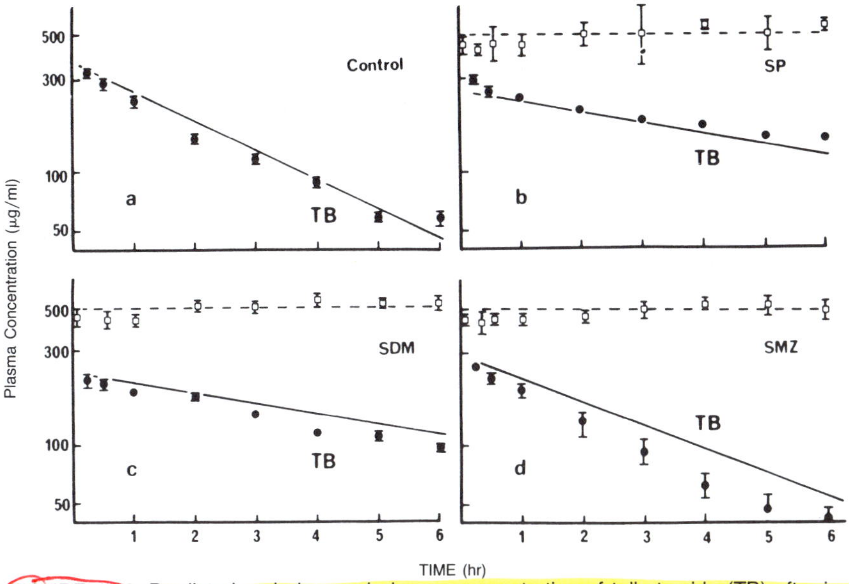

FIGURE 4-20. Predicted and observed plasma concentration of tolbutamide (TB) after intravenous administration of 80 mg/kg in the presence or absence of sulfonamides in rats. Each point and vertical bar represent the mean ± SE of three rats. Left to right from upper left panel: control (tolbutamide alone); tolbutamide (TB) with sulfaphenazole (SP); tolbutamide (TB) with sulfadimethoxine (SDM); and tolbutamide (TB) with sulfamethoxisazole (SMZ). (•) = plasma concentration of tolbutamide; (□) = plasma concentration of the sulfonamide; (——) = predicted concentration of tolbutamide; and (---) = mean concentration of each sulfonamide for a 6-hr constant infusion. Reprinted with permission from Sugita et al. (78). Copyright 1982. Plenum Publishing Co.

amounts. So great are these differences that it is often a matter of pure luck that animal experiments lead to clinically useful drugs (99). Knowledge of such differences, as well as possible variations in the rate at which various reactions occur, may assist in the selection of the most appropriate species for subsequent toxicity studies and provide a more rational basis for the quantitative assessment of risk (90). The search for an ideal animal model with humanlike enzymes has been futile.

Although it is fundamentally important to investigate the pharmacokinetics and metabolism of chemicals, there is no way of being sure that pharmacokinetically equivalent doses are also toxicologically equivalent doses. This discrepancy occurs when the receptors, as well as their sensitivity, are species dependent (79) or when different species form different metabolites. Each species has, by definition, some characteristics of uniqueness. It would be surprising, indeed, if some aspects of this uniqueness were not related to responses to chemical agents (100). Also, there are many potential differences that are not related to differences between species, such as age,

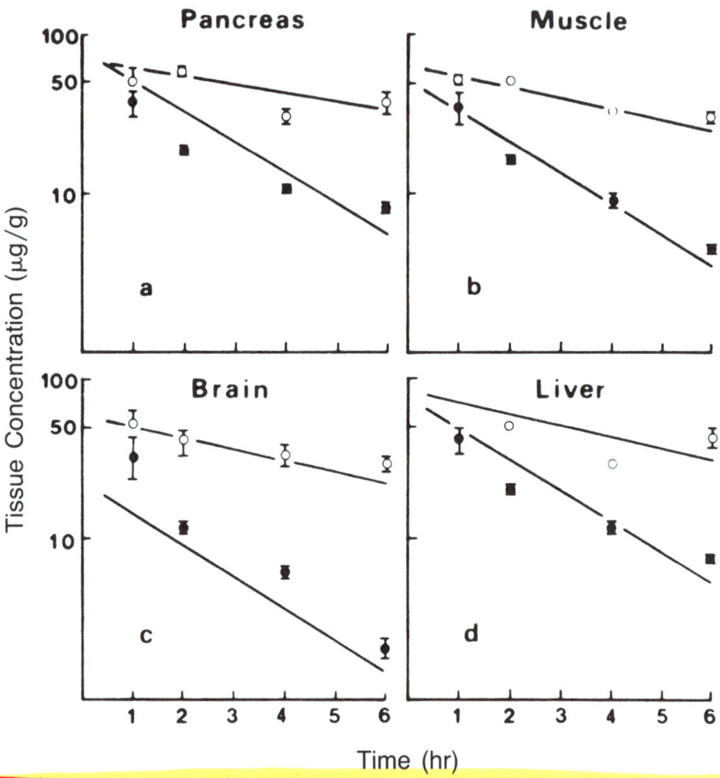

FIGURE 4-21 Predicted and observed tissue concentration of tolbutamide after intravenous administration of 80 mg/kg in the presence or absence of sulfaphenazole (SP) in rats. Clockwise from upper left: pancreas; muscle; liver; and brain. Each point and vertical bar represent the mean ± SE of three rats (●) = tissue concentration of tolbutamide without sulfaphenazole; (○) = tissue concentration of tolbutamide with sulfaphenazole; and (——) = predicted concentration of tolbutamide. Reprinted with permission from Sugita et al. (78). Copyright 1982. Plenum Publishing Co.

polymorphism, size, diet, environment, schedule and route of drug administration, state of health, and extent of supportive treatment (100).

Interspecies scaling (allometric or physiologic) is one method of dealing with the uncertainties of cross-species dose extrapolations in toxicologic risk assessments.

The Allometric Approach

Allometric extrapolation can be used to predict therapeutic, toxic, or lethal doses across species. It is best to know in advance whether average steady-state concentrations, peak concentrations, or area under the concentration-time curve correlate to the therapeutic or toxic effect.

Table 4-3. Pharmacokinetic Parameters Pertinent to an Understanding of Toxicologic Properties of Drugs

Absorption
Extent
Rate
Relationship to route and mode of administration
Distribution
Blood concentrations
Tissue concentrations
Metabolism
Species differences?
Pharmacologically active metabolites?
Toxic metabolites?
Elimination
Route
Rate
Accumulation (chronic administration)

Note: Information from Singhvi et al (87).

If average steady-state concentrations correlate to the therapeutic or toxic effect, then a general equation for predicting equivalent steady-state concentrations is derived as follows:

$$C_{ss} = \frac{(F)(D)}{(\tau)(CL)} \quad \textbf{(42)}$$

where C_{ss} is the steady-state concentration (mg/ml,μg/ml, etc.), F is bioavailability (F is a fraction from 0 (0% bioavailable) to 1 (100% bioavailable)), D is dose (in mg, μg, etc), τ is the dosing interval (minutes, hours, etc.), and CL is clearance (ml/min, ml/hr, etc.). To compare humans to another species, the equations are written as follows:

$$C_{ss,human} = \frac{F_{human}D_{human}}{\tau_{human}CL_{human}} \quad \textbf{(43)}$$

$$C_{ss,animal} = \frac{F_{animal}D_{animal}}{\tau_{animal}CL_{animal}} \quad \textbf{(44)}$$

To obtain equivalent steady-state concentrations in both species (i.e., $C_{ss,animal} = C_{ss,human}$), the equations are related as follows:

$$\frac{F_{human}D_{human}}{\tau_{human}CL_{human}} = \frac{F_{animal}D_{animal}}{\tau_{animal}CL_{animal}} \quad \textbf{(45)}$$

Rearrangement produces the following:

$$D_{human} = D_{animal}\left(\frac{F_{animal}}{F_{human}}\right)\left(\frac{\tau_{human}}{\tau_{animal}}\right)\left(\frac{CL_{human}}{CL_{animal}}\right) \quad \textbf{(46)}$$

The allometric exponent for clearance generally varies between 0.6 and 0.8. If the exact allometric function for clearance is available, it should be used; otherwise, approximations such as $W^{0.7}$ are used. In this derivation, we use $W^{0.7}$ for the estimation of clearance; it is a good compromise between advocates for body surface area ($W^{0.67}$) and advocates for biological flow rates ($W^{0.75}$). Substituting the allometric function for clearance (i.e., $CL = aW^{0.7}$) into equation 46 and assuming the coefficient "a" is the same for both species produces an equation that estimates equivalent doses between species:

$$\begin{aligned} D_{human} &= D_{animal}\left(\frac{F_{animal}}{F_{human}}\right)\left(\frac{\tau_{human}}{\tau_{animal}}\right)\left(\frac{aW^{0.7}_{human}}{aW^{0.7}_{animal}}\right) \\ &= D_{animal}\left(\frac{F_{animal}}{F_{human}}\right)\left(\frac{\tau_{human}}{\tau_{animal}}\right)\left(\frac{W_{human}}{W_{animal}}\right)^{0.7} \end{aligned} \qquad \textbf{(47)}$$

If the time between doses (τ) is the same in the animal and humans (equivalently, keeping the product $C_{ss} \times \tau$ constant in equations 43 and 44) and if bioavailability is 1 (or equivalent) in the two species, equation 47 reduces to the following:

$$D_{human} = D_{animal}\left(\frac{W_{human}}{W_{animal}}\right)^{0.7} \qquad \textbf{(48)}$$

When the allometric exponent for clearance is 0.7 (or any value less than 1.0), the smaller species will require a larger dose (mg/kg) to produce an equivalent steady-state concentration. If the volume of distribution approximates $W^{1.0}$, dosing regimens designed by this approach will produce greater peak-to-trough concentration ratios in the smaller species following bolus administration. It is possible to control the magnitude of the peak-to-trough concentration ratio by changing the dosing interval (τ), i.e., administering smaller amounts of the drug more frequently to the species with the fastest elimination.

The selection of the proper exponent for the clearance term in equation 47 is sometimes difficult. We used 0.7, but every scientist is advised to select an exponent that is most logical for his or her compound or that gives a fairly conservative estimate. Ideally, the exponent should be determined empirically.

Sometimes toxicity occurs only when a particular threshold concentration is surpassed (101); when this occurs, production of a specific peak concentration is more important than the average steady-state concentration. Equivalent peak concentrations for a single dose are determined as follows:

$$\text{peak concentration} = \frac{FD}{V} \qquad \textbf{(49)}$$

where F is bioavailability, D is dose (mg, μg, etc.), and V is volume of where F is bioavailability, D is dose (mg, μg, etc.), and V is volume of distribution (ml, L). To compare human beings to another species, the equations are written as follows:

$$\text{peak concentration}_{\text{human}} = \frac{F_{\text{human}} D_{\text{human}}}{V_{\text{human}}} \quad \textbf{(50)}$$

$$\text{peak concentration}_{\text{animal}} = \frac{F_{\text{animal}} D_{\text{animal}}}{V_{\text{animal}}} \quad \textbf{(51)}$$

For equivalent peak concentrations, the two equations are equated and rearranged as follows:

$$D_{\text{human}} = D_{\text{animal}} \left(\frac{F_{\text{animal}}}{F_{\text{human}}} \right) \left(\frac{V_{\text{human}}}{V_{\text{animal}}} \right) \quad \textbf{(52)}$$

Assuming bioavailability (F) is 1 (or equivalent) and assuming volume of distribution scales as $W^{1.0}$, the dose in human beings is calculated as follows:

$$D_{\text{human}} = D_{\text{animal}} \left(\frac{W_{\text{human}}}{W_{\text{animal}}} \right)^{1.0} \quad \textbf{(53)}$$

When the allometric equation for the volume of distribution is represented by $W^{1.0}$, each species requires the same dose (mg/kg, μg/kg, etc) to produce an equivalent peak concentration. As mentioned earlier, the allometric exponent for volume of distribution is not always one, so it is best to use the actual allometric equation for volume of distribution whenever it is known. Small laboratory animals usually eliminate drugs more rapidly than do human beings; therefore, dosing regimens based on equation 53 will provide identical peak concentrations, but the animal with the highest clearance will have a smaller area under the curve in a 24-hour period if the dosing interval (τ) is the same in both species.

If it is important to keep the area under the concentration-time curve equivalent, the dosing frequency can be adjusted (50). The following relationships are used to determine the number of doses that must be administered each day to produce an equivalent 24-hour area under the curve in each species:

$$\#\text{ doses per day}_{\text{human}} = \#\text{ doses per day}_{\text{animal}} \frac{AUC_{\text{animal}}}{AUC_{\text{human}}} \quad \textbf{(54)}$$

where the area under the surve (AUC) is for one dose. This equation is used to determine the dosing interval (τ, in hours) for any species as follows:

$$\tau = \frac{24 \text{ hours}}{\#\text{ doses per day}} \quad \textbf{(55)}$$

If pharmacokinetic studies have not been performed yet (i.e., CL and area under the curve are not known), one can use the approximation CL $\sim W^{0.7}$ to solve for AUC as follows:

$$AUC = \frac{F\,D}{CL} = \frac{F\,D}{W^{0.7}} \tag{56}$$

Substituting equation 56 into equation 54 produces a general equation for the number of doses to administer for an equivalent area under the curve:

$$\#\text{ doses per day}_{human} = \#\text{ doses per day}_{animal}\left(\frac{F_{animal}}{F_{human}}\right)\left(\frac{D_{animal}}{D_{human}}\right)\left(\frac{W_{human}}{W_{animal}}\right)^{0.7} \tag{57}$$

Alternately, the dosing interval can be obtained by combining equations 47 and 55.

It is tacitly assumed that the pharmacokinetic parameters of the drug in each species remain first order at all dose levels for equations 42 through 57 to be applicable.

Yates and Kugler (40) demonstrated the problems inherent in blindly selecting the allometric exponent for dose extrapolations:

> Using typical allometric relations, what are our options for scaling the dose of a drug from mouse (typical adult weight 20 g) to man (typical adult weight 70 kg)? For the moment we shall suppose that the data for *Homo sapiens* obey the isometry of the other mammals. We could scale between species by setting up ratios of the form below, and knowing either D_{human} (dose in humans) or D_{mouse} (dose in mouse) from clinical or laboratory experience, solve for the other:
>
> $$\frac{D_{human}}{D_{mouse}} = \left(\frac{a_{human}(70)^{b_{human}}}{a_{mouse}(0.02)^{b_{mouse}}}\right) = \left(\frac{70}{0.02}\right)^{b} \tag{58}$$
>
> where D is dose, weight is in kilograms, and a and b are the parameters of the allometric equation. (But the point of allometry is that, for most measures, $a_{mouse} = a_{human}$ and $b_{mouse} = b_{human}$, i.e., that isometry holds).
>
> If we use the allometric coefficients for body volume ($W^{1.0}$), the dose for man should be 3,500 times that for a mouse; if we use metabolic rate ($W^{0.75}$), it would be 400 times greater; if we use surface area ($W^{0.67}$), it would be 200 times greater; and if we use the heartbeat interval ($W^{0.25}$), it would only be 8 times greater. There is an enormous range of possible doses, and this ambiguity is unsatisfactory. Either we need a theory of the allometric coefficient to guide us, or we need to use some formulation that takes into account more than one physiological variable as the basis.

Yates and Kugler propose the transformation of the coordinate space coefficients in an intrinsic geometry for the mammalian body plan. We certainly would like to see pharmacologists pursue this and other alternatives.

Weiss (102) used the theory of biological similarity to study the dependence of pharmacokinetic parameters on body weight. He suggested that renal clearance scales as $W^{0.82}$ (from the allometric equation for glomerular filtration rate), hepatic metabolic clearance scales as $W^{0.73}$ (from the allometric equation for enzyme activity), and blood flow-limited hepatic metabolic clearance scales as $W^{0.75}$ (from allometric equation for blood flow). He recommended the use of these exponents for dose selection when the mechanism of elimination is known; otherwise, he recommended 0.7 as the general dosage scaling exponent.

Collins and co-workers (103) used LD_{10} data from only one animal species (mice) and body surface area to devise an approach for estimating the maximum tolerated dose (mg/m^2) of various antineoplastic agents in humans. The estimation was based on achieving the same plasma drug concentration and an equivalent area under the plasma concentration vs. time curve in each species. Using this approach, the investigators were often successful at predicting the safe starting dose for phase 1 clinical trials.

The allometric approach has been used successfully for extrapolating toxic doses across species. In a retrospective study, toxicity data for 18 antineoplastic agents in six animal species, obtained by numerous investigators using different protocols and endpoints, were compiled in tabular form to make quantitative comparisons (104). The biologic endpoint was the lethal dose in 10 percent of the smaller species (LD_{10}; mice and rats) and the maximum tolerated dose in the larger species (monkeys, dogs, and humans). In the original report, these data were compared on a mg/m^2 basis, and the authors found that the body surface area adjustment was a good method for normalizing the doses. Since body surface area is an indirect allometric comparison (i.e., $W^{0.67}$), these same data were reanalyzed with the allometric approach to determine the actual value for the allometric exponent (50,105). There were enough data to perform regression analysis on 14 compounds. The allometric equation described the antineoplastic toxicity data reasonably well, although it did not apply in every case. The mean value for the exponent was 0.72. Normalization of dose by body surface area (mg/m^2) worked well because the allometric equation for body surface area ($W^{0.67}$) was close to the actual allometric equation for the data ($W^{0.72}$) than total body weight ($W^{1.0}$). Stated a different way, the residual mass exponent for a body surface area correlation was only 0.05, whereas the residual mass exponent for a dose per unit body weight correlation was 0.28.

In general, the exponent on dose (expressed as mg, μg, etc.) is between 0.6 to 0.8, but exceptions are numerous. Because body surface area is approximated by $W^{0.67}$, it is a good surrogate for normalization; however, the use of independent variables does not suggest causation, merely correlative relationships, and any allometric function with the same exponent will work equally well. We do not recommend the use of body surface area because it is too difficult to measure; instead, we recommend the use of an allometric constant, such as $W^{0.7}$.

Sedgwick (106–108) created a very versatile application of allometric scaling to determine therapeutic drug doses and parenteral alimentation requirements for domestic and wild animals. His methods are based on basal metabolic rate (herein called minimum energy cost, MEC) and specific metabolic rate (SMR), where MEC $= KW^{0.75}$, SMR $= KW^{-0.25}$, and K is a constant. The constant K is dependent on taxonomy and is based upon average core body temperature. The values for K are listed as follows: passerine birds, K = 129; nonpasserine birds, K = 78; placental mammals, K = 70; marsupial mammals, K = 49; and reptiles (at preferred temperature), K = 10. The use of this constant facilitates dosage extrapolation outside the class Mammalia which is not possible with equations 42 to 58. According to Sedgwick, the dose in milligrams (D) for the ill animal (subject) is determined from the therapeutic dose used in another species (control) as follows:

$$D_{\text{subject}} = D_{\text{control}}\left(\frac{\text{MEC}_{\text{subject}}}{\text{MEC}_{\text{control}}}\right) = D_{\text{control}}\left(\frac{KW^{0.75}_{\text{subject}}}{KW^{0.75}_{\text{control}}}\right) \qquad \textbf{(59)}$$

The dosing interval (τ) for the ill animal (subject) is determined from the dosing regimen used in another species (control) as follows:

$$\tau_{\text{subject}} = \tau_{\text{control}}\left(\frac{\text{SMR}_{\text{control}}}{\text{SMR}_{\text{subject}}}\right) = \tau_{\text{control}}\left(\frac{KW^{-0.25}_{\text{control}}}{KW^{-0.25}_{\text{subject}}}\right) \qquad \textbf{(60)}$$

Davidson, Parker, and Beliles (109) discuss the application of allometric principles to the extrapolation to humans of dose-tumor incidence data from carcinogenicity bioassays of laboratory animals. The paper reemphasizes the fact that the familiar methods of extrapolation, milligrams per kilogram body weight and body surface area, are simply examples of the power functions $W^{1.0}$ and $W^{0.67}$, respectively. Criteria for the selection of an appropriate base for the transfer of specific biological data from laboratory animals to humans were enunciated in four guiding principles (109):

> *Principle 1.* The biological basis for extrapolation of experimental data from one animal species to another is founded in the overwhelming anatomic, physiologic, and biochemical similarities among species, with the recognition that singular differences may occur within one species and not in others. Morphologic and biologic functions are quantitatively related among species by body weight (W) according to the general allometric equation
>
> $$Y = aW^b$$
>
> where the values of a and the exponent b are distinctive of the biological function Y. Hence, the morphologic and biologic functions themselves are related by the general equation

$$Y = aX^b$$

where Y and X are two functions.

Corollary 1. $W^{1.0}$ and $W^{0.67}$ as bases for extrapolation of experimental data have no unique justification as intrinsic common denominators of biologic similarity among species. Additionally, the traditional terms "mg/kg body weight basis" and "on basis of body surface area" are commonly misunderstood as connoting two qualitatively differing bases of extrapolation, whereas both are encompassed by the general allometric equation, $Y = aW^b$, and differ quantitatively only as $W^{1.0}$ and $W^{0.67}$, respectively.

Principle 2. Intraspecies extrapolations are associated with less intrinsic error than interspecies extrapolations. Numerical scaling of biological data from laboratory animals to human beings most often does not taken into consideration important factors such as age and gender, polymorphism, diet, environment, state of health, or route of chemical administration and scheduling. The two most commonly used bases of extrapolation, $W^{1.0}$ (mg/kg) and $W^{0.67}$ (surface area), for scaling biologic data of laboratory animals (mouse, rat) to human beings, provide scaling factors and hence human equivalent values differing by approximately 10-fold. In contrast, scaling factors derived from bases $W^{0.67}$ (surface area) and $W^{0.75}$ (basal metabolic rate), inclusive, differ by less than twofold, an extent of variance well within the probable error associated with any single one of these bases. The scaling factor derived from any body weight base is particularly susceptible to error due to the variances of body weight among laboratory animals; therefore, the choice of body weight used for extrapolation must be justified from experimental study data.

Corollary 2. When a human equivalent dose is quoted as extrapolated from laboratory animal data, the allometric base for the extrapolation and the body weights used for the human beings and for the laboratory animals should be defined and specified and, in the case of body weight of the laboratory animal, justified from experimental study data.

Principle 3. The allometric equation

$$\text{dose (for a given toxicity)} = aW^b$$

adequately describes quantitative interspecies relationships for acute toxic responses to most xenobiotics (80 to 85%). The power exponent, b, is often observed to be 0.67 (e.g., anticancer agents) and, for the majority of compounds, varies between 0.62 and 0.81, although for a significant number of compounds or toxic endpoints some other exponent may be obtained, including 0 and 1.0. For any given xenobiotic, the probability of the best extrapolation prediction from laboratory animals to human beings is provided by scaling on the base W^b (where b is determined experimentally from four to six species), less well by $W^{0.67}$, and least well by $W^{1.0}$. For any given xenobiotic, the kinetics of body disposition and, in particular, metabolism, are important factors intrinsic to interspecies allometric correlation of toxicologic parameters. Although species differences in pharmacokinetics and metabolism are known to exist for some xenobiotics, in general the kinetic parameters of . . . clearance and hepatic enzyme activity, including P-450 mono-oxygenase system, correlate with interspecies body weight with powers of 0.67 and 0.75.

Collary 3. Extrapolation predictions from laboratory animals to humans based on regression analyses of toxicologic data known for four to six species provide the best estimates of dose for human toxicity, with a difference of calculated response to actual toxic response ranging from 1.5 to 3.4 times, i.e., the error in predicted dose will not be greater than three- to fourfold.

Principle 4. The allometric equation

$$\text{dose (for a given tumor incidence)} = aW^b$$

is appropriate to use for interspecies extrapolation of carcinogenicity bioassay data from laboratory animals to humans. Although reliable interspecies information on the relationship of dosage to carcinogenesis is not available, in general other toxicologic, metabolic, and pharmacokinetic data correlate with interspecies body weight to the power of 0.67 to 0.75 for the majority of compounds studied. In the absence of comparative toxicologic, metabolic, and pharmacokinetic data for a given xenobiotic, the extrapolation base $W^{0.67}$ (i.e., body surface area equivalent dose) is considered to provide the best dose extrapolation prediction, with a greater probability of correctness then the base $W^{1.0}$ (i.e., mg/kg equivalent dose). When adequate toxicologic, metabolic, and pharmacokinetic data are available for a xenobiotic in two or more species of laboratory animals or humans, the experimental data should be used to determine and justify the extrapolation base.

A list of the components in an extrapolation base assessment is given in Table 4-4.

There is no guarantee that the allometric approach will work. Several reasons for the failure of the allometric equation to describe some data include (1) species differences in binding and metabolic pathways, (2) species differences in target cell sensitivity, (3) schedule dependency due to exposure time differences, and (4) laboratory differences in experimental design and techniques (when analyzing data retrospectively). When the metabolism produces active metabolites, the factors considered for the allometric model are not, in many cases, relevant. Indeed, it could be argued that the faster metabolism often associated with small animals will make them more vulnerable (on a mg/kg basis) than humans, because of the relatively higher production of toxic metabolites.

If pharmacokinetic or toxicologic data exist for several animal species and humans, visual inspection of the data usually alerts the investigator when the data are ill conditioned for an allometric analysis; in these instances, extrapolation from animals to human beings would be unwise, and a different approach is advisable. Of course, there is no way of knowing in advance whether human pharmacokinetic behavior will be different from the prediction from the regression line (so called outliers), as in the antipyrine example. Ultimately, judgment is required in the final evaluation of any method of extrapolation, and such judgment must maintain all pertinent data in perspective.

The Physiologic Approach

Conventional risk-assessment models have implicitly assumed linear extrapolation of external (administered) dose, combined with an interspecies factor based on body surface area. By contrast, physiologically based phar-

Table 4-4. Components in Extrapolation Base Assessment

General
What acute toxicologic data (TD_{10}, TD_{50}, etc.) are available for four to six species, including mouse and rat?
What chronic toxicologic data are available for four to six species, including mouse and rat?
What comparative metabolic and pharmacokinetic studies are available for mouse, rat, or other species?
Metabolism
Are data relating oral dose(s) with disposition available for mouse, rat, human, or other species: Amount metabolized? Body burden? Expired unchanged? Urinary excretion?
Are data relating inhalation dose(s) with disposition available for mouse, rat, human, or other species: Amount metabolized? Body burden? Expired unchanged? Urinary excretion?
Are data available on rate(s) of metabolism for mouse, rat, human, or other species?
Is there evidence of different metabolic pathways in mouse, rat, human, or other species? Are the metabolites identified?
Is there evidence of saturation of metabolism: At what concentration for mouse, rat, human, or other species?
Are data available on saturation of detoxification mechanisms? Conjugation with glutathione depletion, etc.?
Kinetics
Are data available for mouse, rat, human, or other species for:
Oral absorption: Extent as percentage of dose? Rate constant? Influence of vehicle? Influence of diet?
Inhalation exposure: Retention values? Relation of increasing ppm in air to steady-state plasma concentration? Blood/gas partition coefficient? Particulate ppm in air to lung uptake?
Tissue distribution: Liver? Adipose tissue? Sites of target organs? Plasma protein binding? Organ tissue binding?
Single dose (iv, oral, inhalation) kinetics: Blood concentration-time profile? Area under the curve? Clearance? Volume of distribution? Terminal phase half-life?
Are the kinetics described by first-order models, nonlinear models, physiologic models?
Covalent binding
Are data available on in vivo macromolecular covalent binding (DNA, RNA, protein) in target organs as indices of mechanisms and tissue damage in mouse, rat, man, or other species: Exposure dose intensity? Comparative tissue binding?

Note: Information from Davidson et al. (109).

macokinetic models permit the calculation of internal doses (total amount of parent or metabolite in body tissue or fluid) through the integration of information on the administered dose, the physiological structure of the mammalian species, and the biochemical properties of the specific chemicals (110). The physiologic approach can be used to describe situations in which nonlinear dynamics occur or in which biological response is not a function of the total or unbound concentration in the plasma. Clewell and Andersen (111) have previously discussed the reasons why the scientific basis (soundness) of the risk assessment process could be improved through the use of physiologically based pharmacokinetic modeling. The following examples highlight the uses of physiologic modeling in risk assessment.

Two chronic bioassays of methylene chloride toxicity in the B6C3F1 mouse produced disparate results: the inhalation bioassay revealed significant increases in lung and liver tumors (112), while the drinking water study failed to show a dose-related increase in the incidence of either type of tumor in this same strain of mouse (113). Andersen and colleagues (110) describe the application of a physiologically based pharmacokinetic model for the risk assessment of methylene chloride. They proposed a model based on a model developed by Ramsey and Andersen (114) and modified to include a distinct, metabolically active lung compartment in addition to the liver because tumors formed in both organs. The model had seven compartments: gas exchange, lung metabolism, richly perfused tissues, slowly perfused tissues, fat, liver, and gastrointestinal tract. On the basis of data about the metabolism of dihalomethanes, they assumed two metabolic pathways for methylene chloride: one dependent on oxidation by mixed function oxidases and the other dependent on glutathione S-transferases. They treated the glutathione S-transferase pathway as a first-order pathway (inhaled concentrations of 10,000 ppm did not saturate the metabolism in rodents) and the mixed function oxidase pathway was modeled using Michaelis-Menten kinetics (saturation occurred at a few hundred ppm in rodents). They used in vitro studies to obtain partition coefficients (e.g., blood to air); and they used literature values, laboratory studies, and allometric scaling to obtain physiological constants such as tissue volumes and blood flows and biochemical constants such as K_m and V_{max}. They validated the model by comparing predictions of blood concentrations with results from experiments on animals and humans. The model gave very good predictions of blood concentration data and to data on the appearance and elimination of metabolites.

The physiologic model was used to obtain the area under the tissue concentration-time curve for methylene chloride in the lungs and the liver and the total amount of the metabolites formed by each pathway in the lungs and liver of B6C3F1 mice under the conditions of the bioassays. The results indicate that the doses at which tumors were caused in the laboratory animals were such that the mixed function oxidase pathway had been saturated, leading to a greater production of the glutathione S-transferase metabolites. The authors concluded that the inhalation and oral dose experiments produced very different results because the oral doses did not saturate the mixed function oxidase pathway. While this pharmacokinetic model does not prove the mechanism of tumorgenicity, the glutathione S-transferase pathway does appear to be somehow related to the increased tumor incidences observed in B6C3F1 mice exposed to methylene chloride. More importantly, this model demonstrates how linear extrapolation to low doses, in which the mixed function oxidase pathway is first order, severely overestimates the response.

Despite the utility of this model, D'Souza and Boxenbaum (57) note that neither this model nor any other risk assessment model can explain why Syrian golden hamsters (which also form glutathione conjugate) exposed to

3,500 ppm methylene chloride for six hours per day (five days per week) did not show a tumorigenic response at any site (115); quite the contrary, exposed animals were healthier than controls and lived longer lives. D'Souza and Boxenbaum (57) suggest that this latter observation probably results from a phenomena termed longevity hermesis—that is, paradoxical life prolongation by relatively low doses of otherwise toxic agents (116).

Ethylene dichloride (1,2-dichloroethane) produces tumors in rats and mice after chronic oral dosing (75 and 150 mg/kg), but not after chronic inhalation exposures (150 ppm for seven hours daily). Ethylene dichloride is metabolized by two competing pathways. One pathway is a saturable pathway that uses mixed function oxidases to produce chloroacetaldehyde; this compound is detoxified by glutathione. The other pathway is a direct conjugation with glutathione to form 2-(s-chloroethyl)-glutathione; it is this conjugate and not the parent compound ethylene dichloride that is believed to be the ultimate carcinogen. Laboratory results showed that the glutathione pathway is first order until high ethylene dichloride doses cause a depletion of glutathione, decreasing the glutathione available to react with ethylene dichloride. A physiologically based pharmacokinetic model was developed to address this route-of-exposure difference by quantifying the amount of 2-(s-chloroethyl)-glutathione conjugate produced in target organs following oral and inhalation exposure (117). The amount of 2-(s-chloroethyl)-glutathione produced in the liver and lung was computed for oral gavage doses of 75 and 150 mg/kg and compared with those that would be produced by a seven-hour inhalation exposure at 150 ppm. Lower amounts of 2-(s-chloroethyl)-glutathione were predicted at the maximum tolerated inhalation dose of 150 ppm, and this observation may be a possible reason that the treatment-related tumors were not seen in the inhalation bioassay, but were observed at both oral doses.

Glutathione generally serves a detoxifying role; compounds such as acetaminophen and vinylidine chloride exhibit greater toxicity when glutathione is depleted. With the halogenated ethylenes like ethylene dichloride, glutathione is involved in the generation of the putative ultimate carcinogenic metabolite; therefore, the depletion of glutathione results in less carcinogen being produced. The physiological pharmacokinetic model developed for ethylene dichloride was extended to describe glutathione tissue turnover and its depletion following ethylene dichloride exposure (118). The glutathione model was necessary to keep track of glutathione concentrations with time, because ethylene dichloride metabolism is affected by glutathione status. Reactions of glutathione with ethylene dichloride and chloroacetaldehyde were defined as second order; steady-state glutathione formation was modeled as zero order; and glutathione loss was modeled as first order. Glutathione rebound effects, following its depletion, were controlled by a glutathione synthetase reaction which allowed a time- and glutathione concentration-dependent feedback for increased glutathione resynthesis. The model was developed for liver glutathione in the rat and was extrapolated to include the lung. Allometric scaling was used to extrapolate the model to other animal species. Experimental observations in the mouse and rat were consistent with model predictions. When these principles are used, a glutathione depletion model can be constructed to provide a prediction of the toxicity of drugs that depend on glutathione for elimination.

Physiologically based pharmacokinetic models have several advantages over the allometric approach. They have the potential of describing situations in which nonlinearities occur and can be used to model more appropriate surrogates in tissue compartments. In addition, physiologic models can be designed to account for differences in route and frequency of administration and have been successful in extrapolating from high to low dose, a source of uncertainty in many models. On the other hand, these are very sophisticated models, requiring skill in their development, use, and interpretation. Furthermore, the data required for the models can quickly run up the expense of doing risk assessments. It would be very useful to develop a set of criteria for deciding when the physiologically based pharmacokinetic model is needed and when simpler models will suffice.

DISCUSSION

The important issues in the design and interpretation of toxicity tests include (1) differences between the dosing regimens and routes of administration used in the laboratory setting in comparison to actual human consumption; (2) target-site dosimetry; (3) species-specific metabolic rates and pathways; (4) acute versus chronic exposure; and (5) the validity of high to low dose extrapolations. Most of the pharmacokinetic literature data base can be used directly to address the assumptions concerning different routes of administration, the target dose relationship to administered dose, and the question of average dose exposure or additivity of multiple exposure; biomarkers can be used to predict toxic endpoints; and quantitative structure activity relationships can be applied to wide based pharmacological effects (85).

Customarily, it is assumed that treatments that produce equivalent average daily tissue exposures of revelant chemical species in target organs will produce equivalent effects on the carcinogenic process in each species (110). When pharmacokinetic equivalency is critical, pharmacokinetic studies can be conducted to ensure that dosage regimens are equivalent in each species. Equivalent dosage regimens may achieve identical peak concentrations in serum and produce the same area under the serum concentration-time curve in a finite time interval (such as 24 hours) or they may produce equivalent steady-state concentrations (without controlling the peak concentration). An animal that clears drugs quickly (such as a mouse or rat) may require more frequent injections to attain a daily area under the curve that is equivalent to that of human beings or to decrease the peak-to-trough ratio for bolus doses. When pharmacokinetic equivalency is the ultimate goal, it is tacitly assumed that pharmacodynamics do not affect the risk-assessment process; if pharmacodynamics have a significant effect, scaling only the pharmacokinetic variables may cause gross error in estimation of toxic doses (110). Factors such as longevity of the various species and latent periods for tumor induction, which may be biologically important, are not always incorporated into the model (110).

Scaling doses to achieve pharmacokinetic equivalence is rather straightforward. Extrapolation of animal data in an attempt to predict the carcinogenic potential of chemicals is somewhat different and dependent upon type of injury, method of repair, length of exposure, threshold versus single-hit theory, dose dependency of metabolic pathways, and validity of high dose to low dose extrapolation (119). It is also dependent on the role of absorption, distribution, metabolism, and excretion in increasing or decreasing carcinogenic activity (119).

The greatest difficulty in projecting data from animals to human beings arises from species differences in biotransformation of certain drugs (99). Not only are different metabolites formed, but, when the same metabolites are formed, they may be formed at different rates from one species to another (100). When a compound is metabolized, the investigator needs to consider (1) the mechanism of biotransformation, (2) the rate of disappearance of the parent compound, (3) the rate of formation and elimination of the metabolite(s), (4) the route of elimination, and (5) the toxicity of each chemical entity. The investigator needs to establish which compound (parent or metabolite) is to be scaled (based on which is the active or toxic compound), and at what concentration the drug or metabolites saturate the transport systems, binding sites, and drug-metabolizing enzymes (94). The metabolism of foreign compounds usually occurs at a higher rate in small rodents than in human beings. This difference in rates of metabolism is apparently caused by several factors, including the higher ratio of liver to body weight, the more rapid circulation time, the larger amount of liver cytochrome P450 (and analogues), and the higher oxygen tension (necessary for the activity of mixed function oxygenases, a major class of enzymes involved in the metabolism of foreign compounds) in small rodents than in human beings (79). These differences may magnify the toxic effects of chemicals in small animals compared to human beings when metabolites are responsible for such effects (79). In other words, when toxic metabolites are formed, the smaller species may require smaller doses (mg/kg) to produce equivalent toxicities (120).

Scaling lethal dose (LD_{10}, LD_{50}, etc.) across species may be easier than scaling discrete toxic effects such as hair loss, neutropenia, rashes, vertigo, peripheral neuropathies, and so on. Several retrospective studies (121, 122) gathered information on the side effects of drugs in various laboratory animals and human beings. Although testing in several animal species provided information on a vast majority of the side effects, no one species predicted all the side effects that were reported in humans; in fact, a few of the side effects that occurred in the laboratory animals never occurred in humans, and vice versa. The generation of false-positive and false-negative findings has hampered extrapolation (81,82). Failure of an animal model to predict trivial side effects is acceptable; however, failure to predict a significant or irreversible side effect is serious. When discussing the difficulties in extrapolating the results of toxicity studies in laboratory animals to human beings, Rall concluded: "The problem of predictability lies primarily in the fact that the stakes are so high and not that the systems are so bad" (100).

Garattini (88) provides these closing thoughts: "The evaluation of toxic effects of chemicals should be not just a checklist of tests, but an individualized process which distinguishes routine from research. Regulatory authorities and industry may have to work in a climate of less certainty, but doubt has always been a powerful tool for progress. When the problem is to avoid the toxic potential of chemicals for human beings, it is very healthy to have a lot of doubts!"

ACKNOWLEDGMENT

The authors wish to thank Drs. Harold Boxenbaum and Ken Bischoff for their helpful comments and suggestions.

REFERENCES

1. W. R. Stahl. Scaling of respiratory variables in mammals. J. Appl. Physiol. *22*, 453–460 (1967).
2. T. A. McMahon and J. T. Bonner. *On Size and Life*. Scientific American Books, New York (1983).
3. W. A. Calder, III. *Size, Function, and Life History*. Harvard University Press, Cambridge, MA (1984).
4. K. Schmidt-Nielsen. *Scaling: Why Is Animal Size So Important?* Cambridge University Press, New York (1984).
5. M. Kleiber. Physiological meaning of regression equations. J. Appl. Physiol. *2*, 417–423 (1950).
6. E. F. Adolph. Quantitative relation in the physiological constitution of mammals. Science. *109*, 579–585 (1949).
7. J. Prothero. Scaling of blood parameters in mammals. Comp. Biochem. Physiol. *67A*, 649–657 (1980).
8. Sarrus and Rameaux. Mémoire addressée à l'Académie Royale. Bull. de l'Acad. Roy. de Méd. *3*, 1094–1100 (1839).

9. S. Brody, J. E. Comfort, and J. S. Matthews. Growth and development with special reference to domestic animals. XI. Further investigations on surface area with special reference to its significance in energy metabolism, University of Missouri College of Agriculture, Agricultural Experiment Station Res. Bull. *115,* 3–60 (1928).
10. M. Kleiber. Body size and metabolism. Hilgardia *6,* 315–353 (1932).
11. M. Kleiber. Body size and metabolic rate. Phys. Rev. *27,* 511–541 (1947).
12. A. S. Iberall. Blood flow and oxygen uptake in mammals. Ann. Biomed. Engineer. *1,* 1–8 (1972).
13. A. A. Heusner. Energy metabolism and body size. I. Is the 0.75 mass exponent of Kleiber's equation a statistical artifact? Respiration Physiol. *48,* 1–12 (1982).
14. H. Bartels. Metabolic rate of mammals equals the 0.75 power of their body weight. Expl. Biol. Med. *7,* 1–11 (1982).
15. H. A. Feldman and T. A. McMahon. The 3/4 mass exponent for energy metabolism is not a statistical artifact. Respiration Physiol. *52,* 149–163 (1983).
16. V. Hayssen and R. C. Lacy. Basal metabolic rates in mammals: Taxonomic differences in the allometry of BMR and body mass. Comp. Biochem. Physiol. *81A,* 741–754 (1985).
17. W. A. Calder. III. Scaling energetics of homeothermic vertebrates: An operational allometry. Ann. Rev. Physiol. *49,* 107–20 (1987).
18. W. R. Stahl. The analysis of biological similarity. Advan. Biol. Med. Phys. *9,* 355–464 (1963).
19. B. Gunther and E. Guerra. Biological similarities. Acta. Physiol. Latinoam *5,* 169–186 (1955).
20. N. A. Edwards. Scaling of renal function in mammals. Comp. Biochem. Physiol. *52A,* 63–66 (1975).
21. W. R. Stahl. Similarity and dimensional methods in biology. Science *137,* 205–212 (1962).
22. S. J. Gould. One standard lifetime. New Scientist, February *8,* 1979, p. 388–389.
23. W. R. Stahl. Similarity analysis of physiological systems. Perspect. Biol. Med. *6,* 291–321 (1963).
24. S. J. Gould. Allometry and size in ontogeny and phylogeny. Biol. Rev. *41,* 587–640 (1966).
25. R. L. Dedrick, K. B. Bischoff, and D. S. Zaharko. Interspecies correlation of plasma concentration history of methotrexate (NSC-740). Cancer Chemother. Reports, Part 1, *54,* 95–101 (1970).
26. S. Brody. Relativity of physiologic time and physiologic weight. Growth *1,* 61–67 (1937).
27. H. Boxenbaum. Interspecies scaling, allometry, physiological time and the ground plan of pharmacokinetics. J. Pharmacokinet. Biopharm. *10,* 201–227 (1982).
28. H. Boxenbaum and R. Ronfeld. Interspecies pharmacokinetic scaling and the Dedrick plots. Am. J. Physiol. *245,* R768–774 (1983).
29. J. Mordenti. Pharmacokinetic scale-up: Accurate prediction of human pharmacokinetic profiles from animal data. J. Pharm. Sci. *74,* 1097–1099 (1985).
30. H. Boxenbaum. Interspecies pharmacokinetic scaling and the evolutionary-comparative paradigm. Drug Metab. Rev. *15,* 1071–1121 (1984), (Marcel Dekker, Inc.).
31. E. Swabb and D. Bonner. Prediction of aztreonam pharmacokinetics in humans based on data from animals. J. Pharmacokinet. Biopharm. *11,* 215–223 (1983).
32. T. Murakawa, H. Sakamoto, S. Fukada, S. Nakamoto, T. Hirose, N. Itoh, and M. Nishida. Pharmacokinetics of ceftizoxime in animals after parenteral dosing. Antimicrob. Agents Chemother. *17,* 157–164 (1980).
33. G. Sacher. Relation of lifespan to brain weight and body weight in mammals. Pages 115–133 in: *CIBA Foundation Colloquia on Aging.* G. E. W. Wolstenholme and M. O'Connor, eds. Churchill, London *5* (1959).

34. H. Boxenbaum and J. Fertig. Scaling of antipyrine intrinsic clearance of unbound drug in 15 mammalian species. Eur. J. Drug Metab. Pharmacokinet. *9,* 177–183 (1984).
35. H. Boxenbaum. Interspecies variation in liver weight, hepatic blood flow, and antipyrine intrinsic clearance: Extrapolation of data to benzodiazepines and phenytoin. J. Pharmacokinet. Biopharm. *8,* 165–176 (1980).
36. H. Boxenbaum, W. Murray, R. Markin, and D. Ciraulo. Benzodiazepine pharmacokinetics: Clinical highlights and interspecies scaling. Pages 93–119 in: *Pharmacokinetics and Pharmacodynamics of Psychoactive Drugs.* G. Barnett and N. Chiang, eds. Biomedical Publications, Foster City, CA (1985).
37. S. J. Gould. *Ever Since Darwin: Reflections in Natural History.* W. W. Norton and Co., New York, (1977).
38. S. J. Gould. *Ontogeny and Phylogeny.* The Belknap Press, Harvard Univ. Press, Cambridge, MA (1977).
39. S. E. Luria, S. J. Gould, S. Singer. *A View of Life.* The Benjamin/Cummings Publ. Co., Menlo Park, CA (1981).
40. F. Yates and P. Kugler. Similarity principles and intrinsic geometries: Contrasting approaches to interspecies scaling. J. Pharm. Sci. *75,* 1019–1027 (1986).
41. H. Boxenbaum and R. D'Souza. Interspecies pharmacokinetic scaling: Reductionist and allometric paradigms. Pages 49–62 in: *Topics in Pharmaceutical Sciences 1987.* D. D. Briemer and P. Speiser, eds. Elsevier Science Publ., Amsterdam (1987).
42. H. Boxenbaum and R. D'Souza. Physiologic models, allometry, neoteny, space-time and pharmacokinetics. Pages 191–214 in: *Pharmacokinetics: Mathematical and Statistical Approaches.* A. Pecile and A. Rescigno, eds. Plenum Press, New York (1988).
43. Y. Sawada, M. Hanano, Y. Sugiyama, and T. Iga. Prediction of the disposition of beta-lactam antibiotics in humans from pharmacokinetic parameters in animals. J. Pharmacokinet. Biopharm. *12,* 241–261 (1984).
44. Y. Sawada, M. Hanano, Y. Sugiyama, H. Harashima, and T. Iga. Prediction of the volumes of distribution basic drugs in humans based on data from animals. J. Pharmacokinet. Biopharm. *12,* 587–596 (1984).
45. Y. Sawada, M. Hanano, Y. Sugiyama and T. Iga. Prediction of disposition on nine weakly acidic and six weakly basic drugs in humans from pharmacokinetic parameters in rats. J. Pharmacokinet. Biopharm. *13,* 477–491 (1985).
46. G. Duthu. Interspecies correlation of the pharmacokinetics of erythromycin, oleandomycin, and tylosin. J. Pharm. Sci. *74,* 943–946 (1985).
47. J. Mordenti. Forecasting cephalosporin and monobactam antibiotic half-lives in humans from data collected in laboratory animals. Antimicrob. Agents Chemother. *27,* 887–891 (1985).
48. M. Yoshimura, J. Kojima, T. Ito, and J. Suzuki. Pharmacokinetics of nipradilol (K-351), a new antihypertensive agent. I. Studies on interspecies variation in laboratory animals. J. Pharmacobio-Dyn. *8,* 738–750 (1985).
49. Y. Sawada, H. Harashima, M. Hanano, Y. Sugiyama, and T. Iga. Prediction of the plasma concentration time courses of various drugs in humans based on data from rats. J. Pharmacobio-Dyn. *8,* 757–766 (1985).
50. J. Mordenti. Dosage regimen design for pharmaceutical studies conducted in animals. J. Pharm. Sci. *75,* 852–857 (1986).
51. D. G. Covell, J. Barbet, O. D. Holton, C. D. V. Black, R. J. Parker, and J. N. Weinstein. Pharmacokinetics of monoclonal immunoglobulin G_1, $F(ab')_2$, and Fab′ in mice. Cancer Res. *46,* 3969–3978 (1986).
52. K. B. Bischoff. Physiologic pharmacokinetics, Bull. Math. Biol. *48,* 309–322 (1986).
53. L. Gerlowski and R. Jain. Physiologically based pharmacokinetic modeling: Principles and applications. J. Pharm. Sci. *72,* 1103–1127 (1983).

54. K. B. Bischoff. Physiologically based pharmacokinetic modeling. Pages 36–61 in: *Pharmacokinetics in Risk Assessment,* Drinking Water and Health. Vol. 8. National Academy Press, Washington, DC (1987).
55. K. B. Bischoff. Some fundamental considerations in the applications of pharmacokinetics to cancer chemotherapy. Cancer Chemother. Rep., Part 1 *59,* 777–793 (1975).
56. R. J. Lutz, R. L. Dedrick, and D. S. Zaharko. Physiological pharmacokinetics: An in vivo approach to membrane transport. Pharmacol. Ther. *11,* 559–592 (1980).
57. R. D'Souza and H. Boxenbaum. Physiological pharmacokinetic models: Some aspects of theory, practice, and potential. Toxicol. Ind. Health. *4,* 151–171 (1988).
58. J. Mordenti. Man versus beast: Pharmacokinetic scaling in mammals. J. Pharm. Sci. *75,* 1028–1040 (1986).
59. J. Wagner, G. Szpunar, and J. Ferry. A nonlinear physiologic pharmacokinetic model. I. Steady-state. J. Pharmacokinet. Biopharm. *13,* 73–92 (1985).
60. M. Rowland. Physiological pharmacokinetic models and interanimal species scaling. Pharmacol. Ther. *29,* 49–68 (1985).
61. M. Andersen. Recent advances in methodology and concepts for characterizing inhalation pharmacokinetic parameters in animals and humans. Drug Met. Rev. *13,* 799–826 (1982).
62. H.-S. Chen and J. Gross. Physiologically based pharmacokinetic models for anticancer drugs. Cancer Chemother. Pharmacol. *2,* 85–94 (1979).
63. K. Himmelstein and R. Lutz. A review of the applications of physiologically based pharmacokinetic modeling. J. Pharmacokinet. Biopharm. *7,* 127–145 (1979).
64. W. J. Jusko and M. Gretch. Plasma and tissue protein binding of drugs in pharmacokinetics. Drug Metab. Rev. *5,* 43–140 (1976).
65. G. R. Wilkinson. Pharmacokinetics of drug disposition: Hemodynamic considerations. Rev. Pharmac. *15,* 11–27 (1975).
66. G. R. Wilkinson. Clearance approaches in pharmacology. Pharmacol. Rev. *39,* 1–47 (1987).
67. G. R. Wilkinson. Prediction of *in vivo* parameters of drug metabolism and distribution from *in vitro* studies. Pages 80–95 in: *Pharmacokinetics in Risk Assessment,* Drinking Water and Health. Vol. 8. National Academy Press, Washington, DC (1987).
68. R. N. Upton, L. Mather, W. Runciman, C. Nancarrow, and R. Carapetis. The use of mass balance principles to describe regional drug distribution and elimination. J. Pharmacokinet. Biopharm. *16,* 13–29 (1988).
69. J. Gallo, F. Lam, and D. Perrier. Area method for the estimation of partition coefficients for physiological pharmacokinetic models. J. Pharmacokinet. Biopharm. *15,* 271–280 (1987).
70. K. B. Bischoff, R. L. Dedrick, and D. S. Zaharko. Preliminary model for methotrexate pharmacokinetics. J. Pharm. Sci. *59,* 149–154 (1970).
71. K. B. Bischoff, R. L. Dedrick, D. S. Zaharko, and J. A. Longstreth. Methotrexate pharmacokinetics. J. Pharm. Sci. *60,* 1128–1133 (1971).
72. D. S. Zaharko, R. L. Dedrick, and V. T. Oliverio. Prediction of the distribution of methotrexate in the sting rays *Dasyatidae sabina* and *sayi* by use of a model developed in mice. Comp. Biochem. Physiol. *42A,* 183–194 (1972).
73. R. L. Dedrick, D. D. Forrester, and D. H. W. Ho. In vitro-in vivo correlation of drug metabolism—Deamination of 1-β-D-arabinofuranosylcytosine. Biochem. Pharmacol. *21,* 1–16 (1972).
74. R. L. Dedrick, D. D. Forrester, J. N. Cannon, S. M. El Dareer, and L. B. Mellet. Pharmacokinetics of 1-β-D-arabinofuranosylcytosine (Ara-C) deamination in several species. Biochem. Pharmacol. *22,* 2405–2417 (1973).
75. P. F. Morrison, T. L. Lincoln, and J. Aroesty. The disposition of Ara-C and its me-

tabolites: A pharmacokinetic simulation. Cancer Chemother. Rep. *59,* 861–876 (1975).
76. L. I. Harrison and M. Gibaldi. A physiologically based pharmacokinetic model for digoxin disposition in dogs and its preliminary application to humans. J. Pharm. Sci. *66,* 1679–1683 (1977).
77. F. G. M. Russel, A. C. Wouterse, and C. A. M. van Ginneken. Physiologically based pharmacokinetic model for renal clearance of phenolsulfonphthalein and interaction with probenecid and salicyluric acid in the dog. J. Pharmacokinet. Biopharm. *15,* 349–368 (1987).
78. O. Sugita, Y. Sawada, Y. Sugiyama, T. Iga, and M. Hanano. Physiologically based pharmacokinetics of drug-drug interaction: a study of tolbutamide-sulfonamide interaction in rats. J. Pharmacokinet. Biopharm. *10,* 297–316 (1982).
79. S. Garattini. Concluding remarks: Extrapolation of toxicological data from animals to man. Pages 201–208 in: Animals in Toxicologic Research. I. Bartosek, ed. Raven Press, New York (1982).
80. M. A. Schneiderman, N. Mantel, and C. C. Brown. From mouse to man—Or how to get from the laboratory to Park Avenue and 59th Street. Ann. NY Acad. Sci. *246,* 237–248 (1975).
81. G. Zbinden. Biopharmaceutical studies, a key to better toxicology. Xenobiotica *18* (Suppl. 1), 9–14 (1988).
82. C. G. Rousseaux. The use of animal models for predicting the potential chronic effects of highly toxic chemicals. J. Hazardous Materials *14,* 283–292 (1987).
83. C. G. Smith, J. W. Poutsiaka, and E. C. Schreiber. Problems of predicting drug effects across species. J. Int. Med. Res. *1,* 489–503 (1973).
84. A. Yacobi, B. L. Kamath, and C. M. Lai. Pharmacokinetics in chronic animal toxicity studies. Drug Metabol. Rev. *13,* 1021–1051, 1982.
85. John F. Young. Potential role of pharmacokinetics in quantitative risk assessment. Acta. Pharm. Jugosl. *37,* 291–311 (1987).
86. *Biological Bases for Interspecies Extrapolation of Carcinogenicity Data,* July 1986. Task Order #4, Contract No. FDA 223-83-2020, Life Sciences Research Office Publication, Federation of American Societies for Experimental Biology, Bethesda, MD.
87. S. M. Singhvi, G. R. Keim, and B. H. Migdalof. Application of pharmacokinetics in drug safety evaluation. Reg. Toxicol. Pharmacol. *5,* 3–17 (1985).
88. S. Garattini. Toxic effects of chemicals: Difficulties in extrapolating data from animals to man. CRC Crit. Rev. Toxicol. *16,* 1–29 (1985).
89. B. Clark and D. A. Smith. Pharmacokinetics and toxicity testing. CRC Crit. Rev. Toxicol. *12,* 343–385 (1984).
90. J. W. Daniel. Safety evaluation: The role of pharmacokinetics and comparative metabolic studies. Pages 115–126 in: *Animals in Toxicological Research.* I. Bartosek, ed. Raven Press, New York (1982).
91. D. V. Parke. Significance of the metabolism of xenobiotics for toxicological evaluation. Pages 127–145 in: *Animals in Toxicological Research.* I. Bartosek, ed. Raven Press, New York (1982).
92. R. Smyth and G. Hottendorf. Application of pharmacokinetics and biopharmaceutics in the design of toxicological studies. Toxicol. Appl. Pharmacol. *53,* 179–195 (1980).
93. E. R. Garrett. The pharmacokinetic basis of biological response quantification in toxicology, pharmacology, and pharmacodynamics. Prog. Drug Res. *21,* 105 (1977).
94. J. R. Gillette. Application of pharmacokinetic principles in the extrapolation of animal data to humans. Clinical Toxicol. *9,* 709–722 (1976).
95. G. Hottendorf, D. Van Harken, H. Madissoo, and B. Cabana. Pharmacokinetic considerations in toxicology. Proc. Eur. Soc. Toxicol. *17,* 255–262 (1976).
96. *Pharmacokinetics in Risk Assessment,* Drinking Water and Health. Vol. 8. National Academy Press, Washington, DC (1987).

97. Edward J. Calabrese. *Principles of Animal Extrapolation*. John Wiley and Sons, New York (1983).
98. *Animals in Toxicological Research*. I. Bartosek, ed. Raven Press, New York (1982).
99. B. B. Brodie. Of mice, microsomes and man. Pharmacologist *6*, 12–26 (1964).
100. D. P. Rall. Difficulties in extrapolating the results of toxicity studies in laboratory animals to man. Environmental Research *2*, 360–367 (1969).
101. H. Nau. Species differences in pharmacokinetics, drug metabolism, and teratogenesis. Pages 81–106 in: *Pharmacokinetics in Teratogenesis*. Vol. 1. H. Nau and W. J. Scott, Jr., eds. CRC Press Inc., Boca Raton, FL. (1987).
102. M. Weiss, W. Sziegoleit, and W. Forster. Dependence of pharmacokinetic parameters on body weight. Int. J. Clin. Pharmacol. *15*, 572–575 (1977).
103. J. M. Collins, D. S. Zaharko, R. L. Dedrick, and B. A. Chabner. Potential roles for preclinical pharmacology in phase I clinical trials. Cancer Treatment Reports *70*, 73–80 (1986).
104. E. J. Freireich, E. A. Grehan, D. P. Rall, L. H. Schmidt, and H. E. Skipper. Quantitative comparison of toxicity of anticancer agents in mouse, rat, hamster, dog, monkey, and man, Cancer Chemother. Rep. *50*, 219–244 (1966).
105. C. Travis and R. White. Interspecies scaling of toxicity data. Risk Analysis *8*, 119–25 (1988).
106. C. J. Sedgwick. Finding the dietetic needs of captive native wildlife and zoo animals by allometric scaling. Pages 149–155 in: Scientific Proceedings of the American Animal Hospital Association, 55th Annual Meeting, Washington, DC (1988).
107. C. J. Sedgwick. Extrapolating rational drug doses and treatment periods by allometric scaling. Pages 156–161 in: Scientific Proceedings of the American Animal Hospital Association, 55th Annual Meeting, Washington, DC (1988).
108. C. J. Sedgwick. Anesthetic and chemical restraint techniques for zoo animals and wildlife. Pages 162–168 in: Scientific Proceedings of the American Animal Hospital Association, 55th Annual Meeting, Washington, DC (1988).
109. I. W. F. Davidson. J. C. Parker, and R. P. Beliles. Biological basis for extrapolation across mammalian species. Reg. Toxicol. Pharmacol. *6*, 211–237 (1986).
110. M. Andersen, H. Clewell III, M. Gargas, F. Smith, and R. Reitz. Physiologically based pharmacokinetics and the risk assessment process for methylene chloride. Toxic Appl. Pharmacol. *87*, 185–205 (1987).
111. H. Clewell III and M. Andersen. Risk assessment extrapolations and physiologic modeling in: *Advances in Health Risk Assessment for Systemic Toxicants and Chemical Mixtures*. Princeton Scientific Publishers, Princeton, NJ (1985).
112. National Toxicology Program (NTP). "NTP Technical Report on the Toxicology and Carcinogenesis Studies of DiChloromethane in F-344/N Rats and B6C3F1 Mice (Inhalation Studies)." NTP-TR-306 (board draft).
113. D. Serota, B. Ulland, and F. Carlborg. Hazelton Chronic Oral Study in Mice, Food Solvents. March 8–9. Workshop I: Methylene Chloride, Bethesda, MD (1984).
114. J. Ramsey and M. E. Andersen. A physiologically based description of the inhalation pharmacokinetics of styrene in rats and humans. Toxicol. Appl. Pharmacol. *73*, 159–175 (1984).
115. J. D. Burek, K. D. Nitschke, T. J. Bell, D. L. Wackerle, R. C. Childs, J. E. Beyer, D. A. Dittenber, L. W. Rampy, and M. J. McKenna. Methylene chloride: A two year inhalation toxicity and oncogenic study in rats and hamsters. Fund. Appl. Toxicol. *4*, 30–33 (1984).
116. P. J. Neafsey. Pharmacokinetic dose-response models of mortality data from chronic toxicity studies. Dissertation for the degree of Doctor of Philosophy, University of Connecticut, Storrs, CT (1987).
117. R. D'Souza, W. Francis, R. Bruce, and M. Andersen. Physiologically based pharma-

cokinetic model for ethylene chloride and its application in risk assessment. Pages 286–301 in: *Pharmacokinetics in Risk Assessment,* Drinking Water and Health. Vol. 8. National Academy Press, Washington, DC (1987).

118. R. D'Souza, W. Francis, and M. Andersen. Physiological model for tissue glutathione depletion and increased resynthesis following ethylene dichloride exposure. J. Pharmacol. Exp. Ther. *245,* 563–568 (1988).
119. R. H. Reitz, J. F. Quast, A. M. Schumann, P. G. Watanabe, and P. J. Gehring. Nonlinear pharmacokinetic parameters need to be considered in high/low dose extrapolation. Arch. Toxicol., *Suppl. 3,* 79–94 (1980).
120. J. C. Ramsey and P. J. Gehring. Application of pharmacokinetic principles in practice. Fed. Proc. *39,* 60–65 (1980).
121. J. T. Litchfield. Forecasting drug effects in man from studies in laboratory animals. JAMA *177,* 34–38 (1961).
122. A. H. Owens. Predicting anticancer drug effects in man from laboratory animal studies. J. Chron. Dis. *15,* 229–236 (1962).

Chapter 5

Some Pharmacodynamic Aspects of Toxicokinetics

Gerhard Levy

Department of Pharmaceutics, School of Pharmacy
State University of New York at Buffalo

It is now well appreciated that pharmacologic and toxicologic studies on animals must be designed with due regard to pharmacokinetic considerations, including aspects of absorption, presystemic biotransformation, distribution, systemic elimination, and metabolic fate. The pharmacodynamic aspects of these studies (i.e., the variables that can modify the body's response to the drug under investigation) must all receive similar attention. These variables include the drug dosing regimen, the method of drug administration, the use of general anesthetics, the pharmaceutical solvent if the drug cannot be administered in purely aqueous solution, physiologic perturbations associated with drug administration and blood sampling (such as hypovolemia, lack of food intake, and hypothermia), and underlying disease states (such as infections associated with fever, and tumors). These factors will be considered here with an emphasis on their role in studies on rats.

DRUG DOSING REGIMEN

The biologic half-life of most drugs is considerably shorter in rodents than in human beings (1), and yet it has been customary to administer drugs to humans in two or three divided doses per day but to rats or mice in one daily dose for drug safety evaluations. Under these conditions, very pronounced fluctuations of drug concentrations can occur in the animals, ranging from the toxic or subtoxic to the inactive. Such temporal patterns can give rise to unrealistic and uninterpretable results. For example, the embryotoxicity (in mg/kg per day) of valproic acid administered to pregnant mice as a bolus dose is about 10 times greater than that observed when the drug is administered as a continuous infusion, probably because the maximum concentrations produced by rapid drug administration were much higher than those obtained by continuous infusion (2). On the other hand, the nephrotoxicity of some aminoglycosides is more pronounced when the kidneys are exposed continuously rather than intermittently to these drugs. Thus, administration of tobramycin (45 mg/kg per day) for 10 days to dogs reduced their glomerular filtration rate by 40 ± 7 percent (mean ± S.D.) when the drug was infused continuously, by 31 ± 14 percent when given every 4 hours, and by only 12 ± 13 percent when given once daily (3).

It has been known for some time that the total infused dose of a drugrequired to elicit a certain pharmacologic endpoint (for example, the dose of a barbiturate required to produce general anesthesia) may depend on the rate of infusion (RI). Thus, the dose of hexobarbital required to reach an electroencephalographic endpoint known as the "silent second" in rats was about 90 mg/kg at an RI of 5 mg/kg per min, about 60 mg/kg at an RI of 15 mg/kg per min, and about 75 mg/kg at an RI of 60 mg/kg per min (4). We have been able to simulate this type of dose vs. infusion rate pattern (i.e., a minimum effective dose at an intermediate infusion rate) by assuming that the site of action is located in a peripheral ("tissue") compartment of a multicompartmental system (Fig. 5-1).

The larger effective doses at the higher infusion rates reflect the initial disequilibrium between the drug in the central compartment and the drug in the tissue compartment (i.e., a transient overshoot of drug concentrations in the central compartment), whereas the larger effective doses at the lower infusion rates are due to partial drug elimination during the period of infusion (5). This means that it may make a difference toxicologically whether a drug is injected intravenously over 30 seconds or over 3 minutes.

METHOD OF DRUG ADMINISTRATION

To minimize unrealistically and undesirably large fluctuations of drug concentrations in experimental animals, slowly dissolving implanted pellets as well as osmotic minipumps have been employed (6). Our own experience with commercially available pellets has been mixed. Some pellets have dissolved at a reasonably constant and predictable rate when implanted subcutaneously in rats; others have dissolved much more rapidly than specified and have ruined a costly experiment. Osmotic minipumps are more flexible and also permit intravascular drug administration. However, both types of devices must be implanted surgically under general anesthesia and have a

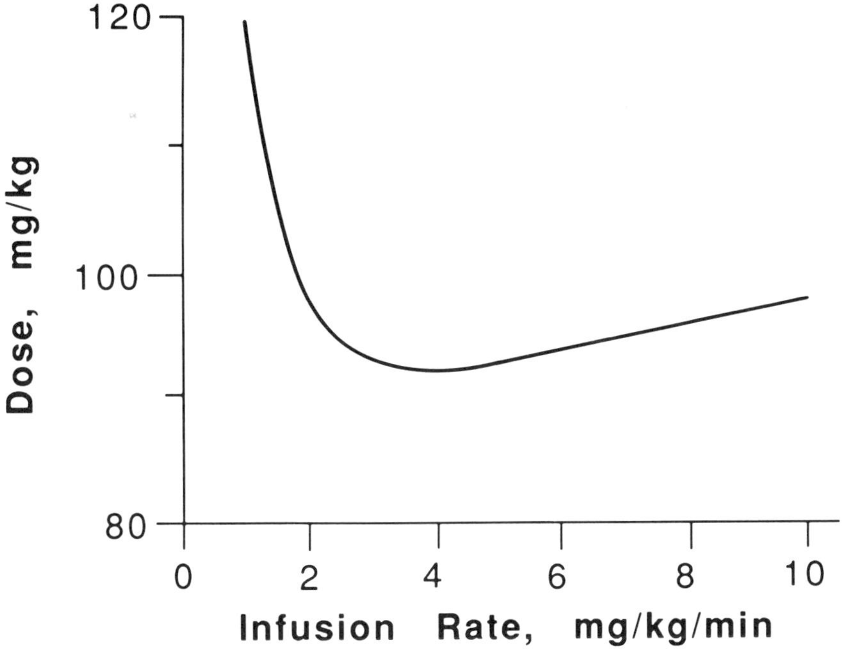

FIGURE 5-1. Simulation of the relationship between infusion rate and amount of drug (threshold dose) required to produce an effective concentration in the peripheral compartment (containing the site of action) of a two-compartment system (5). Reproduced with permission of the copyright holder, the American Pharmaceutical Association.

limited lifetime. At present, not much is known about the effect of repeated surgical implantation of drug-delivery systems on the health and response to drugs of experimental animals. Jarnagin (7) implanted minipumps subcutaneously in rats under ether anesthesia and replaced the devices every two weeks for a total of 20 weeks. The body weight gain, pregnancy rate, litter size, and pup weight of these animals were comparable to those of the control group. We implanted 2-ml-capacity osmotic minipumps filled with water or theophylline solution in rats and found a slightly decreased hematocrit after seven days in the two groups with minipumps, but not in the control group without minipumps (8). There was no evidence of bleeding, and the animals looked and behaved normally. At this point, it is prudent to include suitable controls implanted with drug-free devices as well as controls without implanted devices in toxicologic investigations of drugs that are being administered by minipump or pellet implant.

General Anesthetics

Implantation of drug-delivery systems, cannulation of blood vessels for drug infusion or blood sampling, and certain pharmacologic studies in rodents require general anesthesia. Exposure to some general anesthetics can significantly affect the pharmacokinetic and pharmacodynamic characteristics of drugs. Ether anesthesia reduces the metabolic clearance of acetaminophen (by conjugation) and antipyrine (by oxidation) in intact rats (9), and exposure to ether also inhibits these processes in isolated rat hepatocytes (10). Even brief (5 minute) rather than continuous ether anesthesia causes significant (about 44%) inhibition of acetaminophen clearance in rats (9). Use of implanted delivery system blanks in a control group will, of necessity, include the exposure of these animals to the general anesthetic agent administered to the treatment group. In other cases, a control group specifically for anesthetic exposure may have to be included in the experimental design.

Solvents and Suspending Agents

Apparently, most new drugs are poorly water soluble and require water-miscible organic solvents or solubilizing agents for intravenous administration. Unfortunately, almost all of these substances are pharmacologically active in the dose range required for use as vehicles. Dimethyl sulfoxide, *N, N*-diethylacetamide, glycerin, polyethylene glycol, and polysorbate 80 have skeletal muscle relaxant effects at oral doses of 0.3 to 1.3 g/kg in mice; the corresponding dose for propylene glycol is 2.5 g/kg (11). Very low intravenous doses of ethanol and glycerol (<14 mg/kg) cause transient changes of blood pressure and heart rate in rats (12). Long-term intravenous infusion of polyethylene glycol (about 0.2 mg/kg per hr) reduced seizure frequency in epileptic monkeys and caused loss of appetite and edema of the lower extremities (13). We reasoned that polyethylene glycol 3350 (formerly designated as polyethylene glycol 4000), a polar compound with a relatively large molecular weight, is less likely to penetrate to sites of action in the CNS than is propylene glycol. Though a semisolid, polyethylene glycol 3350 as a 33 percent dispersion in water is a good solvent for many organic compounds, comparable in this respect to 50 percent propylene glycol in water. We found that the latter solvent system, but not the former, potentiated the CNS depressant effect and reduced the systemic clearance of heptabarbital in rats (14) (Table 5-1).

Similar problems with solvents have been encountered clinically. Intravenous administration of phenytoin in a solvent system of 10 percent ethanol and 40 percent propylene glycol has caused cardiovascular collapse and CNS depression, apparently because of the propylene glycol (15). Widely used injectable medications such as Valium, Dilantin, Septra, and Nembutal contain propylene glycol. Patients treated with these preparations had serum concentrations of propylene glycol ranging from 6 to 711 mg/L and only slightly lower concentrations in the cerebrospinal fluid. There was a significant positive correlation between the serum concentrations of propylene gly-

Table 5-1. Effect of Propylene Glycol and Polyethylene Glycol 3350 on the Pharmacodynamics and Pharmacokinetics of Heptabarbital

Parameter	Solvent: Normal Saline	Solvent: 50% Propylene Glycol	Solvent: 33% Polyethylene Glycol
Onset of loss of righting reflex (LRR) min	12.7 ± 1.1	6.5 ± 1.1[a]	12.8 ± 1.5
Drug concentration at LRR (μg/ml)			
Serum	87 ± 11	43 ± 9[a]	91 ± 10
Brain	102 ± 9	55 ± 6[a]	111 ± 10
CSF	39 ± 4	19 ± 2[a]	43 ± 4
Organic solvent (ml/kg)	0	11.1	8.8
Serum clearance (ml/min)	1.56 ± 0.23	1.14 ± 0.27[a]	1.52 ± 0.25
Half-life (min)	70.5 ± 7.4	103 ± 19[a]	72.8 ± 7.4

Note: In the pharmacodynamic study, solvent was infused over 30 minutes. Heptabarbital was then infused in the same solvent. n = 5 per group. In the pharmacokinetic study, solvent (0.1 ml/min) was infused for 30 min before drug administration. The dose of heptabarbital was 12.5 or 25 mg/kg (n = 8–10 per group). All results in this and subsequent tables are expressed as mean ± SD.

[a]Significantly different from normal saline controls. Excerpted from Klockowski and Levy (14).

col and lactate, suggesting that the solvent may be an important cause of lactic acidosis in hospitalized patients (16). Propylene glycol, used as a solvent for an IV solution of nitroglycerin, has also been found to antagonize the anticoagulant effect of heparin under clinical conditions (17).

Even an apparently pharmacologically inert suspending agent such as carboxymethylcellulose (CMC) may present a problem. It increased the mortality of mice treated with adriamycin, 15 mg/kg IP, from about 15 percent (drug in saline solution) to about 80 percent (drug in CMC solution). Apparently, CMC decreases hepatic glutathione levels in mice and thereby enhances the toxicity of adriamycin (18).

STARVATION

Animals that receive drugs in doses large enough to make them feel ill often do not eat. Starvation can modify not only the pharmacokinetics but also the pharmacodynamics (concentration-effect relationship) of drugs. We found a significant increase in the dose and serum, brain and CSF concentrations of phenobarbital required to produce loss of righting reflex in rats starved for 72 hours (19). Interestingly, this decreased sensitivity to a barbiturate was not completely reversed, even after seven days of refeeding. In some studies, there may occur an interaction between body weight loss or starvation and the direct pharmacologic action of the drug under investigation.

BLOOD SAMPLING

Despite their limited blood supply, it is usually desirable to perform pharmacokinetic and pharmacodynamic studies in rats by serial blood sampling rather than risk artifacts of averaging and interindividual variability that arise from single blood sampling of different groups of animals with time. However, excessive blood volume depletion can lead to perturbations of the nervous system (20) and pronounced biochemical changes, including activation of the sympathoadrenal system and increases of plasma insulin, glucagon, and glucose concentrations (21). Withdrawal of 1 ml of blood per hour from rats weighing 250 to 350 g caused a statistically significant decrease of hematocrit and a significant increase of fatty acid concentrations starting at 2 hours, and a significant decrease of albumin and total plasma protein concentrations starting at 10 hours. The plasma protein binding of dicumarol was decreased and its pharmacokinetics and pharmacodynamics were altered by this blood withdrawal schedule (22).

We found that abrupt removal of 30 percent of a rat's blood volume (i.e., about 20 ml/kg) appreciably increased the animal's sensitivity to the CNS depressant action of a barbiturate (23) and a benzodiazepine (24). However, a more gradual withdrawal (over 6 hours) of the same blood volume had very little effect on the pharmacodynamics of phenobarbital (25). Our usual practice of serial blood sampling (i.e., up to 12 samples of less than 0.5 ml each over 6 to 24 hours in rats weighing about 300 g) has not caused us any problems. However, it is not advisable to generalize this conclusion.

BODY TEMPERATURE

Some drugs, when administered in pharmacologic doses, cause hypothermia. Certain disease states, particularly renal failure (26), do the same. Infections and other conditions may cause fever. Body temperature is an important variable in pharmacokinetics and pharmacodynamics. It can change rapidly and markedly in rodents. The body core temperature of mice injected with caffeine (100 mg/kg) decreased by 2° C within 15 minutes and by almost 4° C at 90 minutes (27). Fasted mice treated with a toxic dose (750 mg/kg) of acetaminophen exhibited a lowering of body temperature from the normal 36.5° C to about 29° C; the temperature fell to an average of about 32° C in fed animals (28). Hypothermia of that magnitude has severe effects on many physiologic processes, including biotransformation reactions. For example, the blood clearance of S(−)-acenocoumarol in rats was 3.8 ± 0.4 (mean ± SEM) ml/min at the normal temperature of 37.5° C, decreased to 2.5 ± 0.2 ml/min at 32.5° C, and increased to 4.4 ± 0.4° C at 39.5° C (29).

Heart rate and blood pressure decrease at lower body temperatures (30).

Table 5-2. Renal-Failure-Associated Hypothermia in Rats with Adjuvant-Induced[a] Arthritis: Hypnotic Response to Phenobarbital

Variable	Normothermic	Hypothermic
No. of animals	7	2
Body weight (g)	157 ± 8	180, 180
Rectal temperature (°C)	37.9 ± 0.3	31.0, 32.9
Serum urea nitrogen (mg/dl)	29 ± 22	126, 139
Serum creatinine (mg/dl)	0.27 ± 0.17	2.3, 3.1
SGPT IU/L	7 ± 1	7, 9
Phenobarbital at LRR		
Total dose (mg/kg)	122 ± 8	89, 103
CSF conc. (mg/L)	76 ± 7	47, 54

Note: Reprinted from Wanwimolruk and Levy (32).

[a]Induced with myobacterium butyricum.

Both the plasma clearance of the neuromuscular blocking agent pancuronium and its half-maximum effective plasma concentration (EC_{50}) are reduced to about one-half their normal value when the body temperature of cats is lowered from 38–39° C to 29° C (31). As a consequence of these pharmacokinetic and pharmacodynamic changes, the duration of muscle paralysis produced by a 120 μg/kg dose was prolonged from an average of 60 minutes to 200 minutes. In a recent study in our laboratory of the effect of adjuvant arthritis on the pharmacodynamics of phenobarbital (32), we found that two of the arthritic rats were hypothermic, apparently due to renal dysfunction. Compared to the normothermic rats with arthritis, they were heavier (from water retention) and much more sensitive to the CNS depressant effect of phenobarbital as reflected by the drug concentration in the CSF at onset of loss of righting reflex (Table 5-2). To study certain pharmacodynamic implications of elevated temperature, we produced fever in rats with endotoxin (33). Some of the animals exhibited a temperature increase of about 1.5° C, whereas others showed a less pronounced response to the endotoxin (temperature increase of about 0.4° C). Both groups were significantly more sensitive to phenobarbital, with the more feverish animals showing the largest change (Table 5-3). Similar results were obtained when fever was produced with yeast injection (33).

DISEASE STATES

Even under optimum conditions, some laboratory animals become ill. That illness may alter the pharmacokinetic and pharmacodynamic characteristics of drugs in the affected animal. This is particularly troublesome if the animal shows no overt signs and symptoms of disease. For example, in a recent study of the neurotoxicity of theophylline in rats as a function of age, we

Table 5-3. Effect of Endotoxin-Induced Fever on Concentrations of Phenobarbital at Onset of Loss of Righting Reflex in Rats Receiving Phenobarbital by Slow IV Infusion

Variable	Controls	Endotoxin Treated	
		T < 1° C	T > 1° C
No. of animals	6	6	5
Body weight (g)	187 ± 3	185 ± 5	182 ± 2
Body temp. (°C)			
Before endotoxin		38.4 ± 0.2	38.2 ± 0.2
After endotoxin	38.2 ± 0.4	38.9 ± 0.3[a]	39.7 ± 0.3[a]
Temp. difference		0.4 ± 0.2	1.5 ± 0.1
Phenobarbital infusion time (min)	36 ± 1	29 ± 2[a]	26 ± 1[a]
Total phenobarbital dose (mg/kg)	157 ± 6	129 ± 7[a]	119 ± 3[a]
Serum phenobarbital conc. (mg/L)			
Total drug	243 ± 10	211 ± 22[a]	200 ± 11[a]
Free drug	154 ± 9	130 ± 12[a]	123 ± 8[a]
Brain phenobarbital conc. (mg/kg)	138 ± 6	118 ± 9[a]	111 ± 3[a]
Cerebrospinal fluid phenobarbital conc. (mg/L)	89 ± 7	78 ± 6[a]	73 ± 5[a]

Note: Reprinted from Hisaoka and Levy (33).

[a]Significantly different from control values.

encountered one control animal that was much more sensitive to the drug than the others (34). The body weight, appearance, and biochemical indices of that animal were normal (Table 5-4). Only upon routine dissection at the end of the experiment did it become evident that the liver was substantially enlarged and that it contained tumors. Such tumors occur frequently in old rats.

Table 5-4. Experimental Theophylline Neurotoxicity in Old Rats:[a] Effect of Spontaneous Hepatic Tumor

Variable	Normal Rats	Tumor Rat
No. of animals	4	1
Body weight (g)	364 ± 14	307
Serum total protein (g/dl)	7.49 ± 0.13	7.90
Serum creatinine (mg/dl)	1.02 ± 0.14	0.84
Serum urea nitrogen (mg/dl)	11.6 ± 2.5	16.3
SGOT (IU/L)	46 ± 7	50
SGPT (IU/L)	16 ± 2	20
Liver weight (g/kg)	30.6 ± 1.3	47
Theophylline dose (mg/kg)	206 ± 9	182
Theophylline conc. in CSF (mg/L)	225 ± 4	191

Note: From Yasuhara and Levy (34).

[a]Male Fischer 344 rats 22 months old.

CONCLUSIONS

To prevent or minimize the intrusion of irrelevant or nonspecific variables in preclinical studies and thereby avoid artifacts and misinterpretations, it is necessary to monitor comprehensively the physiologic status of experimental animals. The temporal pattern of drug concentrations should be known and controlled by use of appropriate dosage regimens, if necessary with the aid of suitable delivery systems. There must be an awareness of the potential effects of general anesthetics and nonaqueous solvents on the pharmacokinetics and pharmacodynamics of drugs. Physiologic perturbations such as hypothermia and starvation due to lack of food intake can arise from administration of relatively large doses of drugs; this in turn can cause nonlinear or other unusual pharmacokinetics or pharmacodynamics. Routine dissection of experimental animals at the end of pharmacokinetic-pharmacodynamic experiments may reveal pathologies that explain unusual (outlier) results. The basis of toxicokinetics must be a comprehensive interdigitation of physiologic, pharmacologic, pharmacokinetic, and biopharmaceutic considerations.

ACKNOWLEDGMENT

Research by the author and his collaborators described in this review was supported in part by Grant GM 20852 from the National Institute of General Medical Sciences, National Institutes of Health.

REFERENCES

1. J. Mordenti. Dosage regimen design for pharmaceutical studies conducted in animals. J. Pharm. Sci. *75,* 852–857 (1986).
2. H. Nau. The role of delivery systems in toxicology and drug development. Pharm. Internat. *4,* 228–231 (1983).
3. S. H. Powell, W. L. Thompson, M. A. Luthe, R. C. Stern, D. A. Grossniklaus, D. D. Bloxham, D. L. Groden, M. R. Jacobs, A. O. DiScenna, H. A. Cash, and J. D. Klinger. Once daily vs. continuous aminoglycoside dosing: Efficacy and toxicity in animal and clinical studies of gentamicin, nethilmicin, and tobramycin. J.1 Infect. Dis. *147,* 918–932 (1983).
4. H. B. Bolander, G. Wahlstrom, and L. Norberg. Re-evaluation of potency and pharmacokinetic properties of some lipid-soluble barbiturates with an EEG-threshold method. Acta Pharmacol. Toxicol. *54,* 33–40 (1984).
5. P. M. Klockowski, and G. Levy. Kinetics of drug action in disease states. XXI. Relationship between drug infusion rate and dose required to produce a pharmacologic effect. J. Pharm. Sci. *76,* 516–520 (1987).
6. R. W. Hess, S. L. Hardman, D. Y. Shirachi, and K. A. Taubert. Comparison between osmotic mini-pumps and controlled release pellets in chronic clonidine administration in the spontaneously hypertensive rat. Proc. West. Pharmacol. Soc. *28,* 97–101 (1985).
7. K. Jarnagin, R. Brommage, H. F. DeLuca, S. Yamada, and H. Takayama. 1-but not 24-

hydroxylation of vitamin D is required for growth and reproduction in rats. Am. J. Physiol. *244,* E290–E297 (1983).
8. I. M. Ramzan and G. Levy. Chronic theophylline administration has no apparent effect on theophylline concentrations required to produce seizures in rats. Proc. Soc. Exp. Biol. Med. *182,* 176–180 (1986).
9. W. Johannessen, G. Gadeholt, and J. Aarbakke. Effects of diethyl ether anaesthesia on the pharmacokinetics of antipyrine and paracetamol in the rat. J. Pharm. Pharmacol. *33,* 365–368 (1981).
10. H. Aune, H. Olsen, and J. Morland. Diethyl ether influence on the metabolism of antipyrine, paracetamol and sulphanilamide in isolated rat hepatocytes. Br. J. Anaesth. *53,* 621–626 (1981).
11. R. Budden, U. G. Kuhl, and J. Bahlsen. Experiments on the toxic, sedative and muscle relaxant potency of various drug solvents in mice. Pharmac. Ther. *5,* 467–474 (1979).
12. F. J. Morales-Olivas, E. Rubio, V. Palop, and J. M. Garcia-Diez. Influence of vehicle on the cardiovascular effects of bromocriptine. IRCS Med. Sci. *13,* 1207–1208 (1985).
13. J. S. Lockard, R. H. Levy, W. C. Congdon, and L. L. DuCharme. Efficacy and toxicity of the solvent polyethylene glycol 400 in monkey model. Epilepsia *20,* 77–84 (1979).
14. P. M. Klockowski and G. Levy. Effect of propylene glycol and polyethylene glycol on the pharmacokinetics and pharmacodynamics of barbiturates. Unpublished data. State University of New York at Buffalo, 1986.
15. M. E. Winter and T. N. Tozer. Phenytoin. Page 497 in: Applied Pharmacokinetics. W. E. Evans, J. J. Schentag, W. J. Jusko, and H. Harrison, eds. Applied Therapeutics, Inc., Spokane, WA, 2nd Ed., p. 493–539 (1986).
16. M. J. Kelner, and D. N. Bailey. Propylene glycol as a cause of lactic acidosis. J. Anal. Toxicol. *9,* 40–42 (1985).
17. J. Col, C. Col-Debeys, E. Lavenne-Pardonge, P. H. Meert, L. Hericks, M. C. Broze, and M. Moriau. Propylene glycol induced heparin resistance during nitroglycerin infusion. Am. Heart J. *110,* 171–173 (1985).
18. G. Decorti, F. B. Klugmann, F. Mallardi, R. Brovedani, G. Baldini, and L. Baldini. Enhancement of adriamycine toxicity by carboxymethylcellulose in mice. Toxicol. Appl. Pharmacol. *71,* 288–293 (1983).
19. S. Wanwimolruk and G. Levy. Kinetics of drug action in disease states. XX. Effects of acute starvation on the pharmacodynamics of phenobarbital, ethanol and pentylenetetrazol in rats and effects of refeeding and diet composition. J. Pharmacol. Exp. Ther., *242.* 166–172 (1987).
20. C. G. Peterson, and F. P. Haugen. Hemorrhagic shock and the nervous system. Am. J. Surgery *106,* (1963).
21. H-R. Berthoud, W. B. Laughton, and T. L. Powley. A method for large volume blood sampling and transfusion in rats. Am. J. Physiol. *250,* E331–E337 (1986).
22. M. Hulse, S. Feldman, and J. V. Bruckner. Effect of blood sampling schedules on protein drug binding in the rat. J. Pharmacol. Exp. Ther. *218,* 416–420 (1981).
23. P. M. Klockowski and G. Levy. Kinetics of drug action in disease states. XXIII. Effect of acute hypovolemia on the pharmacodynamics of phenobarbital in rats. Paper J. Pharm. Sci. *77,* 365–366 (1988).
24. P. M. Klockowski and G. Levy. Kinetics of drug action in disease states. XXV. Effect of experimental hypovolemia on the pharmacodynamics and pharmacokinetics of desmethyldiazepam. Paper J. Pharmacol. Exp. Ther. *245,* 508–512 (1988).
25. A. Hoffman and G. Levy. Unpublished data. State University of New York at Buffalo, 1987.
26. G. E. Schreiner and J. F. Maher. *Uremia: Biochemistry, Pathogenesis, and Treatment.* Charles C. Thomas, Springfield, OH (1961), pp. 382–455.

27. J. M. Carney, T. W. Seale, L. Logan, and S. B. McMaster. Sensitivity of inbred mice to mehylxanthines is not determined by plasma xanthine concentration. Neurosci. Lett. *56,* 27–31 (1985).
28. R. M. Walker, T. E. Massey, T. F. McElligott, and W. J. Racz. Acetaminophen toxicity in fed and fasted mice. Can. J. Physiol. Pharmacol. *60,* 399–404 (1982).
29. M. J. A. P. Daeman, H. H. W. Thijssen, H. T. M. Vervoort-Peters, J. F. M. Smits, and H. A. J. Struyker-Boudier. The effect of pentobarbitone anaesthesia and hypothermia on the hepatic clearance of indocyanine green and S(−)-acenocoumarol in the rat. J. Pharm. Pharmacol. *38,* 122–125 (1986).
30. T. Itoh, R. Thomas, B. D. Foltz, and D. H. Dillard. Blood anesthetic levels during surface-induced deep hypothermia under halothane-diethyl ether azeotrope anesthesia. Tohoku. J. Exp. Med. *148,* 103–111 (1986).
31. R. D. Miller, S. Agoston, F. van der Pol., L. H. D. J. Booij, J. F. Crul, and J. Ham. Hypthermia and the pharmacokinetics and pharmacodynamics of pancuronium in the cat. J. Pharmacol. Exp. Ther. *207,* 532–538 (1978).
32. S. Wanwimolruk and G. Levy. Effect of experimental arthritis on the pharmacodynamics of phenobarbital in rats. Unpublished data. State Univ. of N.Y. at Buffalo, 1986.
33. M. Hisaoka and G. Levy. Kinetics of drug action in disease states. IX. Effect of experimental fever on phenobarbital concentrations at onset of loss of righting reflex in rats. J. Pharmacol. Exp. Ther. *232,* 722–724 (1985).
34. M. Yasuhara and G. Levy. Effect of age on neurotoxicity of theophylline in rats. J. Pharm. Sci. 77, 645–646 (1988).

Chapter 6

Role of Pharmacokinetics in Drug Evaluation: Safety-Related Issues

Robert Temple, M.D.

Director, Office of Drug Evaluation I
Center for Drug Evaluation and Research
Food and Drug Administration

A reasonable appreciation of how a drug is absorbed, distributed, metabolized, and excreted is recognized as a necessary basis for intelligent design of clinical trials. Yet it remains true (perhaps less so than in the past) that the pharmacokinetics of drugs is examined most closely late in development—not early—and the logical consequences of pharmacokinetic information are often ignored.

There are many possible reasons for this late attention to pharmacokinetics. Sometimes the precise plasma drug concentration assay needed for good kinetics may be difficult to develop. Or metabolism may be complex, and the matabolites not well characterized early on. In such situations, trials may be initiated before they are ready, or at least before they can be optimally designed pharmacokinetically. Sometimes commercial considerations loom large in determining such choices as dose interval, and the implications of pharmacokinetics may be brushed aside. Pharmacokinetic information may also be perceived as the concern solely of the pharmacokineticist, an area

---

Presented at the First National Meeting of the American Association of Pharmaceutical Scientists (AAPS), Washington, DC, November 3, 1986.

the clinician enters with trepidation and only when it cannot be avoided. Finally, the importance of pharmacokinetics in a given case has much to do with blood level response characteristics (i.e., pharmacodynamics), and these relationships are often poorly characterized, especially for adverse effects and effects other than the main effect of the drug.

Because pharmacokinetic information is often lacking many drugs reach the NDA stage with no clear basis for choice of dose interval, no clear assessment of whether different dosing intervals lead to differences in effectiveness or adverse effects, and no clear assessment of the effect of age, changes in renal function, and so forth, on the kinetics and, therefore, dosing of the drug. This is changing, however, and the changes are both reflected in, and driven by, changes in FDA guidelines; two guidelines in particular are influential: (1) the guideline for the format and content of the clinical and statistical sections of an FDA application and (2) the guideline for studies of drugs in the elderly. Together the guidelines call for the following:

1. An analysis of dose-response information—an integrated analysis of all data, from animal, clinical pharmacology, controlled and uncontrolled studies, that bear on the dose-response relationship of beneficial and adverse effects, the method of dose selection, and the choice of dose interval. Of special interest is the comparison of effectiveness and adverse effect dose responses (the therapeutic ratio).
2. Evidence of different dose-response relationships in age, sex, disease, or other subgroups. Although such differences could reflect true pharmacodynamic differences (i.e., shifts in blood level-response relationships), the most common cause of such differences will, I believe, prove to be pharmacokinetic differences. In any event, subgroups cannot be properly assessed for pharmacodynamic differences until their kinetic characteristics are defined.
3. Eventually, as part of a process set in motion by the development of guidelines for study of drugs in the elderly, we will obtain a wealth of organized data on population pharmacokinetics, the result of systematic steady-state blood level determinations in well-characterized patients in clinical trials (i.e., pharmacokinetic screening).

I have no doubt at all that the guidelines and pharmacokinetic screening data will lead to a drug development world in which pharmacokinetic and dose-response considerations are far more important than they are today.

Good kinetic information is most crucial for drugs with dose-limiting toxicity. If large amounts of drug can be given without increasing toxicity, matters such as dose and dose-interval, or subgroup differences, are not so critical. Beta blockers, for example, cause adverse effects, but they do not appear in most cases to be dose related once substantial beta blockade is attained. It has therefore become common practice to administer these drugs in relatively large doses at dosing intervals several times their half-lives; in this way, an initial high blood concentration is attained so that enough drug will be present at the end of the dosing interval, despite passage of several half-lives. In hypertension, persistence of effect may reflect not only persistence of drug but an effect that remains after blood levels have become inconsequential. If the early high blood concentration has no adverse consequence, it is hard to object to this practice. But the size of the dose needed (e.g., to allow once-daily dosing of a drug with a 4-hour half-life is large, 25 to 50 times the individual doses that would be used in a q4h regimen.

In some situations, beta blockers can have dose-related toxicity. So-called cardioselective agents are not absolutely selective but show a relatively greater effect on cardiac than on bronchial receptors; at larger doses they can fully block the bronchial receptor. In this case, use of a large once-daily dose to produce a longer effect could obliterate cardioselectivity and defeat the purpose of using the selective agent.

Consider the example shown in Figure 6-1 and Table 6-1. The numbers are fictional, but they illustrate the problem.

In this case, to achieve an effective end-dosing-interval blood concentration with a drug with a 4-hour half-life, a large initial dose is used so that after six half-lives an effective 1 mg/ml blood level is still present. Assuming dose proportionality, instantaneous attainment of C_{max}, and a minimum effective blood level of 1 mg/ml, a q8h regimen would allow single doses about 1/16 the size of 64-mg single dose and a total daily dose of about 3/16 the large single dose. Most important, if the selectivity of the drug for heart versus pulmonary receptors is a factor of 10, for more than 8 hours after the single dose, the blood level will be high enough to overcome this selectivity, certainly a serious problem in patients who need that property. I should add also that subtleties such as the dose interval are pertinent only if there has been some attempt to find the appropriate dose has been made. If a cardioselective agent such as atenolol were given in as large an excess dose as nadolol (which is labeled for at least 20 times the needed dose), little cardioselectivity would ever be manifested in clinical use.

Any drug with toxic and therapeutic effects that follow blood level closely can have toxicity at C_{max}, ineffectiveness at trough, or both, if a proper dosing interval is not selected. This is, of course, a particular problem for drugs with very short half-lives, which usually have relatively long (compared to half-life) dosing intervals because intervals of less than 6 hours are impractical; but any drug with a dose interval more than twice its half-life seems to be a candidate for such problems. It is possible that a potentially valuable separation between toxic and beneficial effects can be obliterated by too-infrequent dosing with larger doses, much as cardioselectivity can be.

Recent experience with guanfacine, a long-half-life central alpha agonist,

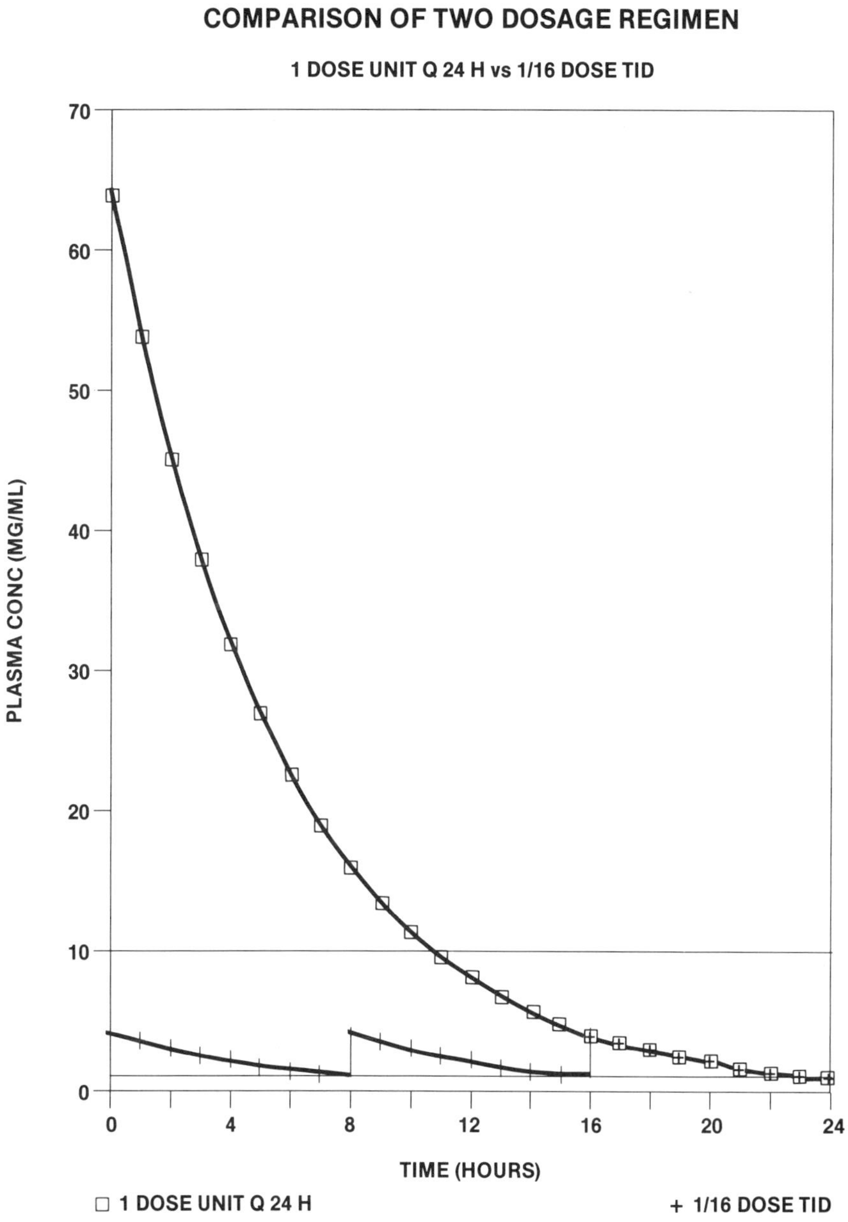
COMPARISON OF TWO DOSAGE REGIMEN
1 DOSE UNIT Q 24 H vs 1/16 DOSE TID
70
60
50
40
30
20
10
0
PLASMA CONC (MG/ML)
0
4
8
12
16
20
24
TIME (HOURS)
□ 1 DOSE UNIT Q 24 H
+ 1/16 DOSE TID

Table 6-1. Relative Cardioselectivity

	Effect of 1 ng/ml on	
	Heart	Bronchi
Usual β blocker	10	10
Selective β blocker	10	1
	Effect of 10 ng/ml on	
	Heart	Bronchi
Usual β blocker	10	10
Selective blocker	10	10

T 1/2 = 4 hours
Effective level = 1 ng/ml, which gives a cardiac effect of 10

suggests that this may have been the case for pharmacologically similar short-half-life drugs such as clonidine. Guanfacine appears to have most of its effect on blood pressure at a dose of 1–2 mg per day. Its main side effects, however, are scarcely present at 1 or even 2 mg but are in full bloom at 3 mg; there is thus apparently a reasonably good separation between the dose needed for desired effect and the dose causing toxicity, a better picture than has been attributed to other drugs of the class. A number of possible reasons may account for this. Guanfacine is given at night so that sedative effects, a major problem, are not disturbing, and it has a half-life of about 12–14 hours, so that peak to trough differences in blood concentration are less than 4 to 1. It also seems possible that the b.i.d. and t.i.d. dosing regimens with the short-half-life drug, clonidine, led to a failure to discern such separation. It is of course possible that the drugs are pharmacologically different, that is, that clonidine has less separation between therapeutic and toxic doses.

A drug with very short half-life with adverse effects at C_{max} might best be introduced as a controlled-release product. Nifedipine, with end-dosing-interval loss of effect in some patients, and excessive peak response in others, has always seemed a potential candidate for such an approach.

Recently, we have seen that the intractable gastrointestinal toxicity of pentoxifylline observed when this very short half-life drug is given as a t.i.d. or q.i.d. regimen could be avoided when the drug is given in a controlled-release formulation. Of course, the blood concentration profiles were so different that new clinical trials were needed for the new regimen.

A proper pharmacokinetic analysis is crucial for any drug with substantial renal excretion, and it is in this setting that pharmacokinetic information today plays its most crucial role in drug safety, particularly for drugs with narrow toxic therapeutic ratios. One need go no further than classic examples of aminoglycosides or digoxin to appreciate the devastation that can ensue when normal doses are given to persons with reduced excretion. There are modern examples, too: The hepatic and renal toxicity of benoxaprofen was probably the result of insufficient dose reduction in renal-impaired people. Labeling for a number of NSAIDs with predominant renal excretion, such as Clinoril, strongly emphasizes the need for reduced dose in renal impairment. It is fairly likely that some of the serious toxicity of captopril resulted from excessive doses, especially in people with renal failure.

Although renal-related differences in kinetics are most prominent, pharmacokinetic differences of other kinds, such as those due to hepatic or circulatory failure, or resulting from other drugs, can also be critical and must be understood. Finally, there is the matter of genetic differences in metabolism or excretion. Relatively few of these are recognized, but there is little reason to doubt that there are many more examples of the kind illustrated by acetylator subtypes, fast and slow debrisoquin metabolizers, or slow succinylcholine metabolizers. In the past these were rarely, if ever, recognized in advance of marketing so that test doses or alternative regimens could be developed. An indication of how fast we are moving to correct this is that the rather complicated case of different encainide kinetics in debrisoquin metabolizer subtypes was worked out before a clinical problem emerged because, at least in the area of antiarrhythmics, in which drugs are relatively toxic, plasma concentration measurements are routinely obtained from many patients, not just a few dozen normal volunteers.

We are, I think, in the middle of a pharmacokinetic revolution. The techniques for doing kinetic analyses have become well developed, and what has been an art form of the kineticist is gradually becoming a widely available clinical tool. Naturally, this has happened where it is most critical, so that clinically usable programs for digoxin or phenytoin dosing preceded many others. But it is spreading rapidly, and the masses of information being collected on new agents will speed the process. It is essential that pharmacokinetic considerations be given proper attention in drug development and that a product not be force fitted into an inappropriate dosing regimen. Variations in kinetics due to genetic, metabolic, and excretion differences should be identified at an early stage. It is also critical to obtain better blood level response data so that kinetics can be properly applied.

Chapter 7

Pharmacokinetics and Adverse Reactions: An Overview

Louis Lemberger, Ph.D., M.D.

Eli Lilly and Company
Lilly Laboratory for Clinical Research
Wishard Memorial Hospital
and
the Departments of Pharmacology, Medicine, and Psychiatry
Indiana University School of Medicine

The importance of the advances contributed by clinical pharmacology and pharmacokinetics to the field of therapeutics cannot be underestimated. A great deal of credit can be attributed to these disciplines for assuring that therapeutics remains a scientific part of medicine.

Striking advances in technology have allowed for the development of instrumentation and methodology such as gas chromatography-mass spectroscopy, mass fragmentography, high pressure liquid chromatography, radioisotopic techniques, radioimmunoassay, and radioenzymic assay. These procedures are capable of measuring minute quantities of a drug and its metabolites in biologic fluids. Likewise, the application of computer technology has allowed for the almost instantaneous manipulation of this data to help assess the pharmacokinetic profile of a drug in patient populations or in experimental studies involving normal volunteer subjects.

In general, many factors can play a role in producing disproportionate responses to what might be expected to be a safe dose of a drug. A variety of these factors may affect the relationship between pharmacokinetics and adverse drug reactions. These include dose administered, route of administration, pharmacogenetics, drug interactions, and concomitant pathologic or disease state. An extremely important factor is the dose administration.

In general, dose-response or dose-effect curves follow a sigmoid curve (Fig. 7-1). A drug's effect exhibits a lag period until it produces its threshold effect. This is followed by its minimally effective dose and finally by a maximally effective dose.

A drug's therapeutic range may be large when the therapeutic and toxic doses are markedly different, or it may have a narrow therapeutic range; that is, the therapeutic dose and the toxic dose are quite close (Fig. 7-2). The plasma concentrations, represented by the minimal therapeutic and maximally tolerated dose, are illustrated in Figure 7-3. The blood levels, and especially the pharmacokinetic curves for these situations, may vary with time, the rate of absorption, the drug's distribution, and its half-life.

Blood or plasma levels may be helpful in the management of patients to prevent the occurrence of adverse reactions or to prevent therapeutic failures. However, because of many factors, such as interindividual and intraindividual variation, these plasma concentrations are not absolute and are thus purposely depicted by the wide ranges and large standard errors from the mean values, as illustrated in Figure 7-3.

A clinical example is seen with the anticoagulant drug Tromexan (1).

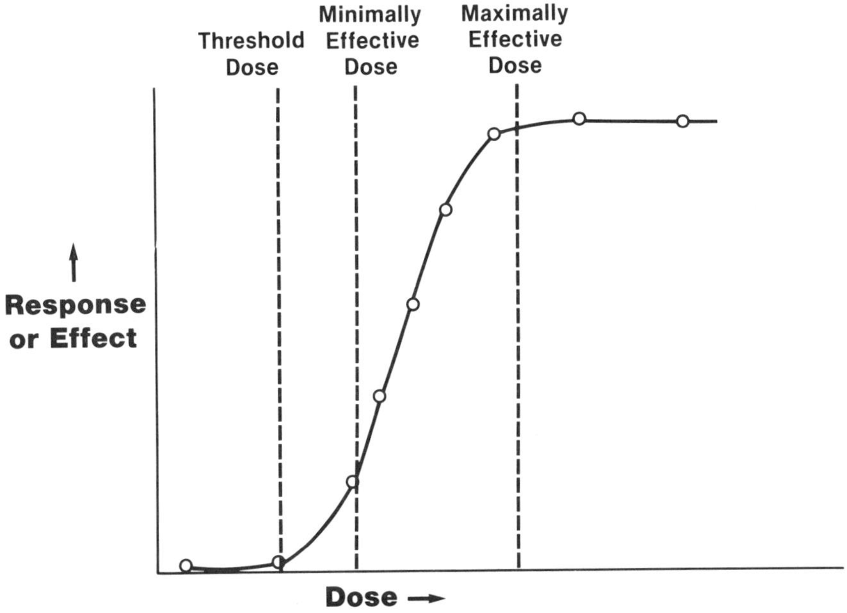

FIGURE 7-1. Depiction of a typical dose-response curve.

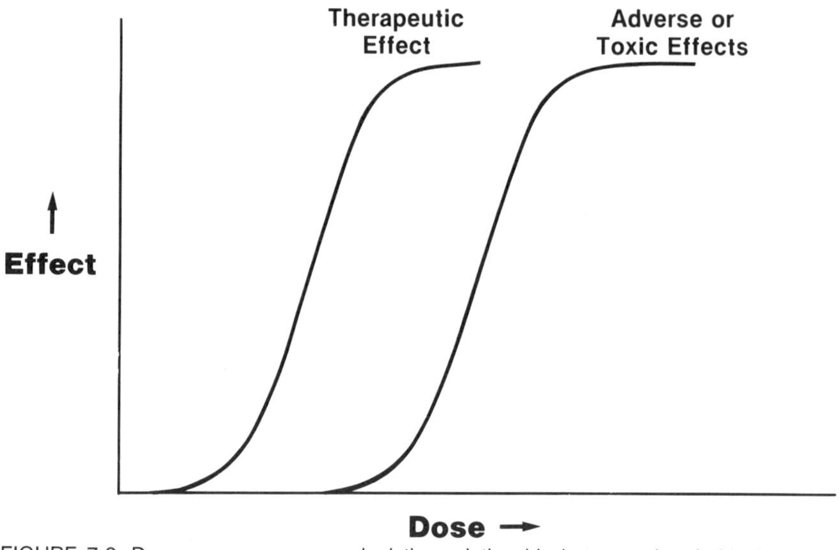

FIGURE 7-2. Dose response curves depicting relationship between threshold effect and toxic effect.

Even after its intravenous administration, on an mg/kg dosage, variations in Tromexan's blood concentrations still exist in different subjects. Similar variations have been reported when relating digitoxin plasma concentrations and toxicity (2). It is clear that different individuals having similar plasma concentrations may exhibit differing levels of toxicity. In two groups of patients having identical plasma concentrations, some patients may exhibit no toxicity, and others may clearly exhibit evidence of digitalis toxicity.

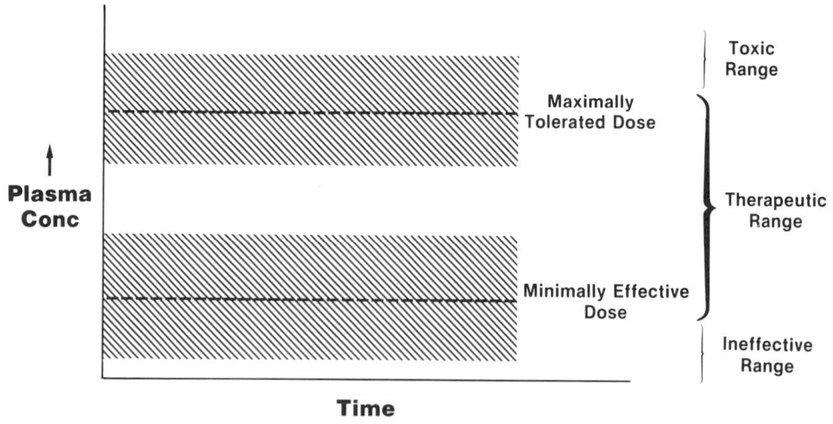

FIGURE 7-3. The relationship between plasma concentration and range of therapeutic and toxic range.

In general, the relationship between an adverse reaction to a drug and its pharmacokinetics is based upon the simple pharmacologic principle of dose-response relationship (Fig. 7-4).

The effect of a drug—whether therapeutic or adverse—is usually related to the dose administered, assuming that dose proportionality exists. Thus, in general, the higher the dose, the higher the plasma and tissue levels and therefore the greater the incidence of adverse effects. This is exemplified by antiarrhythmics. Below a specific dose or plasma concentration, antiarrhythmics are ineffective, but they are capable of suppressing abnormal cardiac conduction within a certain plasma concentration range (3). However, as the plasma concentration exceeds the therapeutic plasma concentration range, the greater is the likelihood for central nervous system side effects, including tremors and convulsions.

Dose proportionality can also be illustrated with the anticonvulsants (4). Diphenylhydontoin is effective in the majority of patients when plasma concentrations are about 10 μg/ml. However, some patients may respond to doses producing levels as low as 3–4 μg/ml, and some severe, relatively refractory cases may require plasma concentrations as high as 40 μg/ml. The degree of toxicity can be correlated with various blood levels.

Another example illustrating dose-related adverse effects involves the drug of abuse—cocaine. After oral administration, cocaine is metabolized rapidly by esterases in the liver and gastrointestinal tract (5). To circumvent this inactivation, drug abusers commonly use cocaine by "snorting" it through the nose, smoking it, using the new, popular form known as crack, or by application to the mucus membranes such as through buccal or sublingual administration. This later mode is common to the natives in the Andes of South America, who claim to use this drug to increase their work perfor-

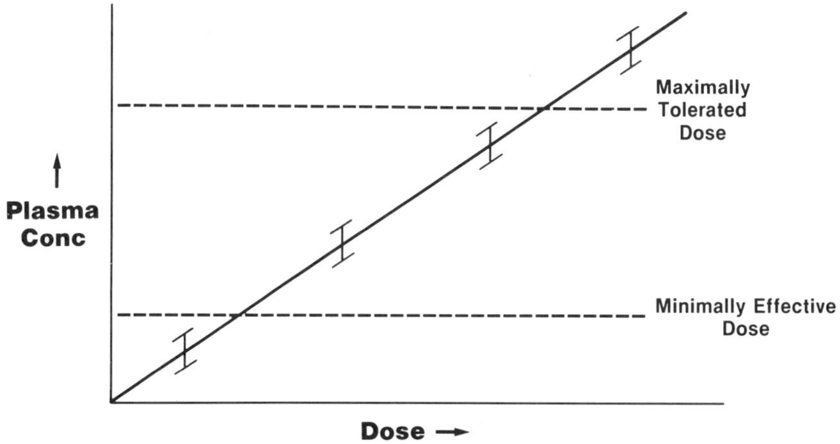

FIGURE 7-4. Correlation between dose and plasma concentrations.

mance. In several instances, drug smugglers have placed large quantities of cocaine in rubber condoms and swallowed them, hoping to avoid detection as they cross international borders. On certain occasions, these condoms have burst, releasing large quantities of cocaine into the gastrointestinal tract and rapidly saturating the capacity of the hepatic esterases, thereby partially avoiding the first-pass phenomenon. This usually results in marked cardiac and central nervous system toxicity and causes death (6).

Another factor involving pharmacokinetics and adverse effects is the route of administration. It is well known that certain of the vinca alkaloids isolated from the plant vinca rosacea possess neurotoxicity. When given intravenously, little of the drug enters the central nervous system. However, if the drug is inadvertently administered by the intrathecal route, large concentrations of the drug are placed in the cerebrospinal fluid, and thus the central nervous system is exposed to toxic concentrations of the drug. This invariably results in damage to the spinal cord (7), which is usually manifested by irreversible sensory and motor deficits and is usually fatal. Similarly, drugs designed to be administered subcutaneously or intramuscularly may be mistakenly administered intravenously or intra-arterially. This also may result in marked toxicity.

The dose and route of administration play very important roles in the relationship of pharmacokinetics to adverse effects. Perhaps the most important factor in the relationship between plasma concentrations and toxic effects is the dose administered. However, other factors can also play a role in producing disproportionate responses to what might be expected to be a safe, therapeutic dose of a drug.

One factor that may affect an individual's response to drugs is pharmacogenetics. The importance of pharmacogenetics as a cause for adverse drug responses was recognized many years ago (8). Many factors can affect and adversely interact with one's genetic constitution and thus with its response to drugs (9).

In certain instances, pharmacogenetic variation in drug responses and adverse effects may be related to pharmacokinetics. In other instances, it is clearly unrelated to blood levels of drug, but is due instead to factors such as differences in response at the receptor site or to altered enzymes. Thus, a drug such as the muscle relaxant succinyl choline, used as an adjunct to general anesthesia, may show exaggerated responses in certain individuals even though they do not have abnormally high peak plasma concentrations of the drug and are receiving doses comparable to those given the general population (10). After succinyl choline administration, these individuals will experience prolonged periods of apnea because of the presence of an atypical pseudocholinesterase that is incapable of metabolizing the drug at the same rate as is expected in the normal population.

A recent example of pharmacogenetics deals with the newly characterized polymorphism of debrisoquine metabolism (11). Debrisoquine, an antihypertensive, is metabolized via the liver microsomal enzymes to 4-hydroxy-debrisoquine. There appears to be a relationship between ethnicity and ability to hydroxylate debrisoquin. About 5 to 10 percent of Caucasians have a form of the enzyme, which results in a decreased capacity to metabolize debrisoquine and an increased possibility of having a greater incidence of adverse effects. These individuals exhibit a longer drug half-life, and with chronic administration, the drug may accumulate. This pharmacogenetic difference may involve a variety of metabolic pathways (12) and drugs of differing therapeutic classes. Therefore, chronic administration of these drugs may result in adverse effects in susceptible individuals.

Isoniazid, hydralazine, and procainamide are also drugs whose metabolism is under genetic control. These drugs are *N*-acetylated. A bimodal distribution occurs in the population for this *N*-acetyltransferase enzyme. Subjects are either slow or fast acetylators, as Evans and colleagues (13) illustrated for isoniazid. This difference in acetylation appears to be related to race, with Orientals being predominantly fast metabolizers, whereas blacks and Caucasians are either fast or slow metabolizers. Some researchers have suggested that individuals who metabolize the drug rapidly may have a decreased therapeutic effect when the drug is given weekly in chemotherapy programs, whereas the slow metabolizers may have a greater chance of developing toxic effects if they also have some degree of renal impairment (14).

With hydralazine and procainamide, systemic lupus erythematosis or an SLE-like syndrome is thought to be associated with the parent compounds and not with the formation of their *N*-acetylated metabolites. Thus, slow metabolizers have a greater potential of developing drug-induced SLE than rapid acetylators (15).

The genetic involvement of specific receptors may also play a role in determining whether or not a dose-response relationship exists for a drug. For example, a small group of individuals has been found to be resistant to warfarin's anticoagulant effects (16). Thus, even increasing the dose and the blood levels of warfarin in these individuals does not result in a therapeutic effect and does not even produce adverse effects. This is also a pharmacogenetic phenomenon, but in this case it is not specifically related to any adverse effect.

Another factor affecting the relationship of pharmacokinetics and adverse effects is drug interactions. Drug combination therapy or environmental exposures may be responsible for interactions that may in turn be manifested as adverse reactions. These reactions may occur at any of the sites involved in the overall physiologic disposition of a drug, including its absorption, distribution, metabolism, or excretion, and they may be secondary to general processes such as enzyme inhibition or enzyme induction. Drug interactions may result in adverse effects when excessive blood concentrations of drug are present after the concomitant administration of two interacting drugs. This occurs when there is an enhanced delivery of one of the drugs to its site of action or a site responsible for an adverse effect.

Enzyme inhibition may be a responsible factor, for example, with the combined administration of sympathomimetics and monoamine oxidase inhibitors. Thus, sympathomimetic drugs such as the nasal decongestants or naturally occurring sympathomimetics such as tyramine, which is a constituent of cheese and wine, may interact with the monoamine oxidase inhibitors, drugs still used in the treatment of depression (17,18). The combination may result in a higher blood level of the sympathomimetic amine, which in turn might be responsible for a high degree of adverse and possibly fatal side effects.

The antithesis of enzyme inhibition is enzyme induction. In this situation, a drug given chronically may enhance the formation of an active metabolite or at times a toxic metabolite from a prodrug. Similarly, if a patient, while hospitalized, receives an enzyme inducer such as the sedatives phenobarbital or chloral hydrate and then requires an anticoagulant such as dicoumarol, the result could be an altered rate of dicoumarol's metabolism. Thus, the potential exists for a bleeding disorder to occur when the enzyme inducer is subsequently discontinued but no dosage reduction for warfarin is instituted (19).

Yet another important factor involving pharmacokinetics and adverse effects is concomitant pathologic states. Various disease states may directly affect the relationship between pharmacokinetics and adverse effects. If a drug is excreted primarily through the kidneys, then any condition associated with decreased renal function might increase that drug's half-life (i.e., decrease its clearance) and thus accumulate with chronic administration. As a result, nomograms have been developed to help in dosage adjustments for certain drugs. These are based upon the patient's degree of renal impairment as determined by creatinine clearance (20,21).

Hepatic impairment may also be an important cause for adverse side effects and toxic events. This can occur in normal subjects when a drug is predominantly metabolized by the liver to nontoxic substances. However, in cirrhotics, the parent drug may accumulate with chronic administration because of the liver's impaired ability to metabolize the drug to nontoxic substances. This could result in increased toxicity and might necessitate reducing the dose administered or increasing the dosage interval.

Several other factors may also relate to the positive relationship, or conversely, the lack of a relationship, between pharmacokinetics and adverse effects. It is well known that tolerance can develop with chronic administration of certain drugs that act on the central nervous system (22). Drugs such as opiates, sedative hypnotics, analgesics, certain antihypertensive drugs, and antiparkinsonism drugs, just to name a few, may produce fewer adverse effects at higher blood levels than they produce at lower blood levels. Drugs like L-dopa and the dopamine agonists used to treat Parkinson's disease may produce nausea, vomiting, and postural hypotension when therapy is first instituted at the lower doses; however, tolerance develops to these adverse effects and at maintenance therapeutic doses corresponding to much higher plasma concentrations, no major problem exists. Likewise, patients receiving chronic therapy for cancer pain with the centrally acting opiate analgesics or addicts using these drugs may not experience respiratory depression, even though the plasma concentrations they achieve would be fatal in nontolerant individuals. Despite the occurrence of very high plasma concentrations, these individuals may have minimal or no adverse effects. If that individual should, however, have some voluntary or involuntary change in compliance and the tolerance diminishes, then the administration of a comparable dose may result in pronounced adverse effects or may even result in death.

In summary, dose administered, route of administration, pharmacogenetics, drug interactions, concomitant pathologic or disease state, and tolerance development may—individually or in combination—play a role in the relationship of pharmacokinetics and adverse effects.

Considering all of these factors, and especially addressing the issue of interindividual variation, it is important to use the *clinical* information available in determining how to care for the patient and what course of action is necessary. Thus a drug's plasma concentration needs to be considered simply another lab test and used in conjunction with all of the clinical data. Although analysis of plasma drug concentrations is a useful and important undertaking and is of consideration when dealing with adverse drug effects, some pitfalls may occur. Therapeutic monitoring can be overemphasized and lead to confusion and, in fact, may even compound the problem. For example, a patient receiving the cardiac glycosides, digitoxin and digoxin, may have what appears to be a high plasma concentration of drug compared to the therapeutic blood level as determined by radioimmunoassay. However, this patient may be clinically undertreated. In contrast, another patient with low plasma concentrations of these drugs may be experiencing signs of digitalis toxicity. Thus, the physician in the first case may be faced with the dilemma of whether to increase the dose in spite of the "high" plasma levels, while the physician in the second case must decide whether to decrease the dose even though the blood levels are in the "therapeutic" range. The physician's clinical judgment still remains the most important determining factor in his or her response to the patient's treatment. Pharmacokinetics and drug plasma concentrations are important laboratory data but should serve only as an aid to the physician, as do other laboratory data, and these must be viewed only in conjunction with the clinical data.

REFERENCES

1. B. B. Brodie, M. Weiner, J. J. Burns, G. Simson and E. K. Yale. The physiological disposition of ethyl biscoumacetate (Tromexan) in man and a method for its estimation in biological material. J. Pharmacol. Exp. Therap., *106,* 453–463 (1952).
2. O. Storstem, V. Hansteen, L. Hatle, H. Leif, and L. Strostein. Studies on digitalis. XIII: A prospective study of 649 patients on maintenance treatment with digitoxin. Am. Heart J. *93,* 434–443 (1977).
3. J. Koch-Weser. Serum drug concentrations as therapeutic guides. N. Engl. J. Med. *287,* 227–31 (1972).
4. H. Kutt. Pharmacodynamic and pharmacokinetic measurements of antiepileptic drugs. Clin. Pharmacol. Therap. *16,* 243 (1974).
5. L. Lemberger and A. Rubin. Cocaine and miscellaneous drugs of abuse. Pages 311–335 in: *Physiologic Disposition of Drugs of Abuse.* E. Vessell and S. Garattini, eds. Spectrum Publications, Inc., New York (1976).
6. C. A. Suarez, A. Arango, and J. L. Lester. Cocaine-condom ingestion, Surgical treatment. J. Amer. Med. Assoc. *238,* 1391–1392 (1977).
7. W. G. Gaidys, J. D. Dickerman, C. L. Walters, and P. C. Young. Intrathecal vincristine: Report of a fatal case despite CNS washout. Cancer *52,* 799–801 (1983).
8. W. Kallow. Pharmacogenetics: Heredity and the response to drugs. Saunders, Philadelphia (1962).
9. E. S. Vessel. Pharmacogenetics—Multiple interactions between genes and environment as determinants of drug response. Amer. J. Med. *66,* 183–187 (1979).
10. W. Kallow and K. Genest. Canad. J. Biochem. Physiol. *35,* 339 (1957).
11. A. Mahgoub, J. R. Idle, L. G. Dring, R. Lancaster, and R. L. Smith. Polymorphic hydroxylation of debrisoquine in man. Lancet *2,* 584–586 (1977).
12. J. R. Idle and R. L. Smith. The debrisoquine hydroxylation gene: A gene of multiple consequence. Pages 148–164 in: Proceedings of the Second World Conference on Clinical Pharmacology and Therapeutics. L. Lemberger and M. M. Reidenberg, eds. Am. Soc. Pharmacol. Exp. Therap. Bethesda, MD (1983).
13. D. A. P. Evans, K. A. Manley, and V. A. McKusick. Genetic control of isoniazid metabolism in man. Brit. Med. J. *2,* 485 (1960).
14. G. L. Mandell and M. A. Sande. Drugs used in the chemotherapy of tuberculosis and leprosy. Pages 1199–1218 in: *The Pharmacological Basis of Therapeutics.* 7th ed. A. G. Gilman, L. S. Goodman, T. W. Rall, and F. Marad, eds. Macmillan, New York (1985).
15. R. L. Woosley, D. E. Drayer, M. M. Reidenberg, A. S. Nies, K. Carr, and J. A. Oattes. Effect of acetylator phenotype on the rate at which procainamide induces antinuclear antibodies and the lupus syndrome. N. Eng. J. Med. *298,* 1157–1159 (1978).
16. R. A. O'Reilly, J. G. Pool, and P. M. Aggeler. Hereditary resistance to coumarin anticoagulant drugs in man and rat. Ann. N.Y. Acad. Sci. *151,* 913–931 (1968).
17. B. Blackwell. Hypertensive crisis due to monoamine-oxidase inhibitors. Lancet *2,* 849 (1963).
18. B. Blackwell, E. Marley, and D. Taylor. Effects of yeast extract after monoamine-oxidase inhibition. Lancet *1,* 1166, (1965).
19. S. A. Cucinelli, A. H. Conney, M. S. Sansur, et al, Drug interactions in man. Lowering effect of phenobarbital on plasma levels of bishydroxycoumarin (Dicumarol) and diphenylhydantoin (Dilantin). Clin. Pharmacol. Therap. *6,* 420–429 (1965).
20. L. C. Dettli. Drug dosage in patients with renal disease. Clin. Pharmacol. Ther. *16,* 274–280 (1974).
21. J. J. Schentag and M. H. Adelman. A microcomputer program for tobramycin consult

services, based on the two-compartment pharmacokinetic model. Drug Intel. Clin. Pharm. *17*, 528–531 (1983).

22. L. Lemberger and A. Rubin. Tolerance. Pages 337–390 in: *Physiologic Disposition of Drugs of Abuse*. E. Vesell and S. Garattini, eds. Spectrum Publications, Inc., New York (1976).

Chapter 8

Clinical Pharmacodynamics of Anticancer Drugs: Concepts and Examples*

William E. Evans, Pharm.D.
John H. Rodman, Pharm.D.

Pharmacokinetics/Pharmacodynamics Section
Pharmaceutical Division
St. Jude Children's Research Hospital
and
Center for Pediatric Pharmacokinetics & Therapeutics
University of Tennessee, Memphis

INTRODUCTION

Drug dose is now well recognized as an important determinant of response to chemotherapy of certain cancers. Within the last five years, it has been demonstrated that the schedule and dose of antineoplastic drugs can signif-

*Supported in part by a Leukemia Program project grant (CA20180), a Cancer Center CORE grant (CA21765), a grant (R37-CA36401) from the National Institutes of Health, The University of Tennessee Centers of Excellence Program, and by the American Lebanese Syrian Associated Charities (ALSAC) icantly influence the efficacy of chemotherapy for a number of drug-sensitive cancers (1–8). Clinical studies have defined the dose administered in several different ways, including percentage of protocol doses administered (e.g., less than 65%, 65–84%, or greater than 85%), or amount of chemotherapy given per unit time (e.g., mg/m^2 per week), often referred to as dose intensity. Patients who received a greater percentage of planned therapy or a higher dose intensity were more likely to have a clinical response to their chemotherapy. For example, Hryniuk (8) demonstrated that the probability of a complete or partial response to etoposide therapy of non-small-cell lung cancer was 20 percent when the dose intensity was 250 mg/m^2 per week vs. 65 percent when the dose intensity was 500 mg/m^2 per week. Although the importance of dose intensity has been demonstrated for several malignancies (8) including breast cancer, Hodgkins disease, small-cell lung cancer, ovarian cancer, acute myelogenous leukemia, and acute lymphocytic leukemia, dose intensity is of therapeutic importance only for cancers that are sensitive to the drugs being given. That is, if the tumor is absolutely drug resistant, the intensity of drug therapy will not be a factor (except as a determinant of toxicity). However, if the tumor is drug sensitive, these data indicate that it is advantageous to design chemotherapy regimens with relatively high dose intensity.

It is well established that the pharmacokinetics of anticancer drugs such as etoposide, methotrexate, teniposide, and doxorubicin are highly variable among patients (9), but the importance of this variability as a determinant of response is less well recognized. Systemic clearance of drugs will vary greatly among patients with corresponding variability in drug concentration. Therefore, even if dose intensity were standardized at the optimal dose level, a three- to fivefold range in drug clearance would yield a wide range of systemic exposure, as reflected by area under the concentration-versus-time curve or steady-state drug concentration, at the same (presumably optimal) dose intensity.

Many variables can intervene between the prescribed dose and the level of tumor exposure to anticancer drugs, even if great care is given to design a protocol with optimal dose intensity. From the schema in Figure 8-1, it is apparent that if a relationship exists between the protocol dose intensity (level A) and the clinical response, the relation between systemic exposure (level D) and the response can be expected to be more precise. If these pharmacodynamic relationships can be defined for individual drugs, they should provide guidelines for designing and adjusting cancer chemotherapy regimes that offer more precision than dose intensity. These pharmacodynamic relationships are particularly useful when multiple drugs are used together, because it is difficult to know which drug among a four-drug combination is being under- or overdosed when the dose intensity is fixed at the population average, but confounded by variability in systemic exposure for

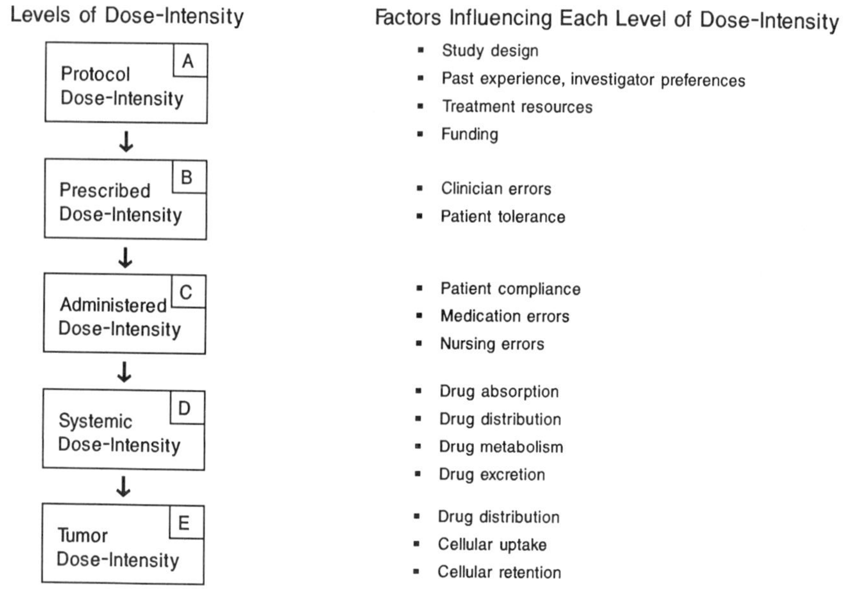

FIGURE 8-1. Scheme of various levels at which dose intensity (DI) can be defined, and the corresponding factors that may influence dose intensity at each level. Level A represents the DI written in any given protocol; level B represents the DI prescribed for the patient; level C represents the DI taken by the patient; level D represents the extent and duration of systemic exposure achieved in the patient (e.g., area under C × T curve in the patients plasma); and level E represents the actual exposure in the tumor cell. If the intracellular target is known (i.e., dihydrofolate reductase for methotrexate), level F (not depicted) might be drug target DI.

each agent. Future research will focus on defining drug delivery to the actual target site (level E).

Recent studies have demonstrated that interpatient variability in the pharmacokinetics of selected anticancer drugs can significantly affect the probability of the efficacy of toxicity of the drugs (10–16). In the next section, we briefly review recent published clinical pharmacodynamic studies with high-dose methotrexate, teniposide, and carboplatin.

Studies in Children with Cancer

During the last eight years, we completed clinical pharmacodynamic studies of two anticancer drugs in two different populations of children. The first study examined high-dose methotrexate (HDMTX) in children with newly diagnosed, previously untreated acute lymphocytic leukemia (ALL). The second study evaluated teniposide pharmacodynamics in children with cancer who had relapsed after initial treatment with conventional chemotherapy.

Childhood ALL is a potentially curable cancer with chemotherapy (more than 60% of cases can now be cured), indicating that it is a highly drug-sensitive cancer and therefore a good model for testing pharmacodynamic principles. Moreover, methotrexate and teniposide are both highly active drugs for this disease; therefore, these clinical pharmocodynamic data should have utility for most treatment regimes for childhood ALL.

High-Dose Methotrexate (HDMTX)

Our prospective study with HDMTX (1,000 mg/m^2) began in 1979 and was limited to children with standard- to intermediate-risk ALL. ALL patients with (1) an initial white blood cell count (WBC) greater than 100,000/μl, (2) E-rossette surface immunoglobulin positive lymphoblasts, (3) lymphoblasts in the CSF, or (4) a thymic mass at diagnosis were considered high-risk cases and were excluded from this protocol. Those patients were treated by a much more intensive protocol. All children meeting the entry criteria (75% of all new cases) were randomized to one of two postremission treatment protocols. One of the two treatment protocols was comprised of 15 HDMTX infusions given over the first 1.5 years of remission, superimposed on conventional therapy with oral, daily mercaptopurine and weekly low-dose methotrexate. The 108 children randomized to this treatment protocol comprise the population for our pharmacodynamic studies. Our diagnostic criteria, chemotherapy administration, patient evaluations, sample collection, and data analysis have been previously reported in detail (10).

An initial analysis of these patients was performed after a median duration of follow-up of two years and was designed to assess the influence of HDMTX clearance on the probability of leukemia relapse. In this early analysis (13), we found that children with rapid HDMTX clearances (>80 $ml/min/m^2$) were more likely to have an early relapse of their leukemia (Fig. 8-2). The influence of HDMTX clearance retained its prognostic importance even when the risk of relapse was assessed in a multivariate analysis that included WBC count at diagnosis, age, and race as known prognostic variables. This finding in our initial analysis of HDMTX pharmacodynamics encouraged us to continue our evaluation and follow-up of these patients to assess the long-term effects of HDMTX disposition on clinical outcome.

In 1986, we reported the results of this study after all 108 patients had completed their HDMTX therapy and the median duration of follow-up was 3.5 years (range 2.2–5.5 yrs) (10). Despite the same dose intensity, interpatient variability in HDMTX clearance yielded steady-state methotrexate serum concentrations that ranged from 9.3 to 25.4 μm (using the median value of 15 measurements in each patient). Thus, there was a 2.7-fold range in systemic exposure (i.e., systemic dose intensity) despite all patients receiving the same dose intensity. When patients with steady-state serum con-

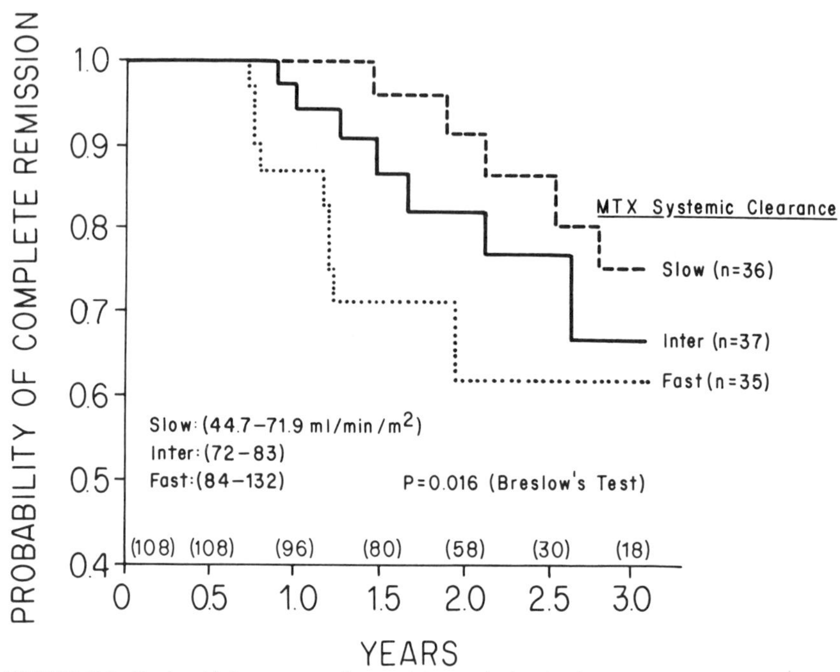

FIGURE 8-2. Kaplan-Meier curves of complete remission in the three groups of patients, divided based on their rates of methotrexate clearance. Numbers in parentheses represent numbers of patients who have reached or exceeded the corresponding time from diagnosis. Reproduced with permission from Evans et al. (13).

centrations of methotrexate below 16 μM ($n = 59$) were compared with those who had concentrations above 16 μM ($n = 49$), an analysis of the Kaplan-Meier curves estimating the probability of complete remission revealed a significant difference between the two groups ($p = 0.046$ by Breslow test), with patients having the lower methotrexate concentrations demonstrating a higher probability of relapse (Fig. 8-3). Likewise, an analysis of the Kaplan-Meier curves estimating the probability of hematologic remission revealed a significant difference between the two groups ($p = 0.024$). Multivariate analysis indicated that patients with methotrexate concentrations of less than 16 μM were three times more likely to have any kind of relapse during therapy ($p = 0.01$) and seven times more likely to have a hematologic relapse during therapy ($p = 0.001$). Stepwise Cox's regression identified leukemic-cell DNA content, methotrexate concentrations, initial white blood cell count and hemoglobin as significant prognostic variables for hematologic relapse ($p = 0.0005$).

This clinical study demonstrated a drug concentration-effect relationship for HDMTX in childhood ALL. Although this study did not attempt to establish a therapeutic range for MTX in ALL (which can be influenced by

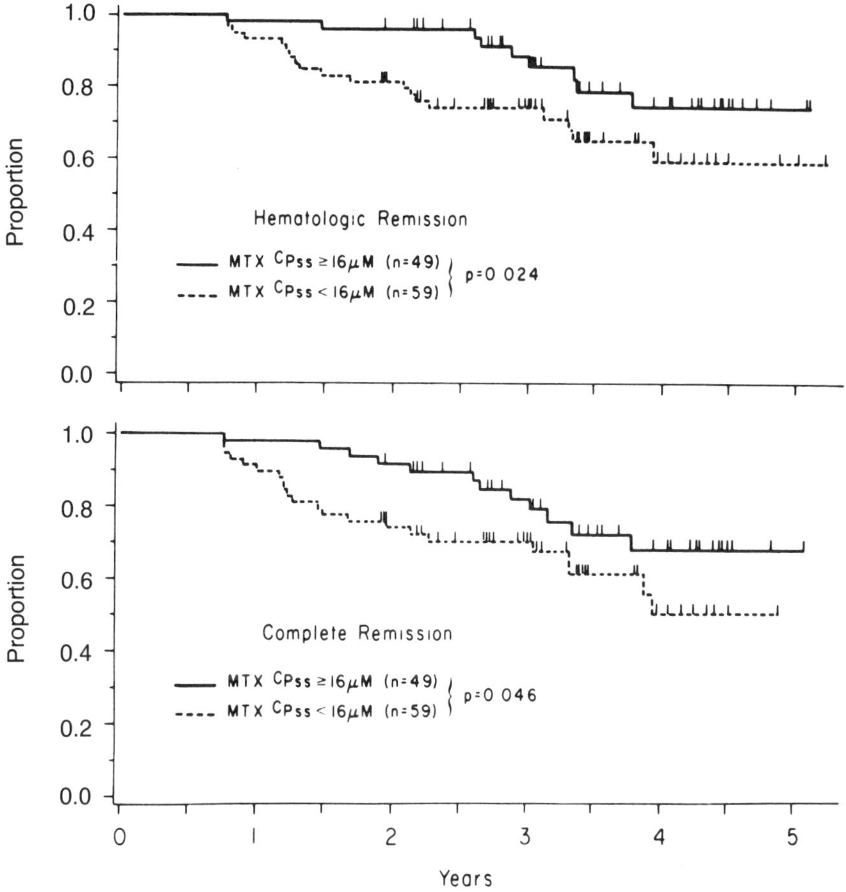

FIGURE 8-3. Kaplan-Meier curves of hematologic remission and complete remission for patients with median steady-state concentrations of methotrexate (MTX Cp_{ss}) <16 μM and ≥ μM *p* = 0.024 by Breslow test of difference between the two hematologic-remission curves; *p* = 0.046 for the difference between the complete remission curves. (Reproduced with permission from Evans et al. (10).

other drug therapy, subtype of ALL, duration of therapy, and so on), it did identify a concentration for 24-hour HDMTX infusions (1,000 mg/M^2), below which therapeutic failure is more likely to occur and that retained prognostic significance after accounting for other known variables influencing outcome.

Teniposide

Teniposide (VM26) is an investigational anticancer drug that has been used in various combination regimens to successfully treat childhood ALL for more than 10 years. Despite clear evidence of antileukemic activity, the most appropriate dosage schedule and drug combinations for teniposide remain to be defined. The majority of protocols use VM26 as a short (i.e., 45-min) intravenous infusion at a dosage of 150–165 mg/m^2 given twice weekly. Our Phase I–II clinical pharmacodynamic study was designed to assess the toxicity and oncolytic effects of VM26, given as a 72-hour continuous infusion.

This study was conducted in children with leukemia and solid tumors who failed initial therapy with conventional drug combinations. Details of the study population, diagnostic criteria, prior therapy, patient evaluations, and data analysis were reported previously (11). A total of 23 children were studied, 17 with leukemia, 1 with lymphoma, and 5 with neuroblastoma. Drug concentration-effect relationships were assessed at maximum dosage levels of 450, 600, and 750 mg/M^2. The clearance of VM26 for all patients averaged 15.3 (±8.9) ml/min/m^2, (range 3.7–43.8). The large interpatient variability in VM26 clearance produced highly variable steady-state drug concentrations (Cp_{ss}) at each dose level and substantial overlap in Cp_{ss} values between the various dosages.

As depicted in Figure 8-4, a subset of patients at the 450 mg/m^2 dose level had Cp_{ss} exceeding those of patients treated at the 750 mg/M^2 level. Moreover, when the patients having an objective oncolytic response (defined as 75% decrease in circulating lymphoblast count for ALL or partial remis-

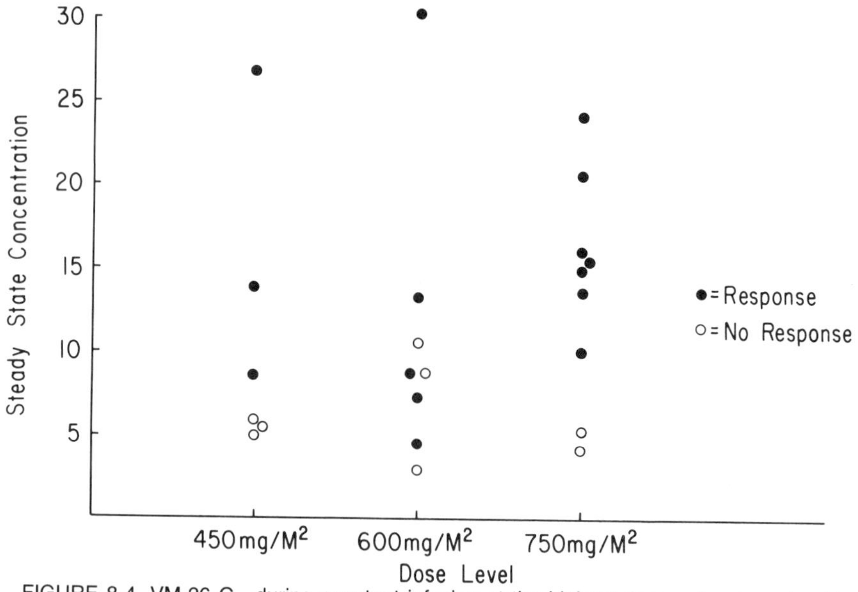

FIGURE 8-4. VM-26 C_{ss} during constant infusion at the highest dosage level received by each patient for whom pharmacokinetic studies were performed. Patients who had responses (●) versus nonresponders (○) are shown at each dose level. Reproduced with permission from Rodman et al. (11).

sion for solid tumors) were compared to nonresponders, there was no statistically significant relationship between dose level and response but a highly significant relationship between C_{ss} and response was demonstrated. The mean C_{ss} for the responding patients was 15.2 mg/L (±7.4) and significantly greater ($p < .005$ by the Wilcoxon rank sums test) than the mean value of 6.2 mg/L (±2.8) measured in the nonresponding patients. Likewise, patients developing toxicity (grade 3–4 gastrointestinal toxicity) had higher mean Cp_{ss} values than patients who did not develop severe toxicity. When the proportion of patients having an oncolytic response and those incurring toxicity was plotted versus VM26 systemic exposure as reflected by the area under the curve, the relationship depicted in Figure 8-5 was obtained. These data clearly suggest that the interpatient variability in pharmacokinetics will be a determinant for both efficacy and toxicity.

These findings further suggest problems inherent in Phase I–II dose-finding studies when interpatient variability in drug clearance is large relative to the magnitude of dosage escalations. This is frequently the case with anticancer drugs, and the number of patients studied at each dosage level is usually relatively small (about three to six patients). In such studies, it would be easy to reach the wrong conclusion about the maximum tolerated dosage

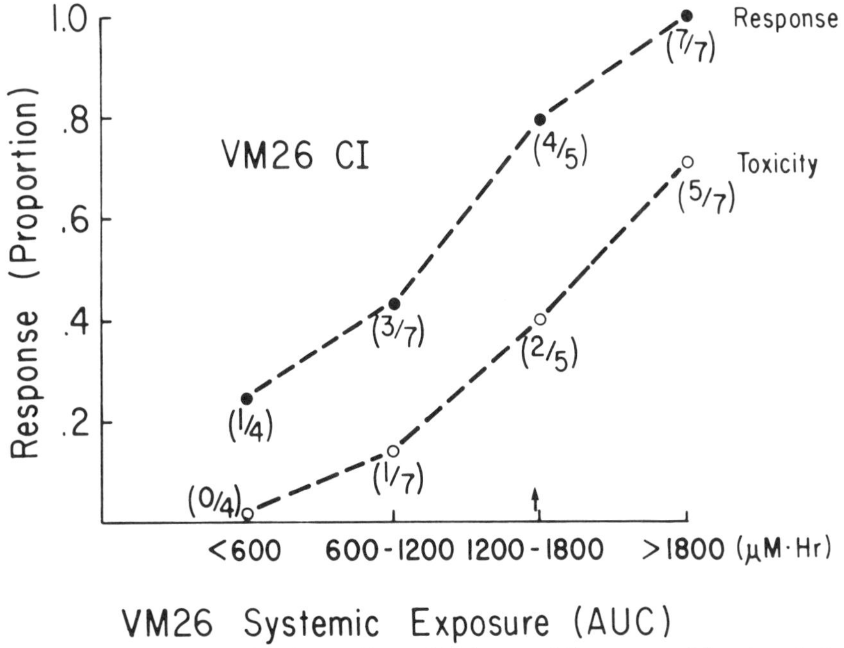

FIGURE 8-5. Proportion of patients with an objective oncolytic response (●) and grade 3–4 gastrointestinal toxicity (○) vs. teniposide systemic exposure in a Phase I–II trial of children with leukemia or solid tumors.

of a new drug (if by chance most patients at a low dose level had slow clearance). Likewise, one could erroneously conclude that a given dose level was more likely to yield a therapeutic response, if one ignores the level of systemic exposure achieved in each patient. A preferred strategy for Phase I–II trials would appear to be based on some measure of systemic exposure (i.e., Cp_{ss}, AUC, C_{max}), instead of just drug dosage. Moreover, Phase I–II studies are often the only opportunity to evaluate the pharmacodynamics of an anticancer drug given as a single agent, as combination drug regimens are usually used for frontline therapy.

Our clinical pharmacodynamic study of VM26 given as a 72-hour infusion demonstrated a clear drug concentration-effect relationship in children with relapsed ALL and neuroblastoma. We have incorporated these findings into our next frontline ALL protocol, which will prospectively assess the importance of these data.

Studies in Adults with Cancer

The clinical pharmacodynamic studies of carboplatin by Egorin and coworkers (12,14) provide an excellent example of systemic exposure being highly correlated with the toxicity of an anticancer drug. In the initial study (12), carboplatin was given to 22 adults with refractory tumors and renal dysfunction. The dosage was 250 mg/m^2 for patients with creatinine clearance (CrCl) above 40 ml/min, and 150 mg/m^2 for patients with CrCl less than 40 ml/min. Toxicities were assessed by weekly clinical and laboratory evaluations; plasma pharmacokinetic studies of ultrafiltrable platinum (assumed active drug) were performed for all patients. In this trial, marrow suppression, primarily thrombocytopenia, was the major toxicity. As depicted in Figure 8-6, the precentage of reduction in platelet count was found to be linearly correlated with the area under the plasma concentration-time curve (AUC) for ultrafiltrable platinum, when patients without extensive prior therapy and heavily pretreated patients were evalauted separately ($r = 0.73$ and 0.89, respectively). For any AUC, the average reduction in platelet count was 17 percent greater in heavily pretreated patients than in patients who had not received extensive prior therapy.

To prospectively test this finding, these investigators used the correlation between AUC and percentage of change in platelet count and the correlation between AUC and CrCl to develop equations for calculating the carboplatin dosage required to produce a specific change in platelet count (14). A total of 38 courses of carboplatin were evaluated in 23 adult patients with CrCls ranging from 32 to 118 ml/min. Eleven patients were heavily pretreated, and 12 had not received extensive prior therapy.

In both groups of patients, the correlation between the predicted change

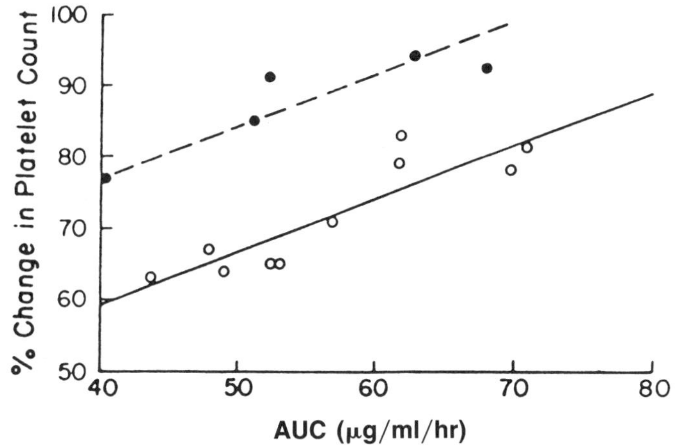

FIGURE 8-6. Relationship between systemic exposure (i.e., AUC) to ultrafilterable platinum and the percentage change in platelet count following carboplatin administration; ●---● = patients who had not received extensive prior therapy; ○---○ = patients who were heavily pretreated. Reproduced with permission from Egorin et al. (12).

and the observed change in platelet count was extremely high (r = 0.94–0.97). Thus, this study prospectively validated the investigators' previous observations and demonstrated that the relation between systemic exposure and drug toxicity could be used to more precisely determine the maximum tolerated dosage of an anticancer drug in an individual patient. This study also demonstrated that drug toxicity could be markedly different in different patients given the same dose intensity, because it was the systemic exposure and not the dosage that correlated with thrombocytopenia. This group of researchers has recently published similar results with the anthracycline menogoril, where a strong relationship was found between the plasma AUC and the percentage of decreases in WBC and absolute neutrophil count (15) and with the differentiating agent hexamethylene bisacetamide, in which the percent decrease in platelet count correlated significantly with plasma AUC (16). These authors advocate comparable pharmacodynamic studies with other anticancer drugs, including those currently used in frontline treatment regimens, as well as Phase I–II investigational agents.

SUMMARY

Clinical pharmacodynamic studies of anticancer drugs can yield concentration-effect relationships for selected antineoplastic drugs. Such pharmacodynamic relationships are potentially of great importance for anticancer drugs because (1) the consequences of undertreatment are severe, (2) toxicities are often lifethreatening, (3) concentrations required for oncolytic effects are often near those that produce host toxicity, and (4) the pharmacokinetics of anticancer drugs are often highly variable from patient to patient. Well-defined pharmacodynamic relationships appear to be particularly useful for drugs used in treatments that are potentially curative in a substantial percentage of patients, as their optimal use could produce a greater number of cures, a lower risk of severe toxicity, or both.

REFERENCES

1. G. Bonadonna and P. Valagussa. Dose-response effect of adjuvant chemotherapy in breast cancer. N. Eng. J. Med. *304*, 10–15 (1981).
2. W. Hryniuk and H. Bush. The importance of dose intensity in chemotherapy of metastatic breast cancer. J. Clin. Oncol. *2*, 1281–1288 (1984).
3. E. Frei III, C. L. Spurr, C. O. Brindley, O. Selawry, J. F. Holland, D. P. Rall, L. R. Waserman, B. Hoogstraten, B. I. Shnider, O. R. McIntrye, L. B. Matthews, and S. P. Miller. Clinical studies of dichloromethotrexate (NSC 29630). Clin. Pharmacol. Ther. *6*, 160–171 (1965).
4. C. O. Brindley, L. G. Salvin, K. G. Potee, B. Lipowska, B. I. Shnider, W. Regelson, J. Colsky. Further comparative trial of triethylene thiophosphoramide and mechlorethamine in patients with melanoma and Hodgkin's disease. J. Chronic. Dis. *17*, 19–30 (1964).
5. P. Carde, F. R. Mackintosh, and S. A. Rosenberg. A dose and time response analysis of treatment of Hodgkin's disease with MOPP chemotherapy. J. Clin Oncol. *1*, 146–153 (1983).
6. M. H. Cohen, P. J. Creaven, B. E. Fosseich Jr., L. E. Broder, O. S. Selawry, A. V. Johnston, C. L. Williams, J. D. Minna. Intensive chemotherapy of small cell bronchogenic carcinoma. Cancer Treat. Rep. *61*, 349–54 (1977).
7. D. Pinkel, K. Hernandez, L. Borella, C. Holton, R. Aur, G. Samoy, C. Pratt. Drug dosage and remission duration in childhood lymphocytic leukemia. Cancer *27*, 247–256 (1971).
8. W. M. Hryniuk. Average relative dose intensity and the impact on design of clinical trials. Seminary in Oncology *14*, 65–74 (1987).
9. W. R. Crom, A. M. Glynn-Barnhart, J. H. Rodman, M. E. Teresi, R. E. Kavanaugh, M. V. Relling, W. E. Evans. Pharmacokinetics *12*, 168–213 (1987).
10. W. E. Evans, W. R. Crom, M. Abromowitch, R. Dodge, A. T. Look, W. P. Bowman, S. L. George, C. H. Pui. Clinical pharmacodynamics of high-dose methotrexate in acute lymphocytic leukemia. N. Engl. J. Med. *314*, 471–477 (1986).
11. J. H. Rodman, M. Abromowitch, J. A. Sinkule, F. A. Hayes, G. K. Rivera, W. E. Evans, Clinical pharmacodynamics of continuous infusion teniposide: Systemic exposure as a determinant of response in a Phase I trial. J. Clin. Oncol. *5*, 1007–1014 (1987).
12. M. J. Egorin, S. J. van Echo, E. A. Tipping, E. A. Olman, M. Y. Whitacre, B. W. Thompson J. Aisner. Pharmacokinetics and dosage reduction of carboplatin in patients with impaired renal function. *Cancer Res 44:5432-5438*, 1984.
13. W. E. Evans, W. R. Crom, C. F. Stewart, W. P. Bowman, C. H. Chen, M. Abramawich, J. V. Simone. Methotrexate systemic clearance influences probability of relapse in children with standard-risk acute lymphocytic leukemia. Lancet 359–362 (1984).
14. M. J. Egorin, D. A. Van Echo, E. A. Olman, M. Y. Whitacre, A. Forrest, J. Aisner.

Prospective validation of a pharmacologically based dosing scheme for carboplatin. Cancer Res. *45*, 6502–6506 (1985).

15. M. J. Egorin, D. A. Van Echo, M. Y. Whitacre, A. Forrest, L. M. Sigman, K. L. Engisch, J. Aisner. Human pharmacokinetics, excretion, and metabolism of the anthracycline antibiotic Menogaril and their correlation with clinical toxicities. Cancer Res. *46*, 1513–1520 (1986).
16. M. J. Egorin, L. M. Sigman, D. A. Van Echo, A. Forrest, M. Y. Whitacre, J. Aisner. Phase I Clinical and Pharmacokinetic study of hexamethylene bisacetamide administered as a five-day continuous infusion. Cancer Res. *47*, 617–623 (1987).

Chapter 9

The Role of Active Metabolites in Drug Responsiveness and Toxicity: Encainide and Propafenone

Grant R. Wilkinson, Ph.D.

Department of Pharmacology
Vanderbilt University

INTRODUCTION

Most compounds developed as therapeutic agents are metabolized, and frequently this process is a major determinant of drug removal from the body. Moreover, considerable intra- and interspecies differences may occur during the process, which, in turn, may be modulated by a variety of factors. Accordingly, knowledge of the qualitative and quantitative fate of a compound is essential in the process of drug development and also in the subsequent assessment of clinical efficacy and toxicity. For many years, drug metabolism was considered to be predominantly a detoxification process, as evidenced by the title of R. T. Williams' classic book, *Detoxication Mechanisms* (1). While this may indeed be the case, many studies over the past 10 to 20 years have established that metabolites can have pharmacological or toxicological activities that may contribute to the drug's biological effects. Certain metabolites may be so chemically reactive that they rapidly and covalently interact with constituents such as proteins and nucleic acids in the cells or organs in which they are formed, and their lifetime in the body is quite short. In many cases, the generation of such reactive metabolites is considered to be a critical step in the drug's irreversible toxic effects (2). However, more stable metabolites may enter the systemic circulation and remain in the body for significant periods after parent drug administration, and elicit reversible responses. With the ever-increasing sophistication and sensitivity of bioanalytical techniques, the formation of this type of metabolite has become routine, at least for those arising from the so-called major pathways of metabolism. The potential involvement of these metabolites in the administered drug's overall effects is, therefore, a particularly relevant question and has been of increasing interest. This chapter describes some general considerations related to active metabolite formation, especially in human beings, and with emphasis on the assessment of the clinical significance of the phenomenon.

GENERAL CONSIDERATIONS

Over the past few years, several reviews have considered the therapeutic role of stable active metabolites with emphasis on specific drugs or classes (3–5) or on conditions (6,7) (e.g., renal failure), in which differences may occur in the ratio of the circulating concentrations of parent drug and metabolite. Such compilations suggest several ways by which the importance of an active metabolite in a drug's effects can be recognized.

Some relevant questions concerning the formation of active metabolites are as follows:

1. What are the pathways of metabolism, and are they likely to generate active metabolites?
2. Does activity correlate with blood and tissue levels of parent compound, of a metabolite, or of both?
3. Is activity modified by altering the rate of metabolism?
4. Is activity different according to the route of administration?
5. If activity is species dependent, is this due to differences in metabolism?

The actual pathway of metabolism appears to be a significant indicator of potential activity. Phase II metabolic pathways, resulting in conjugates, are generally considered to be deactivating; however, the various Phase I reactions, including oxidation, reduction, and hydrolysis, all have the potential to generate active metabolites. It has been noted that of 52 active metabolites formed in human beings from 41 drugs, one-third involved either N- or O-dealkylation, and a further 25 percent were generated by hydroxylation of a cyclic moiety (5). Aliphatic hydroxylation and other types of oxidation, reduction, and deacetylation were less frequently likely to result in metabolic activation. This would suggest that the metabolites produced by these particular pathways are prime candidates to exhibit pharmacological activity and efforts should, therefore, be directed toward assessing their clinical significance.

Several factors need to be considered in such an evaluation. First, and most important, is the evidence indicative of the metabolite's activity and the spectrum of any effects. In the vast majority of instances, the available data are limited to those obtained from in vitro or in vivo animal studies; only in about one in five instances are metabolites directly administered, per se, to human beings (5), and usually late in the drug development process. The limitations and difficulties of extrapolating results from animal studies to human beings are well established; hence, this type of evidence is best considered suggestive rather than definitive. This is also true with respect to the relative potency of the metabolite to the parent drug. Only by administering the metabolite directly to human beings can its pharmacological activity be fully characterized. Importantly, the effects or the disposition of parent drug and metabolite may be sufficiently different to consider developing the metabolite as a drug per se. Accordingly, this type of information should be obtained as early in the drug development process as possible.

Even though a metabolite may demonstrate activity and high relative potency in animal studies, a determining factor of whether it elicits a response is the concentration achieved in the systemic circulation and at the site of action after administration of a parent drug. Numerous examples exist in which active metabolites are generated but never significantly contribute to the drug's response because these levels are too low. On the other hand, a metabolite having low potency may have clinical significance if high concentrations are attained. In this regard, the relative disposition of parent and metabolite are critical, and the pharmacokinetics of metabolite formation and elimination have recently received considerable attention (5,8–11). Unfortunately, appropriate pharmacokinetic characteristics of metabolites are not always established following administration of parent drug and are even more rare after giving the metabolite. This often makes data interpretation and predictions difficult. Particularly important dispositional factors are those affecting the concentration ratio of metabolite to parent drug. For example, the route of administration can have major effects on the drug/metabolite concentration/time profiles, especially when first-pass metabolism is extensive. Similarly, chronic drug administration can lead to the accumulation of active metabolites that exhibit elimination rate–limited kinetics (8,9). Not only does this alter the concentration ratio compared to acute dosing, but additional complications can occur—for instance, product inhibition or autoinduction. Other factors that can alter the formation of an active metabolite include perturbations in drug metabolizing activity caused by other therapeutic and environmental agents, because of enzyme induction or inhibition, and genetically impaired metabolism. In addition, hepatic dysfunction (e.g., cirrhosis), can cause a decrease in the concentration ratio of metabolite to drug by reducing the amount of metabolism. By contrast, renal disease may have an opposite effect since, in many cases, the urinary excretion process is more contributory to the elimination of metabolite than of parent drug (7). Advantage may be taken of strategies that use such perturbations in the metabolite-to-drug concentration ratio to determine the clinical importance of active metabolite formation, as exemplified by recent studies with two investigational agents, encainide and propafenone.

ENCAINIDE

Encainide is an investigational drug that has been shown to be a highly effective and well-tolerated antiarrhythmic agent. In more than 90 percent of patients, the therapeutic effects, especially after chronic dosing, appear to be mediated by active metabolites. It therefore is an excellent example of the phenomenon and also demonstrates the value of appropriate pharmacokinetic studies in the drug development process.

Evidence for the important role of active metabolites in encainide's overall effects was available from some of the earliest clinical trials. First, the drug (4-methoxy-2′-[2-(N-methyl-2-piperidyl) ethyl] benzanilide) was extensively metabolized, and the major oxidative pathway appeared to be O-demethylation to form O-desmethylencainide (ODE), which was subsequently converted to a 3-methoxy metabolite (3-MODE). Importantly, both of these dealkylated metabolites were present at plasma concentrations comparable to, or greater than, those of the parent drug. The latter was particularly noticeable after chronic oral administration (12,13), suggestive of elimination rate-limiting metabolite kinetics because encainide's elimination half-life was short (2–4 hr). The initial oral dose-ranging clinical studies in patients with chronic, high-frequency ventricular arrhythmias also demonstrated considerable variability in the effective dose (50–300 mg per day) as well as the drug's oral clearance (1.35–36.9 L/min) in patients who responded (14). Furthermore, the range of encainide plasma concentrations associated with a return of ventricular ectopic depolarizations (VEDs) following discontinuation of chronic dosing was large (1.3–56 ng/ml). Additionally, the antiarrhythmic effects often persisted long after encainide itself was undetectable in the plasma and drug-induced prolongation of the QRS interval returned toward its baseline value with a half-life of about 6 hr after discontinuing oral therapy. Thus, there was considerable dissociation between the drug's elimination and its pharmacological effects. Finally, the single nonresponder in the initial clinical trial of 11 patients was found to have fivefold higher encainide plasma concentrations and a much longer elimination half-life (7–8 hr) than the other patients. Subsequent HPLC analysis also indicated that this individual failed to form measurable amounts of ODE, whereas this metabolite was readily demonstrable in the plasma of the 10 patients who responded. Additional data suggestive of an important role for ODE in encainide's effects was the finding of a counterclockwise hysteresis relationship between VED suppression and encainide's plasma concentrations after intravenous drug infusion; that is, there was less effect early than late despite plasma levels of encainide being initially high and then falling. On the other hand, an essentially linear relationship was present when ODE levels were considered (15). Furthermore, the strongest association of both antiarrhythmic effect and QRS prolongation after chronic oral administration was with ODE; correlations with encainide or 3-MODE were not statistically significant (15).

These data, therefore, indicated that encainide undergoes a significant first-pass effect following oral administration, and intersubject differences in (hepatic) metabolism give rise to considerable interindividual variability in the drug's disposition and effects. Moreover, it appeared that the generation of ODE, and possibly of 3-MODE, was important in encainide's overall cardiovascular effects, and individuals exist who exhibit aberrant metabolism that may affect clinical responsiveness.

Direct evidence of the activity of encainide's oxidative metabolites also accumulated during the early investigation period. For example, in several different animal models, ODE was found to be a more potent antiarrhythmic agent than encainide (16–18). Similar electrophysiological effects relative to encainide were also produced in Purkinje fibers and cardiac muscle as well as in the intact heart, but at lower concentrations (19–21). On the other hand, 3-MODE and *N*-desmethylencainide (NDE) appeared to be intermediate or equipotent in their activities (16,18–20). Importantly, the antiarrhythmic activity and electrophysiological effects of ODE and 3-MODE have now been directly investigated in humans (22). Both metabolites were found to be potent sodium channel blocking agents, which, after intravenous infusion, suppress arrhythmias at the low concentrations noted during chronic oral therapy with encainide (Fig. 9-1). For example, during withdrawal of encainide, ODE plasma concentrations at the time of arrhythmia recurrence in eight patients was 55 ± 40 ng/ml, while ODE by intravenous infusion was effective at a concentration of 37 ± 15 ng/ml. Similarly, plasma levels of 3-MODE when arrhythmias returned following discontinuation of chronic encainide were 116 ± 35 ng/ml compared to 105 ± 50 ng/ml after 3-MODE infusion. While both drugs prolonged QRS duration, ODE was more potent. On the other hand, 3-MODE prolonged the JT_c interval, whereas ODE shortened it. This difference in the electrocardiographic characteristics of the two compounds, along with the longer elimination half-life (380 ± 304 vs. 212 ± 70 min) and simpler metabolic fate suggests that 3-MODE may warrant further evaluation as an antiarrhythmic agent in its own right.

Because of the important role of ODE and 3-MODE in encainide's effects, disease states that affect either of these compounds' formation or sub-

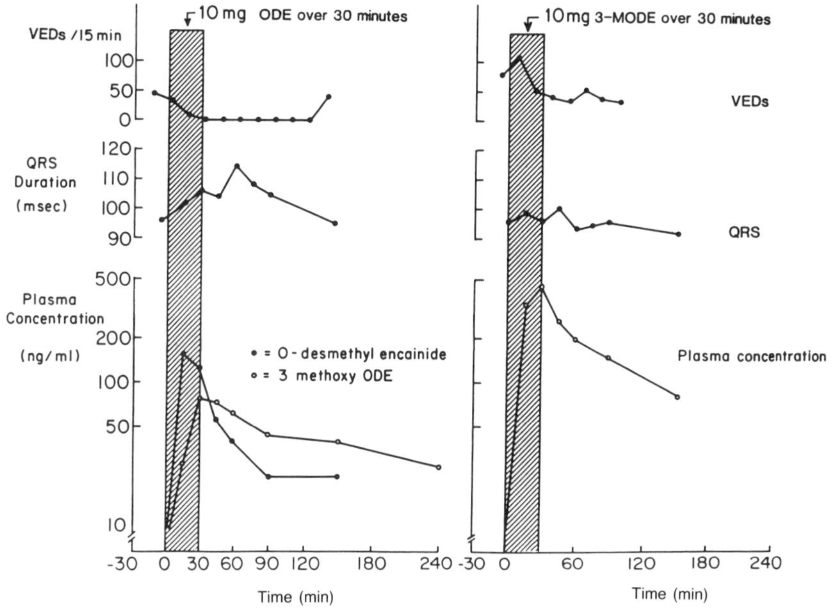

FIGURE 9-1. Effects of a 30-min intravenous infusion of ODE (left) and 3-MODE (right) on arrhythmia frequency and QRS prolongation, and associated plasma concentration-time profiles. Reproduced with modifications from Barbey et al. (22) by permission of the American Heart Association, Inc.

sequent elimination would be expected to alter the clinical response. For example, impaired metabolism, which is possible in patients with hepatic dysfunction, would be predicted to reduce the drug's effects, because lower plasma concentrations of ODE and 3-MODE would be generated. However, studies in patients with chronic cirrhosis showed that the percentage increase in the QRS interval was similar to that observed in normal subjects (23). This occurred despite a significant reduction in drug-metabolizing ability as evidenced by an 85 percent decrement in encainide's oral clearance that resulted in three- to fourfold higher plasma concentrations of parent drug (Table 9-1). The reason for the absence of any change in the pharmacological effect was that the plasma concentrations of ODE and 3-MODE accumulated to a similar extent in the cirrhotics and normal subjects. Since metabolite formation was impaired, this finding suggests that the subsequent elimination of the metabolites was also affected by cirrhosis, and the prolongation of ODE's apparent elimination half-life after discontinuing encainide administration supports this possibility. Studies of encainide's disposition and QRS-prolongation in patients with renal failure also showed the difficulty of predicting the consequences of altered elimination when active metabolites contribute to the overall effects rather than unchanged drug (24). In this case, ODE and 3-MODE plasma levels accumulated two- to threefold higher than in normal subjects, despite the fact that encainide's oral and

TABLE 9-1. Effects of Debrisoquine Phenotype, Renal Disease, and Hepatic Disease on the Disposition of Encainide and Metabolites

	Normal Subjects		Renal Disease	Hepatic Disease
	(EM)[a]	(PM)[b]		
Average plasma level during dosage interval				
Encainide (ng/ml)	18 ± 6	450 ± 57	30 ± 5	63 ± 9
ODE (ng/ml)	115 + 11	12 + 2	207 ± 40	87 ± 18
3-MODE (ng/ml)	94 ± 10	None	252 ± 80	113 ± 81
NDE (ng/ml)	None	80 ± 10	—	—
Bioavailability (%)	30 ± 7	83 ± 9	47 ± 6	78 ± 19
Encainide elimination half-life (hr)	2.3 ± 0.3	11.3 ± 0.3	1.6 ± 0.1	3.7 ± 0.6
Plasma binding (%)	70 ± 2	78 ± 0.6	81 ± 1	76 ± 2
Oral clearance (L/min)	11.7 ± 4.3	0.22 ± 0.3	3.6 ± 0.5	1.7 ± 0.2
Systemic clearance (L/min)	1.9 ± 0.2	0.18 ± 0.02	1.5 ± 0.1	1.2 ± 0.2
Volume of distribution (L)	270 ± 32	172 ± 13	205 ± 12	347 ± 82

Note: Data (mean ± S.E.) presented are after two days of treatment with 50 mg encainide every 8 hr, except in patients with renal disease, who received only 25 mg every 8 hr for two days and in whom the reported plasma levels are double those actually observed.

[a]EM = Extensive metabolizer.

[b]PM = Poor metabolizer.

systemic clearances were unexpectely reduced (Table 9-1). Presumably, such accumulation reflects impaired elimination of the metabolites, and, as might be expected, this resulted in enhanced cardiovascular effects. These investigations, therefore, illustrate the essential need, when active metabolites are involved, to perform studies not only upon the drug's pharmacokinetics, but also that of the metabolites and, most importantly, on the elicited effects. The latter may not be intuitively predicted based solely on the pharmacokinetic parameters.

The single nonresponder of the initial dose-ranging study not only had reduced elimination characteristics for encainide, but also lacked the ability to form ODE in amounts comparable to those in the other patients (14). Subsequently, this individual was found to be a poor metabolizer (PM) of debrisoquine (25), because of a genetic deficiency that gives rise in the population to a polymorphic distribution of drug-metabolizing ability and two different phenotypes: PM and EM (extensive metabolizers). Additional studies (26) confirmed that encainide's oxidative metabolism was linked to the 4-hydroxylation of debrisoquine, probably through a common hepatic cytochrome P-450 (27). Specifically, in normal subjects of the PM phenotype, O-demethylation of encainide was substantially impaired, resulting in several effects (13). First, the fraction of the dose metabolized by this route was reduced, leading to almost 10-fold lower plasma concentrations of ODE (Table 9-1). Since 3-MODE is formed from ODE (22), the levels of this metabolite were also drastically reduced to below the sensitivity of the HPLC assay. The absence in PMs of the O-demethylation pathway resulted in an enhanced role for other metabolic pathways that are minor in the EM. For example, NDE was undetectable in either the plasma or the urine of EMs but was present in significant amounts in PMs. However, this was a shunting rather than a compensatory pathway, and plasma concentrations of unchanged encainide in PMs were much higher than in EMs (Table 9-1). Not unexpectedly, these large, interphenotypic disposition differences were reflected in the pharmacological response; the QRS interval was prolonged in EMs in whom ODE and 3-MODE were formed, but not in PMs in which the plasma concentrations of these active metabolites were essentially negligible. Interestingly, however, this difference in response in normal subjects did not extrapolate to patients with arrhythmias despite the plasma levels of active metabolites being either undetectable or very low in the plasma of PM patients. Encainide was found to be an effective antiarrhythmic agent at doses comparable to those in EMs (15). This was because encainide does, in fact, have intrinsic antiarrhythmic efficacy, although it is less potent that ODE, and the accumulation of 10- to 20-fold higher plasma concentrations of unchanged drug in PMs after chronic oral dosing was sufficient to elicit an effect.

In summary, it is now clear that active metabolites play an important role in the cardiovascular effects of encainide. A variety of direct and indirect studies implicate ODE and 3-MODE but, since less than about 20 percent of the urinary metabolic profile of encainide can be accounted for by these compounds (13), other metabolites may also be contributory. The plasma concentration ratio of metabolite to the parent drug is clearly critical in determining the overall clinical response, and several factors that affect this have been defined. However, it is likely that others remain to be determined, particularly drug-drug interactions involving either induction or inhibition of hepatic drug metabolizing activity. Additional characterization of the clinical pharmacology of ODE and 3-MODE in human beings also appear warranted, particularly the latter, because its disposition appears to be far simpler than that of either encainide or ODE, and it may also have more desirable electrophysiological properties.

PROPAFENONE

Propafenone (2-[2′-hydroxy-3′-propylaminopropoxy]-ω-phenyl-propiophenone) is also an investigational antiarrhythmic agent undergoing clinical evaluation in the United States as well as in Europe. Like many other antiarrhythmics, propafenone undergoes rapid and extensive metabolism in human beings to a large number of metabolites that are excreted unchanged or as their glucuronide/sulfate conjugates in urine or bile (28). The major routes of metabolism appears to be direct glucuronidation and 5-hydroxylation of the phenyl ring, which subsequently is methoxylated; *N*-dealkylation also occurs, but to a lesser extent. Both 5-hydroxypropafenone (5-OHP) and *N*-despropylpropafenone (NDPP) are measurable in the plasma of patients undergoing chronic therapy, but only trace levels of the 5-hydroxy-4-methoxy metabolite are apparently present (29). The average mean steady-state plasma concentrations of 5-OHP and NDPP, however, were only 23 and 18 percent, respectively, of the coexisting propafenone levels (29). Additionally, marked interpatient variability was present in the plasma concentration (64 to 1,044 ng/ml) associated with arrhythmia suppression (29). These findings, coupled with the observations that 5-OHP is twice as potent as propafenone as an antidysrhythmic agent in an aconitine-infused rat model and exhibits greater and more sustained antiarrhythmic activity in coronary-ligated dogs (30) suggests a possible role for this metabolite in propafenone's overall efficacy. The pharmacological effects and antiarrhythmic activity of NDPP have yet to be reported. Importantly, direct evidence in human beings has recently been reported, which suggests a significant role for an active metabolite in the efficacy and toxicity of propafenone (31).

The 5-hydroxylation of propafenone and possible other oxidative pathways appears to be polymorphic and determined in the same genetic fashion by the debrisoquine allele as the O-demethylation of encainide. This has a pronounced effect on the pharmacokinetics of propafenone (32). For example, patients of the EM phenotype had a higher oral clearance (1,115 ± 1,238 vs. 264 ± 48 ml/min), a shorter half-life (5.5 ± 2.1 vs. 17.2 ± 80 hr) and lower average plasma concentrations during the dosage interval (1.1 ± 0.6 vs. 2.5 ± 0.5 ng/ml per mg daily dose) than PM patients. Moreover, 5-OHP was measurable in the plasma of 90 percent of the EMs but was not detectable in PMs. However, as in the case of encainide, such interphenotypic differences did not affect propafenone's efficacy. There was no significant difference between EMs and PMs in the propafenone dosage necessary to suppress arrhythmias or in the frequency of antiarrhythmic response. However, the concentration-response relationship indicated a significant clinical role for propafenone's oxidative metabolites (Fig. 9-2). In those EM patients who responded (>70% VED suppression), the steady-state plasma concentration at the end of the dosage interval showed a 30-fold range (42–1,356 ng/ml), whereas much higher levels (1,408–1,801 ng/ml) were present in PM patients. The lower and widely variable but clinically effective plasma concentrations of unchanged drug in EMs is consistent with the formation of an active metabolite. Also, PM patients were found to have a smaller change in the QRS interval at any given propafenone plasma concentration than were EMs. Thus, it appears that in a fashion similar to encainide, the

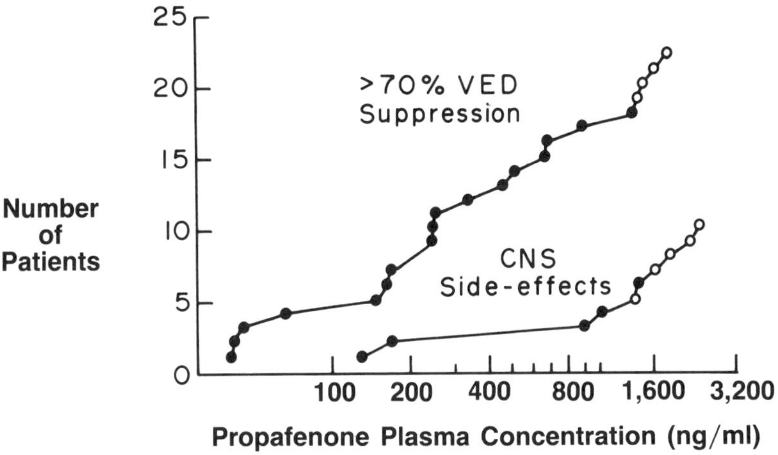

FIGURE 9-2. Cumulative plasma concentration-response curves for arrhythmia suppression and CNS toxicity produced by chronic oral propafenone administration. (Reproduced with modifications from Siddoway et al. (32) by permission of the American Heart Association, Inc.

intrinsic antiarrhythmic activity of propafenone along with its higher plasma levels in PMs offsets the impaired generation of an active metabolite that contributes to the drug's overall activity in EMs. However, there does appear to be one important difference—namely, that the central nervous system side effects of propafenone are more frequent (67% vs 14%) in PMs, presumably as a result of the higher plasma concentrations of unchanged drug (Fig. 9-2).

These early findings strongly suggest that the role of active metabolites (5-OHP and possibly others) in the clinical pharmacology of propafenone requires further investigation and evaluation in a fashion similar to that described for encainide. This will require additional information on the relative plasma concentrations of the known metabolites under a number of conditions in which their formation and subsquent elimination is possibly altered. Further characterization of the specific pharmacological properties of the metabolites will also be required, including studies in human beings.

CONCLUSIONS

Unless specifically designed as a prodrug, it is highly unlikely that a drug candidate will emerge from the discovery process unless it possesses demonstrable intrinsic activity; many pharmacological screening tests are performed under conditions in which the generation of an active metabolite is nonexistent or negligible. Thus, in vivo there is always a balance between the effects produced by a parent drug and those by a metabolite, which depends predominantly on their relative concentrations and potencies. Factors determining this ratio and the resulting effects are not always intuitive (e.g., effects of cirrhosis and renal failure on encainide); thus, empirical studies are necessary.

The critical question is not whether an active metabolite is generated, since this is not an uncommon situation. A more appropriate focus is whether the metabolite is contributory in the clinical situation and to an extent that requires adequate definition and characterization of factors determining its disposition; in many instances, this will not be the case. The latter is a more difficult question to answer, requiring measurements of pharmacological effects as well as disposition profiles. The described findings with encainide and propafenone indicate some, but not all, of the investigational approaches applicable to human beings that may provide useful insights into this problem. In particular, direct investigation of the metabolite's clinical pharmacology appears to be the ultimate means of addressing the question, even though the inherent problems in such an approach are formidable. On the other hand, several examples exist in which a metabolite has been developed as a drug in its own right, because it possesses different or more desirable pharmacokinetic or pharmacodynamic properties. One such characteristic is the likelihood of a less complex elimination profile and more uniformity in disposition, which could result in reduced interpatient variability in response.

Undoubtedly, the formation of putative active metabolites will continue to be of scientific and regulatory interest. It must be recognized, however, that increasing analytical sophistication that allows the measurement of increasingly smaller concentrations of drug and metabolite has, to a large extent, outstripped our capabilities to evaluate their importance. Nevertheless, increased awareness and the recognition of experimental approaches to evaluate the clinical importance of such metabolites are developing and should allow more rigorous study of the phenomenon.

ACKNOWLEDGMENTS

This work was supported in part by USPHS grants GM-31304 and RR-00095.

REFERENCES

1. R. T. Williams. *Detoxication Mechanisms*. John Wiley and Sons, Inc., New York, 1947.
2. M. W. Anders. *Bioactivation of Foreign Compounds*. Academic Press, New York, 1985.
3. J. E. Brown and D. G. Shand. Therapeutic monitoring of antiarrhythmic agents. Clin. Pharmacokin. *7*, 125–148 (1982).
4. D. E. Drayer. Pharmacologically active metabolites of drugs and other foreign compounds. Clinical, pharmacological, therapeutic and toxicological considerations. Drugs *24*, 519–542 (1982).

5. T. A. Sutfin and W. J. Jusko. Compedium of active drug metabolites. Pages 91–159 in: Drug Metabolism and Disposition: Considerations in Clinical Pharmacology. G. R. Wilkinson and M. D. Rawlins, eds. MTP Press, Lancaster, England (1985).
6. D. E. Drayer. Pharmacologically active drug metabolites: Therapeutic and toxic activities, plasma and urine data in man, accumulation in renal failure. Clin. Pharmacokin. *1*, 426–443 (1976).
7. R. K. Verbeeck, R. A. Branch, and G. R. Wilkinson. Drug metabolites in renal failure: Pharmacokinetic and clinical implications. Clin. Pharmacokin. *6*, 329–345 (1981).
8. L. P. Balant and J. McAinsh. Use of metabolite data in evaluation of pharmacokinetics and drug action. Pages 311–371 in: *Concepts in Drug Metabolism*. Part A. P. Jenner and B. Testa, eds. Dekker, New York (1980).
9. J. B. Houston. Drug metabolite kinetics. Pharmac. Ther. *15*, 521–552 (1982).
10. J. B. Houston and G. Taylor. Drug metabolite concentration-time profiles: Influence of route of drug administration. Br. J. Clin. Pharmac. *17*, 385–394 (1984).
11. K. S. Pang. A review of metabolite kinetics. J. Pharmacokin. Biopharm. *13*, 633–662 (1985).
12. R. E. Kates, D. C. Harrison, and R. A. Winkle. Metabolite accumulation during long-term oral encainide administration. Clin. Pharmacol. Ther. *31*, 427–432 (1982).
13. T. Wang, D. M. Roden, H. T. Wolfenden, R. L. Woosley, A. J. J. Wood, and G. R. Wilkinson. Influence of genetic polymorphism on the metabolism and disposition of encainide. J. Pharmacol. Exp. Ther. 228, 605–611 (1984).
14. D. M. Roden, S. B. Reele, S. B. Higgins, R. F. Mayol, R. E. Gammans, J. A. Oates, and R. L. Woosley. Total suppression of ventricular arrhythmias by encainide: Pharmacokinetic and electrocardiographic characteristics. N. Eng. J. Med. *302*, 877–882 (1980).
15. E. L. Carey, H. J. Duff, D. M. Roden, R. K. Primm, G. R. Wilkinson, T. Wang, J. A. Oates, and R. L. Woosley. Encainide and its metabolites: Comparative effects in man on ventricular arrhythmia and electrocardiographic intervals. J. Clin. Invest. *73*, 539–547 (1984).
16. A. W. Gomoll, J. E. Byrne, and R. F. Mayol. Comparative antiarrhythmic actions of encainide and its major metabolites. Arch. Intern Pharmacol. Therap. *281*, 227–297 (1986).
17. D. M. Roden, H. J. Duff, D. Altenbern, and R. L. Woosley. Antiarrhythmic activity of the O-demethyl metabolite of encainide. J. Pharmacol. Exp. Ther. *221*, 552–557 (1982).
18. M. J. Kerr, J. D. Allen, D. W. G. Harron, and R. G. Shanks. The effects of encainide and its major metabolites, O-demethyl encainide and 3-methoxy-O-demethyl encainide, on experimental cardiac arrhythmias in dogs. J. Cardiovasc. Pharmacol. *7*, 449–457 (1985).
19. V. Elharrar and D. P. Zipes. Effects of encainide and metabolites (MJ 14030 and MJ 9444) on canine cardiac Purkinje and ventricular fibers. J. Pharmacol. Exp. Ther. 220, 440–447 (1982).
20. P. E. Dresel. Effect of encainide and its two major metabolites on cardiac conduction. J. Pharmacol. Exp. Ther. *228*, 180–186 (1984).
21. D. M. Roden, A. K. Dawson, H. J. Duff, R. L. Woosley, and R. F. Smith. Electrophysiology of O-demethylencainide in a canine model of sustained ventricular tachycardia. J. Cardiovasc. Pharmacol. *6*, 588–595 (1984).
22. J. T. Barbey, K. A. Thompson, D. S. Echt, R. L. Woosley, and D. M. Roden. Antiarrhythmic activity, electrocardiographic effects and pharmacokinetics of the encainide metabolites O-desmethyl encainide and 3-methoxy-O-desmethyl encainide in man. Circulation *77*, 380–391 (1988).
23. R. H. Bergstrand, T. Wang, D. M. Roden, G. R. Avant, W. W. Sutton, L. A. Siddoway, H. Wolfenden, R. L. Woosley, G. R. Wilkinson, and A. J. J. Wood. Encainide disposition in patients with chronic cirrhosis. Clin. Pharmocal. Ther. *40*, 148–154 (1986).
24. R. H. Bergstrand, T. Wang, D. M. Roden, W. J. Stone, H. T. Wolfenden, R. L. Woos-

ley, G. R. Wilkinson, and A. J. J. Wood. Encainide disposition in patients with renal failure. Clin. Pharmacol. Ther. *40*, 64–70 (1986).
25. R. L. Woosley, D. M. Roden, G. Dai, T. Wang, D. Altenbern, J. Oates, and G. R. Wilkinson. Co-inheritance of the polymorphic metabolism of encainide and debrisoquin. Clin. Pharmacol. Ther. *39*, 282–287 (1986).
26. C. B. McAllister, H. T. Wolfenden, W. S. Aslanian, R. L. Woosley, and G. R. Wilkinson. Oxidative metabolism of encainide: polymorphism, pharmacokinetics and clinical considerations. Xenobiotica *16*, 483–490 (1986).
27. L. M. Distlerath, P. E. B. Reilly, M. V. Martin, G. G. Davis, G. R. Wilkinson, and F. P. Guengerich. Purification and characterization of the human liver cytochromes P-450 involved in debrisoquine 4-hydroxylation and phenacetin O-deethylation, two prototypes for genetic polymorphism in oxidative drug metabolism. J. Biol. Chem. *260*, 9057–9067 (1985).
28. H. G. Hege, M. Hollmann, S. Kaumeier, and H. Lietz. The metabolic fate of ^{2}H-labelled propafenone in man. Eur. J. Drug Metab. Pharmacokin. *9*, 41–55 (1984).
29. R. E. Kates, Y. G. Yee, and R. A. Winkle. Metabolite accumulation during chronic propafenone dosing in arrhythmia. Clin. Pharmacol. Ther. *37*, 610–614 (1985).
30. S. J. Connolly, R. E. Kates, C. S. Lebsack, D. C. Harrison, and R. A. Winkle. Clinical pharmacology of propafenone. Circulation *68*, 589–596 (1983).
31. G. v. Philipsborn, J. Gries, H. P. Hofman, H. Kreiskot, R. Kretzschmar, C. D. Müller, M. Raschak, and H. J. Teschendorf. Pharmacological studies of propafenone and its main metabolite 5-hydroxypropafenone. Arzneim. Forsch./Drug Res. *34*, 1489–1497 (1984).
32. L. A. Siddoway, K. A. Thompson, C. B. McAllister, T. Wang, G. R. Wilkinson, D. M. Roden, and R. L. Woosley. Polymorphism of propafenone metabolism and disposition in man: Clinical and pharmacokinetic consequences. Circulation *75*, 785–791 (1987).

Chapter 10

Nitrogen Oxidation and Toxicity

Arthur K. Cho, John F. Brady, and Judith N. Burstyn

University of California, Los Angeles, Department of Pharmacology, School of Medicine and the Jonsson Comprehensive Cancer Center Center for the Health Sciences

Many relatively unreactive organic compounds are susceptible to biotransformations that generate products capable of forming covalent bonds with tissue macromolecules. The resultant changes in molecular structure of the macromolecule can alter its function and result in lesion formation or mutagenesis. This metabolism-dependent toxicity is often difficult to predict because it depends on enzyme systems that are nonselective, are modified or induced by other chemicals, and that exhibit heterogeneity among species. A classic example of activation to a toxic intermediate is the oxidation of polycyclic aromatic hydrocarbons by cytochrome P450 monooxygenase to highly reactive arene oxides that are carcinogenic (1). These unstable epoxides are usually converted to nontoxic substances that are eliminated, but, under circumstances permitting a high concentration, reactions with cellular constituents result in toxic manifestations. A similar toxicological activation has been demonstrated for bromobenzene (2). This chapter briefly describes mechanisms of activation of nitrogen functions to covalent bond-forming groups and studies in our laboratories that relate to these processes.

Nitrogenous functionalities, commonly found in drugs and industrial chemicals such as dyes, are also potential sites for biotransformation to reactive intermediates (3–5). Amines and amides, for example, are oxidized to hydroxylamines that can form sulfate esters by the action of sulfotransferases. These N-hydroxysulfate esters are highly electrophilic and are readily attacked by nucleophilic groups on proteins and nucleic acids to form adducts (6). Such reactions may result in a modification of DNA and may be the initial step in chemical carcinogenesis. Hydroxylamines can also be oxidized to nitroso compounds that form covalent bonds with tissue nucleophiles (7–8) and double bonds (9). For example, 2-nitrosofluorene reacts with double bonds in membrane lipids to form a highly reactive hydroxylamine that readily undergoes oxidation to the nitroxide. The formation of this nitroxide results in a change in the conformation of the fatty acids that destabilizes the membrane. In addition, the nitroxide is a relatively stable free radical that can generate other reactive species such as peroxy radicals that have been shown to cleave DNA (10). Thus, the hydroxylamine function is the key intermediate from which the reactions occur. Examples of nitrogen compounds in which the nitrogen functional group is involved in the toxicity are summarized in Table 10-1. All of the compounds listed are aromatic nitrogen compounds; aliphatic compounds do not appear to exhibit this kind of metabolism-dependent toxicity.

The preceding examples of activation of nitrogen functionalities all involve the oxidation products of amines. The relationship between the different oxidation states of nitrogen in these compounds is summarized in Figure 10-1.

Nitrogen-containing xenobiotics can occur in any of these oxidation states and can be interconverted by enzymatic reduction or oxidation (5,11). Typically, these enzymes interact with neutral substrates, so the state of ionization of the substrate is important. Aliphatic amines generally have high pK_a values (approximately 9–10) and exist predominantly in the ionized form at physiological pH. The positively charged species does not interact with cytochrome P450 monooxygenase (12), and is relatively unreactive toward electrophiles. Aromatic amines, on the other hand, are essentially neutral at pH 7 (pK_a approximately 4–5) and are available for interaction with the oxidase in high concentration. The hydroxyamino group is weakly basic, and the nitroso and nitroxyl groups are neutral. Once formed, these functions

Table 10-1. Examples of Toxic Organo Nitrogen Compounds

Compound	Toxicity	Investigators
2,6-Dinitrotoluene	Carcinogen	(37)
2-Acetoxyaminofluorene	Carcinogen	Miller and Miller, 1977 (6)
Aromatic amines	Methemoglobinemia	(38)
Nitrosobenzene	Hemolysis	(39)
Chloramphenicol	Aplastic anemia	Murray et al., 1982 (10)
Acetaminophen	Hepatotoxin	(41)
Procaine amide	Immunotoxin	(40)

are present in the biological milieu as the neutral species that can be further oxidized or can participate in reactions with nucleophilic functions.

Hydroxylamines are formed metabolically by oxidation of amines or by reduction of nitroso or nitro compounds. The oxidation has been shown to be mediated, for the most part, by two enzyme systems: the flavin monooxygenase (13), and cytochrome P450 (14). However, prostaglandin H synthase (15,16) and peroxidase (17) have also been shown to effect N-oxidation reactions. The first two enzyme systems are present in hepatic endoplasmic reticulum, but the relative contribution of each to N-oxidation is highly species and substrate dependent. The cytochrome P450 monooxygenase is very nonspecific and oxidizes substrates in a manner that reflects their chemical reactivity (18,19) instead of chemical structure. The overall reaction catalyzed by cytochrome P450 is

$$O_2 + RZH + NADPH \rightarrow RZOH + NADPH + H_2O \quad (1)$$

where Z can be C, N, or S.

Most products of the reaction contain functional groups that participate in Phase II, or conjugation, reactions, but some can be very unstable and can react with available nucleophilic centers. When these reactive intermediates react with nucleophilic sites on essential macromolecules, they can render them nonfunctional, resulting in a biochemical lesion. The toxicity of compounds acting by these mechanisms depends on the reactivity of the intermediate and the availability of secondary pathways of metabolism. Studies of the enzymatic interconversion of nitrogen functions have shown that a number of different enzymes are involved. As indicated above, the key intermediate is the hydroxylamine function.

Early work studying the enzymology of the interconversion used pharmacological evidence to demonstrate the participation of cytochrome P450 in the oxidation of nitrogen functions to hydroxylamines. This enzyme is induced by drugs such as phenobarbital and inhibited in vitro by carbon monoxide. N-Hydroxylation of some substrates was shown to respond to these agents in a manner consistent with P450 participation. However, the oxidation of nitrogen functions also has been demonstrated directly by re-

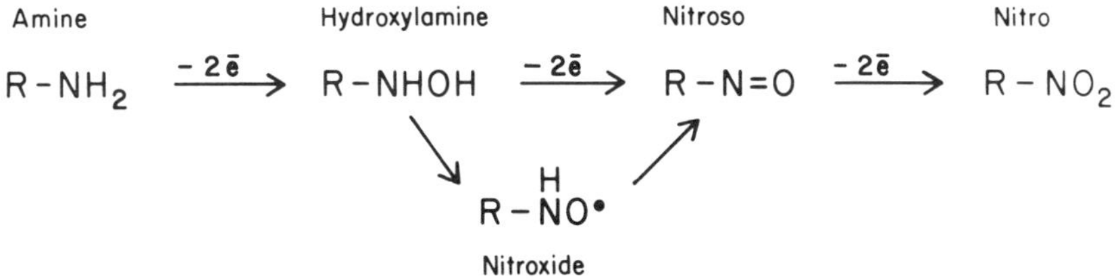

FIGURE 10-1. Oxidation States of Nitrogen

constituting the enzyme system from purified components (14,20–22). The reduction of nitiro groups to hydroxylamines is catalyzed by several enzymes including cytochrome P450 and the flavoprotein, cytochrome P450 reductase (23).

The hydroxylamine is readily oxidized in air (24) to the reactive nitroso state, but there is also evidence that this reaction can be enzymatic (25). The one electron oxidation product of hydroxylamines, the nitroxyl radical, can also be generated biochemically (26). This radical function reacts with glutathione, and its toxicity is thought to involve similar reactions with essential thiols in the cell.

Our laboratory has been studying the oxidation of aliphatic and aromatic amines by cytochrome P450. We have focused on the biochemistry of N-hydroxylation of amines and the formation of metabolic intermediate complexes (MI complex), (27,28) by nitroso derivatives of some of these compounds. These complexes result from binding of the nitroso function to the Fe(II) heme (29) and, once formed, inhibit the catalytic activity of the monooxygenase. Complex formation from amines, hydroxylamines, and nitroso compounds was investigated because it can occur by a sequence of cytochrome P450-mediated oxidation reactions with all of these functions. The effect of the complex on cytochrome P450 function has also been examined as a method of evaluating the stability of the complex and its pharmacological or toxicological significance.

The studies were conducted with microsomal and reconstituted preparations. The microsomal preparations contain the elements of the enzyme system in their native membrane state, whereas the reconstituted systems contain a single cytochrome P450 isozyme in an artificial phospholipid vesicle. Thus, the microsomal preparations contain several cytochrome P450 isozymes and effect a wider variety of oxidations. Since aliphatic amines are not commonly associated with metabolism-dependent toxicity, it was of interest to us to compare aliphatic and aromatic amines for differences in their interaction with cytochrome P450. The compounds used in the studies were amphetamine, phentermine, and *p*-chloroaniline, as shown in Figure 10-2.

A comparison of the N-hydroxylation of aliphatic and aromatic amines by microsomal preparations and reconstituted systems revealed quantitative differences. The presence of a geminal dimethyl group at the alpha carbon of aliphatic amines such as phentermine resulted in higher rates of N-

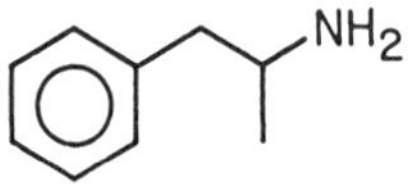

1

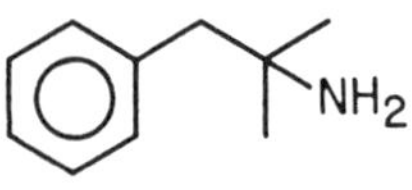

2

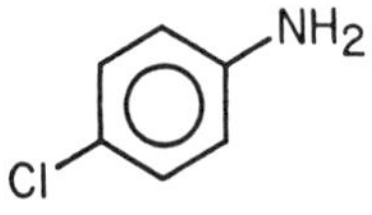

3

FIGURE 10-2.

Table 10-2. N-Hydroxylation of Amines by Rabbit Liver

	Microsomes	P450 LM_2
Amphetamine	0.39 ± 0.06	0.22 ± 0.02
Phentermine	1.20 ± 0.24	1.50 ± 0.14

Note: The substrates (5 m*M*) were incubated with microsomes from phenobarbital-pretreated animals or with a reconstituted cytochrome P450 system containing isozyme LM_2 from rabbit liver. The data are expressed as nmol × min^{-1} × nmol $P450^{-1}$ (34).

hydroxylation than for the alpha monomethyl derivative amphetamine (Table 10-2). This difference was more marked in reconstituted than in microsomal preparations and was attributed to the isozymes responsible for the N-hydroxylation of the two substrates. The presence of the geminal dimethyl group in an aliphatic amine appears to enhance the N-hydroxylation by isozyme LM_2. The rates of N-hydroxylation of aromatic amines appeared to be substantially greater (Table 10-3). The stoichiometry, evidenced by the ratio of NADPH oxidized to substrate oxidized, shows that the aliphatic amines have a very low efficiency for N-hydroxylation. The theoretical ratio is 1.0 and is approached by reactions such as the N-demethylation reaction. Thus, the N-hydroxylation of aliphatic amines catalyzed by cytochrome P450 is an extremely inefficient reaction. Aromatic amines, on the other hand, are much better substrates, generating higher levels of hydroxylamines. This quantitative difference between the two types of amines may contribute to their greater toxicity.

We have studied metabolic intermediate (MI) complex formation from amines, hydroxylamines, and nitroso compounds. These complexes are characterized by an absorption band at approximately 455 nm (the exact position appears to vary with the substrate) so that their formation is readily detected.

The relative rates of MI complex formation for a series of amphetamine

Table 10-3. Efficiency of N-Hydroxylation

Substrate (pK_a)	Rate of NOH[a] Formation	Rate of NADPH[b] Consumed	Ratio NADPHR/NOH
Amphetamine (10.0)	0.21 ± 0.10	7.7 ± 0.2	20
Phentermine (10.0)	0.27 ± 0.005	8.7 ± 0.3	10
4-Cl-aniline (3.98)	3.2 ± 0.15	11.9 ± 0.3	2

[a]This rate (nmol × nmol $P450^{-1}$ × min^{-1}) was determined in an incubation at a substrate concentration of 1.0 m*M* with rabbit liver microsomes in the presence of an NADPH generating system.

[b]This rate (nmol NADPH consumed × min^{-1} × nmol $P450^{-1}$) and the ratio of NADPH to product were determined under conditions of limiting NADPH. Incubation conditions were otherwise identical.

Table 10-4. Rates of MI Complex Formation by Aliphatic Amines and Hydroxylamines

$PhCH_2CHRNHX$ *R*	*X*	V_m
Methyl	H	1.6
	OH	187.0
Ethyl	H	3.6
	OH	144.0
i-Prop	H	10.8
	OH	223.0
t-Butyl	H	10.2
	OH	131.0

Note: The substrates, at different concentrations, were incubated with microsomes from phenobarbital-pretreated rats and the rates of MI complex formation determined spectrophotometrically. Values of maximal velocity were determined kinetically and are expressed as change in absorbance min^{-1} mM^{-1} P450 (25).

analogues were determined with amine or hydroxylamine as substrate. The values of the maximal velocity (Table 10-4) show that the hydroxylamine is 10 to 100 times faster in forming the complex than the amine, indicating that N-hydroxylation is a slow process compared to the second oxidation to the nitroso state. Complex formation from the amines was preceded by an induction period, consistent with the postulate that the amine had to undergo the slower N-hydroxylation reaction before nitroso formation. Metabolic intermediate complex formation appears to have steric constraints, as N-hydroxyphentermine and *t*-butylamine, with their hindered alpha, alpha dimethyl-substituted carbon, do not form it (30). The inability of N-hydroxyphentermine or its nitroso analogue to bind to the heme alters the catalytic cycle of cytochrome P450 so that it acts nonproductively to reduce oxygen to superoxide (31), acting as a peroxidase. Studies of this reaction revealed additional complexities; the superoxide converted N-hydroxyphentermine to the nitroxide, which was oxidized ultimately to the nitro state (24,31). Thus, by aborting the normal catalytic cycle of the monooxygenase, a chemical reaction between hydroxylamine and superoxide takes place within close proximity of the active site.

Studies have also been performed with aromatic hydroxylamines and nitroso compounds. 4-Substituted aromatic nitroso compounds with their trigonal carbons, may not present a hindered nitrogen to the heme, but 2-substituted nitroso compounds do. As expected, 2-substituted aromatic nitroso compounds are much less effective in forming MI complexes. There is a mechanistic difference between the complexes formed by aliphatic and aromatic nitroso compounds. The complex with aliphatic nitroso compounds forms only after the reduction of cytochrome P450 to the Fe(II) state. In contrast, aromatic nitroso compounds form the complex directly with oxidized P450 in the absence of added NADPH, although complex formation requires the reduction of the Fe(III) to Fe(II). Although the chemical mechanism is still unknown, this reaction appears to be an internal (within the protein) oxidation-reduction reaction (32).

In a more pharmacological study, the MI complexes from aromatic and aliphatic nitrogen compounds were compared for their ability to inhibit drug metabolism. This could be an important consequence of MI complex formation, because it suggests that the ability of the host to eliminate foreign substances would be compromised. The approach taken was to determine the effects of preincubation of liver microsomes with the amine or hydroxylamine on benzphetamine demethylation, a common and highly efficient cytochrome P450 reaction. This reaction is rapid and, in livers from phenobarbital-treated rabbits, 90 percent of demethylation activity appears to reside with a particular isozyme (LM_2) (33). The rationale was that preincubation would activate the amine or hydroxylamine to the nitroso state and allow complex formation to take place before introduction of the demethylation substrate. The control, which was not preincubated, would reflect primarily the ability of the inhibitor to act competitively. Preincubation of both the amine and the hydroxylamine corresponding to amphetamine and 4-chloroaniline resulted in an inhibition of demethylation greater than that of the non-preincubated mixture (Table 10-5).

The hydroxylamine from amphetamine was a more effective inhibitor than the amine (Table 10-5). These data are consistent with those of Table 10-4 that show complex formation to be faster from the hydroxylamine. The data also show that complex formation is required for inhibition. The smaller difference between preincubated and non-preincubated inhibition for *p*-chloro-N-hydroxyaniline is thought to reflect the rapid air oxidiation of N-hydroxyanilines. The lower level of inhibition by *p*-chloro-N-hydroxyaniline may be due to the lower affinity of the arylnitroso compound for cytochrome

Table 10-5. Effect of MI Complexes on Benzphetamine N-Demethylation

	Control Demethylation	
Inhibitor	No Preinc (%)	Preinc (%)
Amphetamine	106	78.4
Phentermine	105	91
4-Cl-aniline	86	38
NOH amphetamine	86	28
NOH phentermine	108	104
NOH 4-Cl-aniline	75	63

Note: In the preincubation experiments, the inhibitors (0.1 m*M*) were incubated with rabbit liver microsomes for 5 minutes before addition of benzphetamine (final concentration 1.0 m*M*). The rates obtained without preincubation were used to determine the competitive inhibitory actions of the complex forming compounds.

P450. Neither phentermine nor N-hydroxyphentermine forms the complex, and they appear to be weak competitive inhibitors.

Table 10-6 shows that the MI complex can be selective, because N-hydroxy amphetamine did not inhibit all cytochrome P450 reactions. Amphetamine deamination, a cytochrome P450-mediated oxidation, was not affected under conditions that resulted in substantial reduction of phentermine N-hydroxylation and benzphetamine demethylation (Tables 10-5, 10-6). Thus, the MI complex appears to form with particular isozymes and inhibit their catalytic cycle. In more recent work (36) N-hydroxy-methylenedioxyamphetamine has proven to be a very general inhibitor, completely blocking cytochrome P450 function after complex formation.

Other studies examined the relationship between structure and the enzymatic constants, K_m and V_{max}. Results from experiments with a series of alpha-substituted phenylethylamines indicated that lipophilicity was the determining factor for the maximal rate of N-oxidation (25). Cytochrome P450 is a membrane-bound enzyme so that substrates have to penetrate the lipid matrix of the enzyme to undergo oxidation. This feature of the enzyme should be manifested in a correlation between lipid solubility and the apparent K_m for different substrates. Such a correlation was observed for N-demethylation (34), but not for N-oxidation of aliphatic amines (25). This property of the N-oxidation reaction was generalized to aromatic amines in a study of the N-oxidation of a series of 4-substituted anilines. The maximal rates of reaction (V_{max}), but not K_m, correlated with π, the hydrophobic substituent parameter, for the 4-substituent (35). These results were interpreted to indicate that the rate-limiting process for N-hydroxylation differs from C-hydroxylation reactions catalyzed by cytochrome P450 and involves transfer of the substrate from a hydrophilic to a hydrophobic region. Thus, this non-specific enzyme system appears to be able to effect reactions that proceed through different mechanisms.

Thus far, these studies have shown quantitative but not qualitative differences in the oxidation of aromatic and aliphatic nitrogen functions by cytochrome P450. The differences in these reactions and in the chemical properties of the products could account, in part, for the greater toxicity

Table 10-6. Effect of N-Hydroxy Amphetamine-Generated MI Complex on Cytochrome P450 Reactions

Substrate	Reaction	Control Levels (%)
Amphetamine	Deamination	97
Phentermine	N-hydroxylation	36

Note: N-Hydroxyamphetamine (0.1 m*M*) was preincubated with rabbit liver microsomes in the presence of NADPH. Three minutes later, the substrate (1 m*M*) was added, and incubation continued for 10 minutes.

associated with aromatic nitrogen compounds. The higher proportion of neutral substrate, in the case of aromatic amines, and the greater efficiency of their N-hydroxylation result in higher yields of hydroxylamine. The resulting high levels of these compounds may allow them to diffuse away from their sites of formation in significant concentrations, where they can then form highly reactive sulfate conjugates and bind irreversibly to tissue nucleophiles. Alternately, they can be oxidized to the nitroso compounds that react with double bonds on biologically important structures to form covalent bonds and disrupt their function.

In contrast, the aliphatic amines are much less reactive toward N-hydroxylation. This is due, in part, to the small proportion of free base that exists at physiological pH. In addition, however, their N-hydroxylation by cytochrome P450 is slow and inefficient, and the hydroxylamine generated is less reactive than an aromatic hydroxylamine. Aliphatic hydroxylamines are converted to nitroso compounds enzymatically, but, because of the low levels of hydroxylamine, only relatively small amounts are available for reaction with tissue macromolecules. However, aliphatic amines do form MI complexes with cytochrome P450 after N-oxidation, and this complex can inhibit the metabolism of drugs and other xenobiotics and delay their elimination.

ACKNOWLEDGMENTS

The work performed in this laboratory was supported by the National Institutes of Health (GM 26024, CA 9030), the National Institute of Drug Abuse (DA 02411, DA 04026), and the California Institute for Cancer Research. The technical assistance of Joon Dokko and Marco Iskandar is gratefully acknowledged.

REFERENCES

1. D. M. Jerina, H. Yogi, D. R. Thakker, R. E. Lehr, A. W. Wood, W. Levin, and A. H. Conney. Bay-region activation of polycyclic aromatic hydrocarbons to ultimate mutagens and carcinogens. Pages 1041–1049 in: *Microsomes, Drug Oxidations, and Chemical Carcinogensis*. Vol. 2. M. J. Coon, A. H. Couney, R. W. Estabrook, H. V. Gelboin, J. R. Gillette, P. J. O'Brien, eds. Academic Press, New York (1980).
2. B. B. Brodie, W. D. Reid, A. K. Cho, G. Sipes, G. Krishna, and J. R. Gillette. Possible mechanism of liver necrosis caused by aromatic organic compounds. Proc. Nat. Acad. Sci. *68*, 160–164 (1971).
3. C. Y. Quon. Clinical pharmacology and drug metabolism. Pages 132–160 in: *Biotransformation of Organic Nitrogen Compounds*. Vol. 1. A. K. Cho and B. Lindeke, eds. S. Karger AG, Basel.
4. R. A. Prough, J. M. Erikson, and P. Wiebkin. Nitrogen oxidation in toxicity. Pages 161–183 in: *Biotransformation of Organic Nitrogen Compounds*. Vol. 1. A. K. Cho and B. Lindeke, eds. S. Karger AG, Basel.

5. J. W. Gorrod and L. A. Damoni. Eds. Biological oxidation of nitrogen in organic molecules. Ellis Horwood, Chichester (1985).
6. J. A. Miller and E. C. Miller. The concept of reactive electrophilic metabolites in chemical carcinogenesis: Recent results with aromatic amines, safrole and aflatoxin B_1. Pages 6–24 in: *Biological Reactive Intermediates*. D. J. Jollow, J. J. Kocsis, R. Snyder, and H. Vainio, eds. Plenum Press, New York (1977).
7. G. J. Mulder, L. E. Umnruh, F. E. Evans, B. Ketterer, and F. F. Kadlubar. Formation and identification of glutathion conjugates from 2-nitrosofluorene and N-hydroxy-2-aminofluorene. Chem.-Biol. Interactions *39*, 111–127 (1982).
8. R. A. Floyd, L. Soong, M. A. Stuart, and D. L. Reigh. Free radicals and carcinogenesis. Some properties of the nitroxyl free radicals produced by covalent binding of 2-nitrosofluorene to unsaturated lipids of membranes. Arch. Biochem. Biophys. *185*, 450–457 (1978).
9. A. B. Sullivan. Electron spin resonance studies of a stable arylnitroso-olefin adduct free radical. J. Org. Chem. *31*, 2811–2817 (1966).
10. T. Murray, K. M. Downey, and A. A. Yunis. Degradation of isolated deoxyribonucleic acid mediated by nitroso-chloramphenicol. Biochem. Pharmacol. *31*, 2291–2296 (1982).
11. A. K. Cho. Metabolic disposition of nitrogen functionalities. Pages 184–212 in: *Biotransformation of Organic Nitrogen Compounds*. Vol. 1. A. K. Cho and B. Lindeke, eds. S. Karger AG, Basel.
12. A. K. Cho and G. T. Miwa. The role of ionization in the N-demethylation of some N,N-dimethylamines. Drug Metab. Disp. *2*, 477–483 (1974).
13. D. M. Ziegler. Microsomal flavin-containing monooxygenase: Oxygenation of nucleophilic nitrogen and sulfur compounds. Pages 201–230 in: *Enzymatic Basis of Detoxication*. Vol. 1. W. B. Jakoby, ed. Academic Press, New York (1980).
14. E. F. Johnson, D. S. Levitt, U. Muller-Eberhard, and S. S. Thorgeirsson. Catalysis of divergent pathways of 2-acetylaminofluorene metabolism by multiple forms of cytochrome P450. Cancer Res. *40*, 4456–4459 (1980).
15. J. A. Boyd and T. E. Eling. Evidence for a one-electron mechanism of 2-aminofluorene oxidation by prostaglandin H Synthase and horseradish peroxidase. J. Biol. Chem. *22*, 13885–13896 (1984).
16. P. Hilavica and I. Golly. N-oxidation of 4-chloroaniline by the microsomal prostaglandin synthetase system: Redox cycling of a nitroxide intermediate. Pages 320–326 in: *Biological Oxidation of Nitrogen in Organic Molecules*. J. W. Gorrod and L. A. Damani, eds. Ellis Horwood, Chichester (1985).
17. P. J. O'Brien and B. Gregory. The peroxidase catalysed N-oxidation and activation of N,N′,N,N′-tetramethylbenzidine. Page 337 in: *Biological Oxidation of Nitrogen in Organic Molecules*. J. W. Gorrod and L. A. Damani, eds. Ellis Horwood, Chichester (1985).
18. P. R. Ortiz de Montellano. in: *Cytochrome P450*. P. R. Ortiz de Montellano, ed. Plenum Press, New York (1986).
19. G. T. Miwa and J. S. Walsh. Cytochrome P450 in nitrogen metabolism. Pages 27–62 in: *Biotransformation of Organic Nitrogen Compounds*. Vol. 1, A. K. Cho and B. Lindeke, eds. S. Karger AG, Basel.
20. P. D. Lotlikar and K. Zaleski. Ring and N-hydroxylation of 2-acetamidofluorene by rat liver reconstituted cytochrome P450 enzyme system. Biochem. J. *150*, 561–564 (1975).
21. S. S. Thorgeirsson, D. J. Jollow, H. A. Sasame, I. Green, and J. R. Mitchell. The role of cytochrome P450 in N-hydroxylation of 2-acetylaminofluorene. Mol. Pharm. *9*, 398–404 (1973).
22. J. D. Duncan and A. K. Cho. N-Oxidation of phentermine to N-hydroxy-phentermine by a recoinstitued cytochrome P-450 oxidase system from rabbit liver. Mol. Pharmacol. *22*, 235–238 (1982).
23. D. S. Hewick. Reductive metabolism of nitrogen-containing functional groups. Pages

151–171 in: *Metabolic Basis of Detoxication. Metabolism of Functional Groups.* W. B. Jakoby, J. R. Bend, and J. Caldwell, eds. Academic Press, New York (1982).

24. J. M. Fukuto, E. W. di Stefano, J. N. Burstyn, J. S. Valentine, and A. K. Cho. Mechanism of oxidation of N-hydroxyphentermine by superoxide. Biochemistry *24,* 4161–4167 (1985).
25. B. Lindeke, U. Paulsen-Sorman, G. Hallstrom, A. H. Khuthier, A. K. Cho, and R. C. Kammerer. Cytochrome P-455-nm complex formation in the metabolism of phenylalkylamines. VI. Structure-activity relationships in metabolic intermediatry complex formation with a series of a α-substituted 2-phenylethylamines and corresponding N-hydroxylamines. Drug Metabol. Disp. *10,* 700–705 (1982).
26. E. J. Rauckman, G. M. Rosen, and J. Cavagnaro. Norcocaine nitroxide. A potential hepatotoxic metabolite of cocaine. Molecular Pharmacology *21,* 458–463 (1981).
27. M. R. Franklin. Inhibition of mixed function oxidations by substrates forming reduced cytochrome P450 metabolic intermediate complexes, Pharmacol. Ther. Part A. Chemother. Toxicol. Metabol. Inhibitors *2,* 227–245 (1977).
28. J. Jonsson and B. Lindeke. On the formation of cytochrome P450 product complexes during the metabolism of phenylalkylamines. Acta Pharm. Suec. *13,* 313–320 (1976).
29. D. Mansuy, P. Gans, J. C. Chottard, and J. F. Bartoli. Nitrosoalkanes as Fe(II) ligands in the 455 nm absorbing cytochrome P450 complexes from nitroalkanes in reducing conditions. Eur. J. Biochem. *76,* 607–615 (1977).
30. B. Lindeke and U. Paulsen-Sörman. Nitrogenous compounds as ligands to hemoporphyrins—The concept of metabolic-intermediatry complexes. Pages 63–102 in: *Biotransformation of Organic Nitrogen Compounds.* Vol. 1. A. K. Cho and B. Lindeke, eds. S. Karger AG, Basel.
31. J. D. Duncan, E. W. Di Stefano, G. T. Miwa, and A. K. Cho. Role of superoxide in the N-oxidation of N-(2-methyl-1-phenyl-2-propyl)hydroxylamine by the rat liver cytochrome P-450 system. Biochemistry *24,* 4155–4161 (1985).
32. J. M. Fukuto, J. F. Brady, J. N. Burstyn, R. Van Atta, J. S. Valentine, and A. K. Cho. Direct formation of complexes between cytochrome P-450 and nitrosoarenes. Biochemistry *25,* 2714–2719 (1986).
33. D. A. Haugen, T. A. van der Joeven, and M. J. Coon. Purified liver microsomal cytochrome P-450, separation and characterization of multiple forms. J. Biol. Chem. *250,* 3567–3570 (1975).
34. J. D. Duncan, G. Hallstrom, U. Paulsen-Sörman, B. Lindeke, and A. K. Cho. Effects of α-carbon substituents on the N-demethylation of N-methyl-2-phenethylamines by rat liver microsomes. Drug Metab. Disp. *11,* 15–20 (1983).
35. J. N. Burstyn, M. Iskandar, J. F. Brady, J. M. Fukuto, and A. K. Cho. Mechanistic Studies of N-Oxidation by Microsomal Cytochrome P450. Fed. Proc. *46* Abs. 184 (1987).
36. N. Patel, M. Iskandar, J. Dokko, S. Chakrabarti and A. K. Cho. (1988) The inhibition of cytochrome P450 reactions by methylenedioxymethamphetamine (MDMA) derivatives. FASEB J. *2,* A1141.
37. J. A. Popp and T. B. Leonard (1983) Hepatocarcinogenicity of 2,6-dinitrotoluene (DNT) Proc. Am. Assoc. Cancer Res. *24,* 91.
38. M. Kiese (1966). The biochemical production of ferrihemoglobin-forming derivatives from aromatic amines and mechanisms of ferrihemoglobin formation. Pharmacol. Rev. *18,* 1091–1161.
39. K. Hirota and H. A. Itano (1978) Influence of ring substituents on the binding of nitrosobenzene by ferrohemoglobin. J. Biol. Chem. *253,* 3477–3481.
40. N. C. Henningsen, A. Cederberg, A. Hauson and B. W. Johansson (1975) Effects of long range treatment with procaine amide. Acta Med. Scand. *198,* 475–482.
41. L. F. Prescott, L. Park and A. T. Proudfoot (1976) Cysteamine, L-methionine and D-Penicillamine in Paracetamol poisoning. J. Int. Med. Res. *4,* (suppl 4) 112–117.

Chapter 11

Comprehensive Evaluation of the Central Nervous System Effects of Cimetidine: A Role for Toxicokinetics, Toxicodynamics, and Clinical Studies in Volunteers, Animal Models, and Patients

Jerome J. Schentag, Pharm.D., Patricia L. Ebbeling, Pharm.D., John A. Ziemniak, Ph.D., Lynda S. Welage, Pharm.D., Harold Bernhard, M.D.

The State University of New York at Buffalo, School of Pharmacy, and The Department of Medicine and The Clinical Pharmacokinetics Laboratory, Millard Fillmore Hospital, NY

CASE REPORTS OF CNS EFFECTS ASSOCIATED WITH CIMETIDINE

Introduction

Numerous case reports suggest an association between treatment with H_2 antagonists and central nervous system (CNS) toxicity. The majority of these cases involve cimetidine. However, since ranitidine was introduced, it too has been implicated in causing adverse CNS effects. Famotidine, the newest H_2 antagonist released in the United States, has not had published case reports to date. Case reports aid in characterizing the nature of a mental status change and in designing studies to differentiate whether cimetidine is a precipitating agent in patient subpopulations. We have reviewed and analyzed the available cases to aid in identifying subpopulations that may be more susceptible to CNS changes. Elements common to the cases may also point to the mechanism of CNS toxicity due to H_2 antagonists, and in this manner foster the initiation of specific toxicokinetic studies in a variety of animal and human models.

Cases

The majority of cimetidine cases describe patients who experienced effects ranging from mild confusion and delirium to stupor and coma (1–29). In addition, there have been several case reports of psychiatric complications, such as depression or paranoia (29–38). Tremors, peripheral neuropathy, and extrapyramidal signs have also been associated with cimetidine (39–44). These cases were reviewed to derive a rating scale useful for prospective analysis of patients who have symptoms.

Mental Confusion

A typical patient experiencing mental status changes associated with cimetidine may experience a variety of signs and symptoms, including restlessness, confusion, disorientation, agitation, hallucinations, myoclonic twitching, seizures, and unresponsiveness progressing to periods of apnea (45). A review of those descriptor words in the 39 cases reported revealed that symptoms of confusion, disorientation, agitation, hallucinations, coma, drowsiness, dizziness, twitching, and seizures were frequently reported. The data are reported in Table 11-1.

Individual patients usually exhibited one to four of these symptoms in various combinations; however, five patients (6,11,19,23) progressed from mild confusion, lethargy, agitation, or disorientation to total unresponsiveness. Coma or unresponsiveness was the presenting symptom in four patients (19,21,26). In general, confusion may consist of the following: decreased alertness, decreased attentiveness, decreased ability to grasp all elements of the immediate situation, inadequate perception, and forgetfulness. These findings are consistent with the progression of symptoms found in confusion with various etiologies. Irritability may or may not be present, and paranoid features such as suspicion, as well as demanding and aggressive behavior, may be present. Decreased responsiveness may be observed as the severity of confusion increases. This may progress to stupor with

Table 11-1. Description of CNS Symptomatology in 39 Cases Associated with Cimetidine, and Frequency of Various Descriptors

	Symptoms		Miscellaneous Symptoms
	Number	Percent	(n = 15, 38.5%)
Confusion	22	56.4	Belligerent
Disorientation	9	23.1	Irrational behavior
Agitation	9	23.1	Insomnia
Hallucinations	8	20.5	Lightheadedness
Drowsiness	4	10.3	Memory loss
Dizziness	3	7.7	Respiratory arrest
Flushing	3	7.7	Somnolence
Unmanageable	3	7.7	Combative
Delirium	3	7.7	Incoherent
Lethargic	3	7.7	Unsteadiness
Seizures	3	7.7	Frightened
Slurred speech	3	7.7	Loss of concentration
Sweating	2	5.1	Suspicious
Restlessness	2	5.1	Visual or hearing impairment
Aggressiveness	2	5.1	
Headache	2	5.1	
Twitching/Myoclonic contractions	2	5.1	

hallucinations and finally to coma (46). All of these symptoms occur in patients with mental status changes associated with cimetidine.

Analysis of time to the onset of symptoms associated with changes in mental status revealed that 68.3 percent of patients experienced symptoms within 72 hours of initiating treatment. Symptoms in 41.5 percent began within the first 24 hours, as shown in Table 11-2.

Close surveillance of patients in high-risk subpopulations for the first few days after cimetidine is started may detect most cases early after the onset of symptoms. After reduction in dosage or discontinuation of cimetidine therapy, 39 percent of patients experienced a complete reversal of symptoms within 24 hours. Another 34.2 percent returned to their baseline mental sta-

Table 11-2. Time to Onset of Symptoms After Initiation of Cimetidine

Time	Number	Percentage
<24 hours	17	41.5
<48 hours	5	12.2
<72 hours	6	14.6
>72 hours	8	19.5
Unknown	5	12.2
Total	41	100

Table 11-3. Time to Disappearance of Symptoms After Stopping Cimetidine

Time	Number	Percentage
<24 hours	16	39.0
<48 hours	9	22.0
<72 hours	5	12.2
>72 hours	5	12.2
Unknown	6	14.6
Total	41	100

tus within 72 hours, with 12.2 percent requiring greater than 72 hours for their symptoms to disappear (Table 11-3). The cimetidine was reduced in four of the cases (13,19,20,23). Symptoms disappeared within 48 hours after dosage reduction in two patients, while symptoms persisted in one patient. The fourth patient died shortly after the dosage change. Thus, confusion can be effectively managed and potentially reversed with appropriate dosage adjustment. Rechallenges with cimetidine were attempted in four of the cases (13,20,23,27). In all patients, symptoms of confusion recurred when therapy with cimetidine was reinstituted. These cases provide distinct evidence for cimetidine-associated toxicity. In patients who have previously experienced confusion while on this drug, recurrence of these same symptoms can be expected if cimetidine is reinstituted.

Age is commonly associated with increased risk. In case reports, the median age of patients was found to be 61.5 years; 34 patients (83%) were found to be over 50 years of age. Table 11-4 illustrates the age-frequency distribution of these patients. It is not clear whether this data illustrates increased risk due to aging, or simply that most cimetidine-treated patients in hospital critical-care units are elderly. Of the patients who experienced cimetidine-related CNS changes, 26 were males and 13 were females; the gender of two patients was not reported.

If these results are a reasonable reflection of the distribution of the incidence of CNS effects in the true adult population, then we can conclude

Table 11-4. Age vs. Mental Status Changes

Age (years)	Number	Percentage
31–40	2	4.9
41–50	3	7.3
51–60	13	31.7
61–70	5	12.2
71–80	9	22.0
Not reported	2	4.9
Total	41	100

that this toxicity is more frequent in the elderly. Thus, increasing age can be a predisposing factor to CNS toxicity. A second possibility is that decreased renal function associated with increased age may result in increased serum concentrations of cimetidine, and these values may be associated with increased CNS toxicity. In addition, other disease states may predispose patients to CNS toxicity because of alterations in blood or brain positioning, and it is these diseases that may be seen more commonly in elderly patients.

In the attempt to define subpopulations that may demonstrate increased CNS susceptibility due to organ dysfunction, patients in each case were placed into subgroups according to whether they had normal renal and hepatic function, renal disease, hepatic disease, or multiple organ disease. The distribution of patients within these subgroups can be seen in Table 11-5.

In a large number of cases (36.6%), the renal and hepatic functions of patients receiving cimetidine were not reported. Of those that were reported, 15 patients (36.6%) had some degree of renal impairment, one patient had hepatic impairment only, and four patients were reported to have multiple organ failure. It is significant to note that in six of these cases, patients reportedly had normal renal and hepatic function (14,15,23,24,26,27). Since many of the reports do not provide direct measures of organ function, Table 11-5 may not be a good approximation of the distribution of toxicity incidence between these subgroups. Even so, it is possible that some degree of organ failure may increase the incidence or predispose the individual to CNS effects. It has been suggested that increased serum cimetidine concentration may increase CNS toxicity. Cimetidine is eliminated from the body primarily by renal excretion (47,48) as well as by hepatic metabolism (49). Thus, decreased renal or hepatic function, or both, can lead to increased serum cimetidine concentrations if dosage adjustments are not made. Because of this risk, we reviewed relative dosages received by the patients based on estimates of organ function. In the subgroup of renal disease (n = 15), 10 patients received the usual recommended dose of cimetidine (1.0–1.2 per day), while only four patients were given an appropriately reduced dose (dosage was not reported in one patient). Of those patients with multiple organ failure (n = 4), two received the usual dosage, one had a dosage reduction, and one received a dose significantly higher than normal rec-

Table 11-5. Association of Underlying Disease State and Mental Status Changes

Subgroup	Number	Percentage
Normal	6	14.6
Renal disease	15	36.6
Hepatic disease	1	2.4
Multiple organ failure	4	9.8
Not reported	15	36.6
Total	41	100

ommended dosages. The patient with hepatic failure was given a normal dosage.

Concurrent drug administration is important to examine in cases of adverse effects associated with any drug. Concomitantly administered drugs may increase the susceptibility of patients to CNS effects of cimetidine, or the CNS effects may simply be due to the other drug alone. Cimetidine may enhance the CNS effects of the concurrent drug, either by inhibiting its metabolism and thereby increasing its serum concentration or by enhancing the susceptibility of the patient to the CNS effects of this drug. In the reported cases, a variety of drugs were administered concurrently with cimetidine to many patients. A large number of these patients received CNS-active drugs during treatment with cimetidine. Five patients were receiving a CNS drug concurrently with cimetidine (10,16,20,24,27). In eight other patients (6,14,15,22,23,28,29), centrally acting drugs were given to treat cimetidine-induced symptoms. Symptoms persisted in all cases.

Psychiatric Complications with Cimetidine

Aside from mental confusion, cimetidine has been reported to cause psychiatric complications. In the 12 cases, symptoms of depression (30–34) or paranoia (29,35,46) have occurred. Mania occurred in two patients (37). Another patient was described as having acute panic attacks that subsequently evolved into symptoms of depression (38). These cases were quite different from cases of mental confusion. The median age of the patients was found to be 51.5 years, with the range being from 35 to 81 years of age. Only 50 percent of patients were 50 years of age or older, in contrast to the patients who had mental confusion. The time course of these psychiatric complications also differs from that of mental confusion. Only three patients developed symptoms within 72 hours. In the remaining patients, symptoms appeared within five days to over a period of several months. Symptoms resolved after discontinuation of cimetidine within 72 hours in five patients, although a few days to as long as three weeks were required in six patients for resolution of symptoms. In one patient with depression, no improvement was seen after discontinuation of cimetidine and treatment of the depression with imipramine; however, the depression worsened when imipramine was withdrawn. Dosage reductions in two patients resulted in improvement of symptoms. Symptomatology was not altered upon dosage reduction in a third patient, although symptoms did resolve with discontinuation of cimetidine (30). Rechallenges with cimetidine in three patients (32,34,37) resulted in recurrence of their depressive or manic symptoms. Hepatic and renal function was normal in six of the 12 patients, and although these conditions were not reported in the remaining six cases, there was no reason to expect abnormalities from the available case reports. Of the 12 patients, 11 were receiving a usual therapeutic dosage of cimetidine, and one a reduced dosage. Medications were administered concurrently with cimetidine in only six of these patients. Of these, four patients received agents that produced CNS activity. A preexisting psychiatric illness was present in only 3 of the 12 patients. Preexisting psychiatric illnesses or simultaneous treatment with psychotropic medications may predispose individuals to cimetidine-associated CNS toxicity, although it is not necessarily a prerequisite. A variety of miscellaneous symptoms have been associated with cimetidine in an additional 10 patients. These include motor neuropathy in four patients (39,40). Chorea was experienced in one patient, and upon rechallenge with cimetidine in this patient, symptoms of chorea did recur (41). Postural and action tremor has been described in three case reports (42). In all three cases, tremor returned upon rechallenge and resolved with the administration of propranolol. Another case report implicates cimetidine in inducing an extrapyramidal and cerebellar syndrome with acute encephalopathy (43). In addition, prolonged postoperative somnolence occurred while a patient received cimetidine as well as a variety of anesthetic agents (44). Since these reports of adverse effects are isolated cases, either such toxicity occurs only very rarely, or the effects may be related to factors other than the cimetidine.

Summary

When cimetidine was first marketed, the incidence of CNS toxicity was reported to be less than 1 percent (50). CNS toxicity was usually manifested as mild symptoms of dizziness, headaches, or somnolence. Postmarketing surveillance has been conducted in the general population, with similar incidence found (51–53). However, numerous case reports demonstrate that significant cimetidine-associated confusion does occur. It is clearly more frequent in certain subpopulations than anticipated. A likely high-risk population is patients in intensive-care units, since these were not included in the formal postmarketing surveillance studies but are frequently implicated by spontaneous reports. As with many adverse reactions, the critically ill patient is a frequent source of occurrence. Although they are only a small fraction of the overall treated population, these patients account for the majority of adverse events.

CASE REPORTS OF CNS EFFECTS ASSOCIATED WITH RANITIDINE

During worldwide clinical trials with ranitidine conducted between 1979 and 1981, adverse CNS effects were not noted (54). Thus, when ranitidine was first introduced, it was advocated for patients at high risk for mental confusion and for patients with renal failure when drug accumulation could possibly predispose the patient to CNS toxicity (55). Flind and Rowley-Jones (56) subsequently pointed out that rare adverse effects may be detected only after widespread use of the drug and collation of several spontaneous reports. They recognized that the type of population treated influences the ability to detect and define risks of drug therapy. Accordingly, they maintained that ranitidine may not demonstrate adverse CNS effects for several years in the general public. Since that time, at least five case reports have implicated ranitidine in association with adverse CNS reactions (57–61). Since the introduction of intravenous ranitidine, further increases in the number of cases may be reported, as ranitidine usage increases in populations identified at high risk for cimetidine CNS toxicity.

Supporting lack of CNS effects with ranitidine as compared to cimetidine are three case reports. In each case report, adverse CNS effects associated with cimetidine did not recur when these patients were treated with ranitidine (62–64). Bories reported (62) that cimetidine-associated mental confusion in one patient did not recur when ranitidine was substituted. Criticisms of this report were made by Sharpe and Burland (65). They pointed out that the dosage of cimetidine, even after having been decreased, was greater than that recommended for use in renal failure, while an appropriate dosage of ranitidine was used. In addition, the patient apparently had varying degrees of renal function, and no information on renal function at the time of ranitidine administration was provided.

In the second case by Pedrazzoli and colleagues (63), the patient became nonresponsive after 19 days on a constant infusion of cimetidine at 4.0 g per day for the treatment of Zollinger-Ellison syndrome. Cimetidine was slowly tapered and ranitidine at 0.6 g per day was started. Within six days, the patient recovered and was fully alert. Benzodiazepine medications were not used during this period of time, and the patient's renal and hepatic function remained stable throughout. These authors failed to mention how long the infusion of ranitidine was continued without reappearance of symptoms. It could be argued that because 19 days elapsed before cimetidine-associated CNS symptoms were manifested, a similar period of time may be required for manifestations of ranitidine-induced CNS toxicity to be exhibited in this patient.

Smith and colleagues (64), in an unpublished report, demonstrated that ranitidine was well tolerated and effective for duodenal ulcer in a patient with advanced cirrhosis who was unable to tolerate cimetidine without development of mental confusion. A 69-year-old female developed mental confusion and tremors while on cimetidine 300 mg qid, and the relationship to cimetidine administration was confirmed with rechallenge. Reduced dosages were attempted, and the maximum tolerated dosage without symptoms of encephalopathy was 150 mg bid. This regimen was ineffective in a subsequent recurrent duodenal ulcer. Consequently, cimetidine was discontinued and ranitidine was started at a dose of 150 mg bid. No symptoms of encephalopathy occurred during the course of ranitidine therapy. Throughout this period, the hepatic status of the patient remained stable, and her serum creatinine remained normal.

These studies do not prove that ranitidine is free of CNS toxicity in patients who develop CNS symptoms when given cimetidine. Interestingly, in one case of ranitidine-associated toxicity, symptoms resolved when cimetidine was substituted for ranitidine (57). Also, two patients experienced CNS symptoms in association with both cimetidine as well as ranitidine (58,59). Thus, the relative potential for inducing ranitidine-adverse CNS effects as compared to cimetidine has yet to be determined.

To compare the profiles of ranitidine-induced to cimetidine-induced CNS toxicity, we compiled and analyzed ranitidine case reports in the same manner as those with cimetidine. Overall, the profile was similar to that of the cimetidine cases. Confusion was reported for all five patients, and disorientation was reported in three. Agitation, hallucinations, and delusions were also manifested. The time from ranitidine administration to onset of symptoms was 72 hours or less in four of the five cases. In two patients, symptoms disappeared within 72 hours after discontinuation of ranitidine, and two patients required longer than 72 hours for resolution. In the last case, the time for resolution was not reported.

All patients experiencing symptoms were 50 years of age or older. Hepatic disease was reported in three patients, while in the remaining two patients organ function was not reported. Thus, patients have the same risk factors of advanced age and hepatic dysfunction that have been identified in cases of cimetidine toxicity. All patients received dosages recommended by the manufacturer (150 mg bid). In one patient, an attempt to reduce the ranitidine dosage resulted in some improvement of symptoms (5). Rechallenge was undertaken in one patient, which resulted in the reappearance of adverse CNS symptoms (61). As with cimetidine, management of these patients can involve either a dosage reduction or discontinuation of the drug. Resolution of these symptoms would be expected within a few days with either option.

Other medications were given with ranitidine in three of five cases. In two patients, CNS-active agents were administered concurrently. In addition, both of these subjects received CNS medications to treat symptoms once they were manifested (haloperidol, diazepam). These medications could possibly predispose patients to additional adverse CNS symptoms and may only have exacerbated them. No patient was reported to have any history of psychiatric illness.

In summary, CNS toxicity may also be expected in association with ranitidine. Reports of toxicity with ranitidine are similar to those previously reported with cimetidine. Patients with risk factors for cimetidine toxicity may also be at risk for ranitidine toxicity. The relative potential for ranitidine versus cimetidine toxicity is not known. Both drugs have been associated with CNS toxicity in a few patients. In others, when one is substituted for the other, symptoms did not recur. It may be reasonable, in cases in which an H_2 antagonist is needed, to switch between these agents when CNS symptoms are encountered.

CASE REPORTS OF CIMETIDINE TOXICITY IN OVERDOSAGE

Case reports describe instances in which large quantities of cimetidine have been ingested in intentional overdosage. A number of these report ingestion followed by few effects. However, three instances of significant toxicity were reported.

Minimal signs of cimetidine toxicity were seen in four cases reported by Illingworth and Jarvie (66). The amount of cimetidine ingested in this series of four cases ranged from 28 to 98 tablets. The patients involved ranged from 26 to 42 years of age. Only in one patient was slight drowsiness reported after ingestion of 16 g of cimetidine, along with 30 mg nitrazepam, and 10 tablets of aluminum hydroxide. Drowsiness could be attributed to the concurrent ingestion of nitrazepam.

Cimetidine plasma concentrations obtained from these victims were in the range of 36–57 mg/L within 1–3.5 hours after overdose (Table 11-6).

The usual peak serum concentrations of cimetidine after a single 400-mg

Table 11-6. Case Reports of Cimetidine Overdosage with Plasma Concentration Measurements

Patient		Substances Ingested	Dose	Time After Ingestion (hrs)	Plasma Cimetidine Conc. (mg/L)	Ref.
Age	Sex					
26	M	Cimetidine	16.0 g	3.2	57.0	(66)
		Nitrazepam	30.0 mg	4.5	40.0	
		Aluminum hydroxide	10 tabs	23.33	3.0	
42	M	Cimetidine	19.6 g	2.0	36.0	(66)
				11.5	2.3	
26	M	Cimetidine	5.2 g	2.0	37.0	
37	M	Cimetidine	6.0 g	10.0	4.5	(66)
		Beer	2 pints	12.0	2.9	
Not reported		Cimetidine	20.0 g	3.5	45.8	(68)
35	M	Cimetidine	24.0 g	8.0	18.7	(71)
				15.0	2.6	

dose are approximately 2.36 mg/L at 1.5 hr (67). Within 12–24 hours, serum concentrations fell to near-normal values.

Meredith and Volans (68) report four children and 14 adults who were admitted after a cimetidine overdose. All children were reported to be symptom free and were discharged well. Of seven adults who ingested cimetidine as a single agent, five remained symptom free, one had a sinus tachycardia, and one experienced mild abdominal discomfort. Three of an additional four patients who ingested alcohol along with cimetidine experienced either drowsiness or dizziness. The remaining patients had either no symptoms or exhibited symptoms that could be attributed to concomitantly ingested drugs. A cimetidine plasma concentration was taken in one patient who remained symptom free after ingestion of 20 g of cimetidine. The serum concentration was markedly elevated to 45.8 mg/L at 3.5 hr postingestion. In all of these cases, adverse effects in temporal association with the overdose cannot be attributable with certainty to cimetidine.

One accidental overdosage of cimetidine was reported by Gill (69). This middle-aged male patient ingested approximately 12 g per day for five days without untoward effects.

In contrast, Wilson (70) described a case in which respiratory depression may have been a complication of cimetidine overdosage. This case involved a 46-year-old chronic schizophrenic who ingested approximately 60 cimetidine tablets. The patient was being treated with 2 mg trifluoperazine twice daily and 25 mg hydroxyzine twice daily. Within one-half hour after acute ingestion of cimetidine, the patient became drowsy but arousable, and his respirations became slow and shallow. After gastric lavage, his condition improved rapidly. These symptoms are most likely associated with cimetidine, as evidenced by the time course of events.

Van Rijthoven (71) reported a 35-year-old male with normal renal and hepatic function who became unconscious in association with ingestion of 24 g of cimetidine concurrently with 400 mg of oxazepam. The patient was admitted unconscious to the hospital and exhibited restlessness, with brisk reactions to painful stimuli and shaking movements of the extremities. Treated with gastric lavage and forced diuresis, the patient slowly regained consciousness after the overdosage. At 8 hr postingestion, a plasma cimetidine concentration was reported at 18.7 mg/L. In this case, it is not possible to separate the adverse effects of cimetidine from those associated with oxazepam.

An additional case report (72) describes a 25-year-old man who ingested 12 g of cimetidine. At 4 hr postingestion upon admission to the hospital, he exhibited slurred speech. Gastric lavage was performed. There was no evidence that alcohol or other drugs had been taken. Within another 5 hours, he became agitated and disoriented. Indices of hepatic and renal function remained normal throughout his admission. By the following day, he had recovered from these symptoms and was lucid. The signs and symptoms exhibited by this patient are similar to adverse CNS toxicity reported in association with the therapeutic use of cimetidine.

Summary

Cimetidine was associated with significant toxicity in a small number of overdosage cases. In many of these cases, adverse symptoms may be attributable to concomitantly ingested drugs. Two of the cases presented are exceptions; in these cases, toxic signs and symptoms were exhibited when only cimetidine had been ingested. Respiratory depression appeared within a short period of time after an acute ingestion of cimetidine as the sole agent (5). In the second case, symptoms similar to cimetidine-associated CNS toxicity appeared late after the overdose event (72).

Subpopulations of subjects that may be more susceptible to cimetidine toxicity cannot be identified from the available overdosage cases. In all cases, the victims were relatively young and had no reported organ dysfunction.

CNS toxicity associated with therapeutic cimetidine use is thought to be influenced by elevated plasma concentrations (45,73,74). Measurements taken in these cases (66,68,71) demonstrated concentrations as high as 10 times those normally seen with therapeutic dosages, without signs of toxicity. In an additional case (71), cimetidine serum concentrations were still markedly elevated even after the patient had regained consciousness. This may suggest that the exhibited toxicity was more likely due to the concomitantly ingested drug. These observations raise the question why CNS toxicity is not seen more often in acute overdosages. Although plasma concentrations were greatly elevated shortly after cimetidine overdosage, they quickly fell to usual concentrations within 12–24 hours (Table 11-6). With therapeutic cimetidine use, CNS toxicity reportedly occurs within 24–48 hours after initiation of therapy. Accordingly, CNS toxicity may be time dependent as well as plasma concentration dependent. Time may be required for significant concentrations of cimetidine to be reached in the brain. This may be what is reflected in the case reported by Nelson (72), in which nine hours elapsed before symptoms of agitation and disorientation began. Longer exposure to elevated serum concentrations may be required to produce adverse CNS effects. However, the patient of Gill (69) reportedly ingested 12 g of cimetidine daily for five days without effects.

NORMAL VOLUNTEER STUDIES OF THE CNS EFFECTS OF H_2-ANTAGONISTS

A limited number of controlled studies have been conducted to evaluate possible effects of H_2 antagonists in normal subjects. Various means have been used to evaluate CNS function in these studies, including electronystagmography, a computer-assisted Romberg test, and a variety of psychomotor function tests.

In view of the associated reports of dizziness, Paazian and colleagues (75) investigated the effect of cimetidine on tests of vestibular function. These researchers studied subjects with normal vestibular function and a second group of subjects with a post-traumatic unilateral vestibular lesion. The investigators found small differences from baseline on electronystamography at 5 and 15 min after the intravenous administration of 200 mg of cimetidine. By 30 min after dosing, all changes had returned to baseline. None of the changes were found to be statistically significant, and dizziness was not reported by the volunteers. Unfortunately, a reference agent capable of altering these tests was not included for comparison. Therefore, it is not possible to determine the sensitivity of electronystamography to vestibular response changes caused by cimetidine.

A computer-assisted Romberg test was used by Brynskov and his colleagues to assess changes in CNS function due to the H_2 antagonists cimetidine (76) and ranitidine (77) in normal subjects. This method determines postural stability measured as a change in sway. There was a significant increase in sway in normal males as compared to placebo at 10- and 20-min postintravenous infusion of 400 mg of cimetidine. At 10 and 20 min after infusion of 100 mg of ranitidine, there was a smaller increase in sway, and these changes were not significant. Notably, there can be a wide variation in percentage changes in sway between volunteer subjects. This study was not double blinded or randomized, and patients were not crossed over between the various treatment groups. These investigators also did not use a reference drug known to alter these tests, so further exploration of this approach in a more carefully controlled fashion will be needed before conclusions can be drawn.

Szabadi in 1983 (78) compared the effects of ranitidine and cimetidine on psychomotor function. Thioridazine, which has documented effects on psychomotor function (79), was used as a positive control in these experiments. A battery of tests was utilized to determine effects on psychomotor function. The tests included visual analog mood scales, digit symbol substitution, symbol copying, digit cancellation, critical flicker fusion frequency, wire maze tracing, and tapping. Thioridazine caused a decrease in alertness, change in mood, and a significant decrease in performance in the paper and pencil as well as instrumental tests. In contrast, ranitidine and cimetidine did not adversely affect either the subjective or the objective tests. Although Szabadi did demonstrate a change in the performed tests by thioridazine, it is not known whether these tests are sensitive enough to detect subtle changes in CNS function caused either by cimetidine or ranitidine in the normal population, or whether normal volunteers (as opposed to patients) are suitable to demonstrate the subtle CNS effects of H_2 antagonists.

The available single-dose studies do not provide evidence for significant CNS effects of H_2 antagonists in normal subjects. However, the studies do not guarantee that these agents are free of CNS effects in the normal population. In all of the studies, single doses of H_2 antagonists were evaluated in normal volunteers, and the effect of chronic dosing needs to be studied. Alteration of CNS function may be time dependent, as CNS effects usually appear only after 24–48 hours of therapy. It may ultimately be necessary to study patients as opposed to healthy volunteers, since the absence of an effect in volunteers or less seriously ill patients does not prove that the effect will not occur in more severely ill subpopulations of patients.

PROSPECTIVE STUDIES OF CIMETIDINE IN THE INTENSIVE CARE UNIT PATIENT

We conducted a blinded, prospective study of the association between cimetidine treatment and altered mental status in 217 surgical intensive-care (ICU) patients (74). Over a 14-month period, 217 general surgical ICU admissions were designated by their attending physicians to either receive or not receive cimetidine. All patients not given cimetidine were given antacids to suppress acid effects. Patients were entered 24 to 48 hours after ICU admission, after the effects of general anesthesia had dissipated and when most no longer required mechanical ventilation. One-hundred and twenty-four patients received cimetidine; 93 did not. Other than assigning the patients to cimetidine or control groups, there was no difference in the type of care they received. All 217 patients were followed daily for seven days. At the end of the seven-day study period, no further interventions were performed.

At the time of entrance into the study, patients were stratified into one of four disease groups, depending on the presence of renal or hepatic dysfunction or both. Renal dysfunction was defined as a 24-hour creatinine clearance of less than 25 ml/min; hepatic dysfunction was defined as a serum bilirubin of at least 4.0 mg/dl, with accompanying hepatic enzyme elevations. The end result was an eight-cell stratification based on the presence or absence of renal or hepatic dysfunction or both, and the use or nonuse of cimetidine. A summary of the initial patient stratification is presented in Table 11-7.

Cimetidine was given intravenously at 300 mg q6h in the absence of renal and liver dysfunction, and 300 mg q12h in the presence of renal or hepatic dysfunction. When antacids were used, the dose was 30 ml hourly via the nasogastric tube. Blood chemistries were assessed at the time of entrance into the study and daily for the next seven days.

Mental status was evaluated daily by nurse clinicians who were blinded

Table 11-7. Final Patient Stratification by Clinical Group and Use or Nonuse of Cimetidine in 217 Patients

Group Number	Description	Number of Patients	
		Cimetidine[a]	No Cimetidine
1	No liver or renal dysfunction	42	49
2	Renal dysfunction	26	17
3	Liver dysfunction	30	18
4	Liver and renal dysfunction	26	9

[a]Cimetidine IV dose: Group 1, 300 mg q6h; groups 2, 3, and 4, 300 mg q12h. From Cerra et al. (74), with permission.

to stratification, chemistries, clinical data, and concurrent medications. Twenty-five mental status characteristics ranging from disorientation to coma were evaluated daily in each patient using a standardized table of descriptors with point rankings based on severity. This is shown as Table 11-8. Each mental status characteristic was awarded a numerical rating consistent with the de-

Table 11-8. Mental Status Assessment Criteria and Rating Points for Quantitative Comparison

Mental Status	Rating
Respiratory arrest	5.0
Periods of apnea	4.5
Generalized seizures	4.5
Unresponsive to either voice or pain	4.0
Responsive to pain only	3.5
Focal twitching (myoclonic)	3.5
Hallucinations	3.0
Belligerent	2.0
Agitated	2.0
Restless	1.0
Disoriented	1.0
Paranoid	1.0
Angry	1.0
Tremors	1.0
Responsive to voice and pain	1.0
Noisy	1.0
Oriented	1.0
Irritable	0.5
Anxious/Nervous	0.5
Uncooperative	0.5
Lethargic	0.5
Restrained	0.5
Apprehensive	0.3
Depressed	0.1
Sedated	−0.5

Note: Reprinted from Schentag (73), with permission.

gree of aberration from normal (45). The presence or absence of each mental status descriptor was recorded. In addition to the type of mental status change, a prospective mental status score was calculated from the daily total. A graph of typical data in a patient with CNS changes is shown in Figure 11-1.

Cimetidine peak and trough levels were drawn on study days 3 and 5. These values were presumed to represent steady state. The postdistributive peak was drawn two hours after the cimetidine dose, while the trough level was drawn just prior to the next dose. In selected patients, a complete serum concentration vs. time profile was obtained for pharmacokinetic analysis. A cerebrospinal fluid (CSF) sample was taken only when a spinal tap was necessary for clinical diagnostic purposes. These CSF samples were obtained and analyzed for cimetidine in 21 cases. Cimetidine was assayed by high-pressure liquid chromatography (80).

Data were evaluated using analysis of variance by the one-, two-, and three-way *F*-tests and evaluating mental status change relative to drug dose,

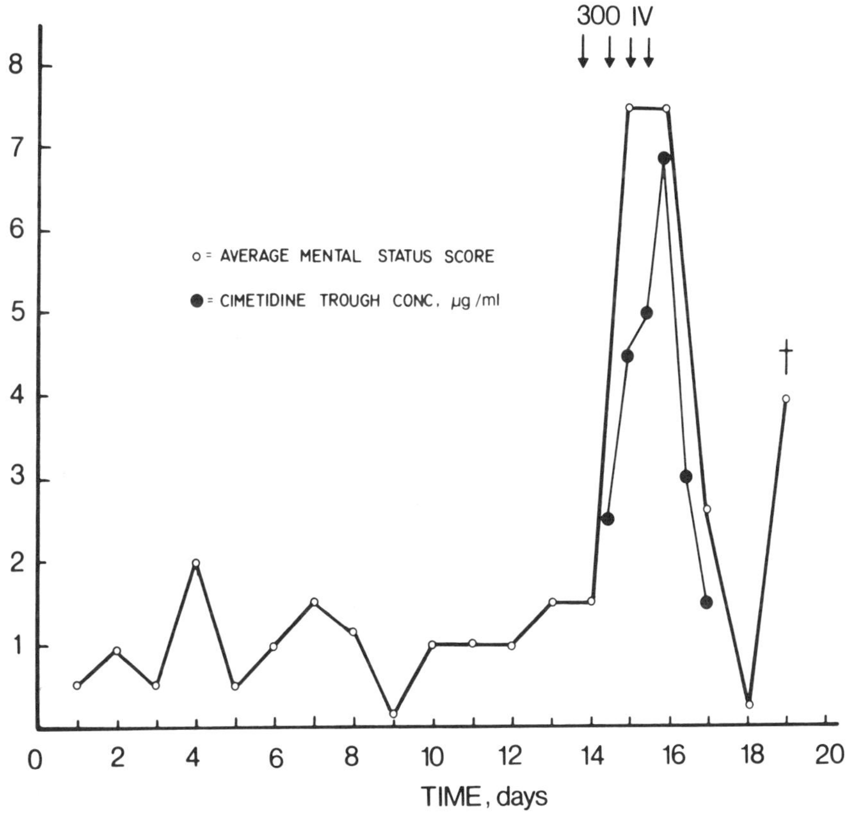

FIGURE 11-1. Cimetidine dosing, mental status score (○), and cimetidine trough concentrations (●) vs. time in a patient with severe symptoms. The patient was given 300 mg intravenously every 6 hr. Reprinted from Schentag (73), with permission.

Table 11-9. Mental Status (MS) Changes in Relation to Both Disease and Serum Trough Concentrations: Two-Way Analysis of Variance

Clinical Group[a]	Description	Mean Trough Concentration[b] With MS Changes	Without MS Changes	All Patients
1	Normal (N = 18,21)	1.00 ± 1.2	0.38 ± 0.19	0.89 ± 1.5
2	Renal disease only (N = 10,7)	1.90 ± 1.1	0.50 ± 0.13	1.24 ± 1.1
3	Liver disease only (N = 27,8)	0.50 ± 0.3	0.40 ± 0.30	0.46 ± 0.3
4	Renal and liver disease (N = 17,9)	2.50 ± 2.5	1.90 ± 2.50	2.30 ± 2.5
Mean ± SD		1.25 ± 1.6	0.69 ± 1.20	1.00 ± 1.5

[a]Significant differences in blood level as an effect of disease ($p < 0.01$).

[b]Significant differences in trough concentration with MS changes, versus without MS changes ($p < 0.05$). No significant interaction, meaning disease alters blood levels, whether or not there are MS changes.

day of administration, and disease group. The populations were normally distributed; significance was defined as $p < 0.01$. (See table 11-9.)

Results

During the seven days of the study, there were no differences in physical examination between each cimetidine and noncimetidine group. On any given study day, there were also no differences in exposure to penicillins, cephalosporins, aminoglycosides, chloramphenicol, inotropic agents, bronchodilators, insulin, vasodilating or vasoconstricting agents, diuretics, antihypertensive drugs, immunosuppressants, steroids, narcotics, sedatives, or antiarrhythmic agents. The use of tranquilizer drugs on days 1 and 2 of groups 3 and 4 who received cimetidine increased.

Prospective mental status scores (PMS) were obtained daily on all patients in all eight subgroups. An example of plotted data is shown as Figure 11-1. Compared to control patients, the data show the cimetidine-associated PMS differential as significant on day 2 and each day thereafter. The differences were borderline in patients with renal dysfunction. There were no differences in lab data that would account for the PMS scores of cimetidine-treated patients consistently above the respective control patients.

The prospective mental status data were statistically evaluated using each individual characteristic and also by the cumulative (PMS) score. The PMS score was then analyzed for an effect arising from the presence of cimetidine in each clinical group and on each study day.

One-, two-, and three-way F-tests were performed (group, day, dose). In all analyses, there was a strong correlation between PMS score and the use of cimetidine ($p < 0.0001$). In those patients in whom the drug was stopped (8%), mental status improved within 24 hours.

Cimetidine Mental Status Changes vs. Blood Levels

The effects of cimetidine were then studied in relation to cimetidine blood levels. There were no significant correlations between the plasma cimetidine peak, trough, or mean levels, and lab values such as BUN, creatinine, creatinine clearance, bilirubin, SGOT, LDH, or alkaline phosphatase. Also there was little relationship between the raw PMS score and the peak, trough, or mean level of cimetidine, except in the group with liver and renal dysfunction, in which 20 percent of the variation in PMS could be accounted for by the mean plasma cimetidine level ($r^2 = 0.20$).

To simultaneously assess the disease effects on blood level and on mental status changes, a two-way analysis of variance was performed. The results are shown as Table 11-9. These data show significant effects of disease on serum trough concentration, with the highest serum trough concentrations associated with renal or combined renal and hepatic disease ($p < 0.01$). In each group except liver disease patients, changes in mental status were associated with higher cimetidine trough concentrations ($p < 0.01$). Toxicity thus appeared to be related to higher concentrations, but the absolute numbers were obviously not predictive unless disease was also considered. This explained why we were not able to correlate cimetidine concentrations with CNS effects in the entire population and suggested that normalizing for disease effect might overcome this difficulty.

Because of the disease-specific nature of the mental status changes, we then normalized the PMS score for baseline and control group to arrive at the normalized PMS score. Each patient's PMS score on each intervention after day 1 was subtracted from day 1 and then divided by the day 1 score to arrive at the percent change in mental status for each intervention. Within each disease group, the percent change in PMS score of the patients receiving cimetidine was subtracted from the score of the corresponding control group, thus deriving the *net* percent change in PMS score for each group. There was a relationship between this normalized PMS score and the steady-state cimetidine trough concentration, as shown in Figure 11-2. The figure shows liver-disease patients to have the lowest blood levels and also a low degree of net change in PMS.

Liver- and renal-failure patients have elevated cimetidine trough concentrations and greater degrees of net change in PMS score.

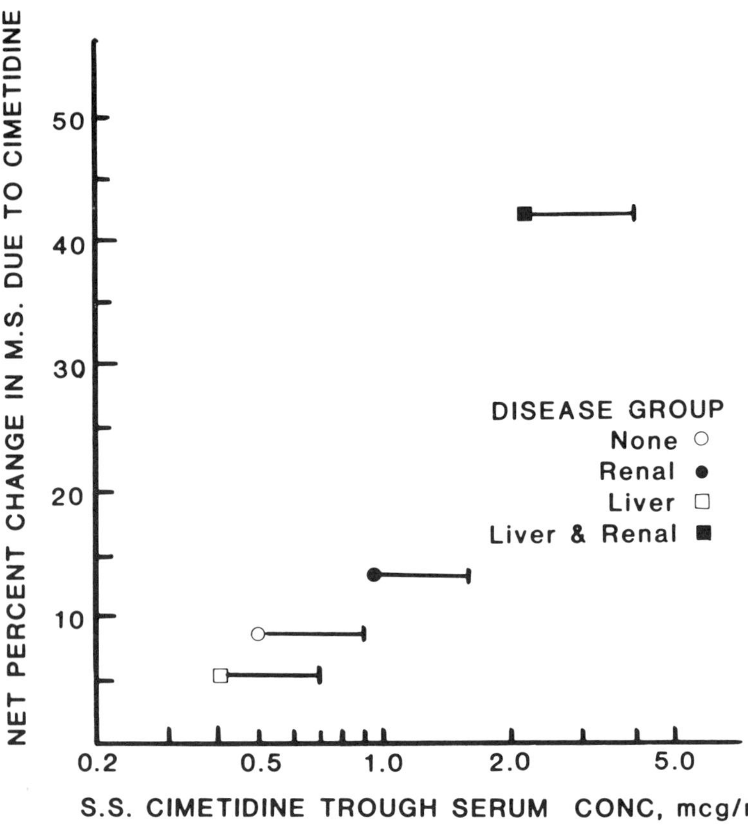

FIGURE 11-2. The net percent change in mental status by groups correlates with the log steady-state serum cimetidine concentration. A disease-specific effect is present with patients who have both renal and hepatic dysfunction manifesting the greatest net change in mental status in the face of the highest serum concentration. Reprinted from Cerra et al. (74) with permission.

CIMETIDINE PHARMACOKINETICS IN PATIENTS

Thirty-one study patients ranging in age from 17 to 90 had complete kinetic profiles (81). Details of this analysis are reported here. All patients were at steady state at the time of the study. Blood and cumulative urine samples were obtained throughout the 9- to 12-hour period between two doses. All samples were analyzed by a modification (80) of the high-pressure liquid chromatography (HPLC) method of Randolph and co-workers (82). The 31 kinetic study patients met the criteria for one of four clinical disease groups we have established (45,74). Six had no impairment of renal or metabolic function, and five had renal disease only. Twelve had liver disease but normal renal function, and eight had both renal and liver disease. Renal function was assessed by 24-hr creatinine clearance. Liver disease was determined by biopsy in most cases, and function was also evaluated by clinical criteria, based on elevation of serum bilirubin or liver enzymes. All patients were assigned to disease groups before blood sampling or kinetic evaluation.

Pharmacokinetic Analysis

Serum concentration vs. time data were fitted to a two-compartment open model using the computer program NONLIN (83). The A and B intercepts were corrected for infusion time by the equations of Loo and Riegelman (84). The slope and corrected intercepts were used to calculate cimetidine volumes of distribution in the central compartment (Vc) and at steady-state (Vdss). Total clearance was calculated from dose/area under the curve (AUC), while renal clearance was determined from the amount recovered in urine divided by serum AUC. The microconstants for distribution and elimination in the model (k_{12}, k_{21}, k_{10}) were also determined from standard equations (84). Cimetidine distribution and elimination variables were assessed in terms of age, disease, and renal function.

To provide perspective to our results in critically ill patients, we fitted the normal subject data of Walkenstein et al (85) to the same two-compartment model.

Results

Table 11-10 compares mean demographic and kinetic data for the patients in each of our groups (81) as well as of Walkenstein's subjects (85). Besides the presence of disease, there were substantial differences in age between the healthy subjects and our patients. Renal function differences are consistent with clinical group, and cimetidine total clearance was highly dependent on creatinine clearance. Serum half-life ($t - 1/2$) increased as total clearance declined, while central and steady-state distribution volumes were influenced little by disease.

Effects of Renal Function

Figure 11-3 shows the dependence of cimetidine total clearance on creatinine clearance in a more explicit manner ($r = 0.87$). Both the slope and intercept values are very similar to those in the literature (86). Most of the variance was in the patients with both renal and liver disease.

Table 11-10. Patient Characteristics and Kinetic Parameters in Patient Groups

Group	Age	Creatinine Clearance (ml/min)	*Vc* (L/kg)[a]	*Vdss* (L/kg)[a]	$C1_B$ (ml/min)	Half-Life (hr)	$C1_R$ (ml/min)	Percent Unchanged[b]
Normal patients ($N = 6$)	46 ± 21	89 ± 18	0.4 ± 0.28	1.1 ± 0.4	511 ± 93	2.3 ± 0.7	305 ± 123	62 ± 20
Renal disease ($N = 5$)	63 ± 13	6 ± 2.5	0.4 ± 0.20	0.9 ± 0.2	193 ± 24	4.8 ± 3.0	30 ± 11	16 ± 4
Liver disease ($N = 12$)	56 ± 14	73 ± 27	0.4 ± 0.21	1.4 ± 0.6	463 ± 145	2.9 ± 1.1	327 ± 119	68 ± 15
Renal and liver disease ($N = 8$)	73 ± 12	15 ± 10	0.3 ± 0.15	1.1 ± 0.4	182 ± 110	6.7 ± 6.0	68 ± 57	36 ± 27
Healthy subjects ($N = 12$)	26 ± 3	108 ± 22	0.4 ± 0.15	1.0 ± 0.2	583 ± 140	1.9 ± 0.3	451 ± 123	77 ± 6

Note: Reprinted from Schentag et al. (81), with permission.

[a]Volumes expressed as liters per kilogram ideal body weight.

[b]Percentage of dose recovered in urine.

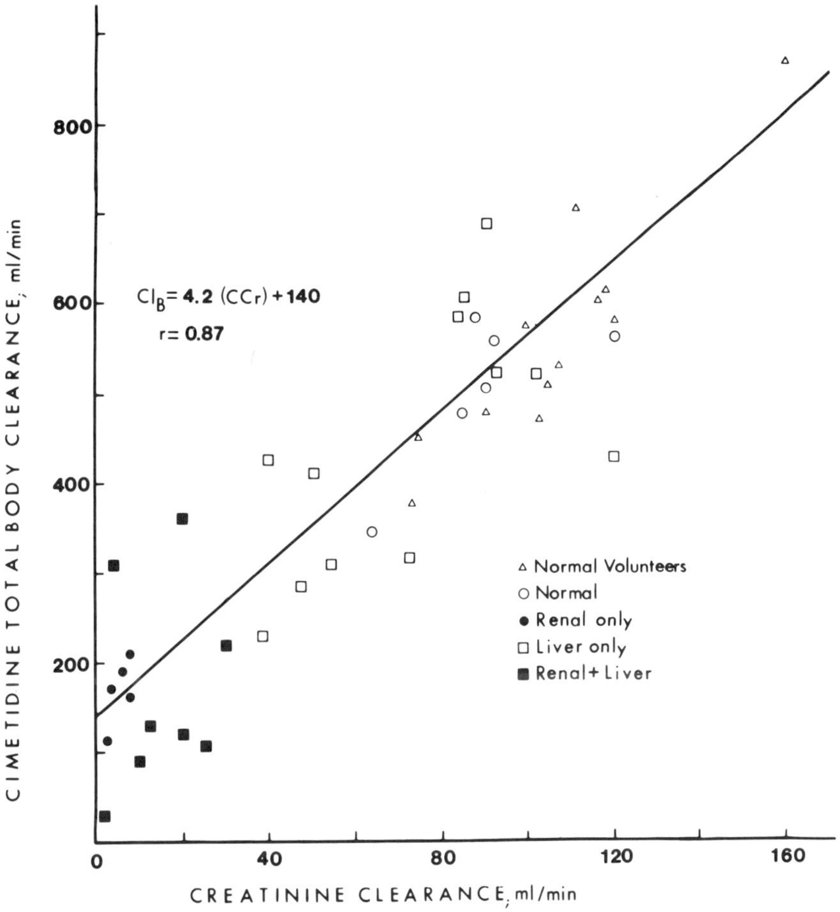

FIGURE 11-3. Cimetidine total body clearance versus creatinine clearance, with individual values given based on disease group. Symbols for normal volunteers represent the 12 subjects evaluated by Walkenstein (85). Reprinted from Schentag et al. (81), with permission. Correlation was strong ($r = 0.87$); the relation between CCr and $C1_B$ is defined by the regression $C1_B = 4.2(\mathrm{CCr}) + 140$.

Cimetidine serum half-life and creatinine clearance correlated ($r = 0.87$) (Fig. 11-4). Although the lower half of Figure 11-4 resembles a previous single-dose study (87), our study of this relationship identifies a large increase in half-life below creatinine clearances of 10 ml/min. The $t - 1/2$ ranged from 4 to 20 hr in the group with renal and metabolic failure, presumably because $t - 1/2$ was dependent on the capacity of the liver to eliminate cimetidine. The relation between cimetidine serum $t - 1/2$ was dependent of the capacity of the liver to eliminate cimetidine. The relation between cimetidine serum $t - 1/2$ and creatinine clearance (CCr) was bi-

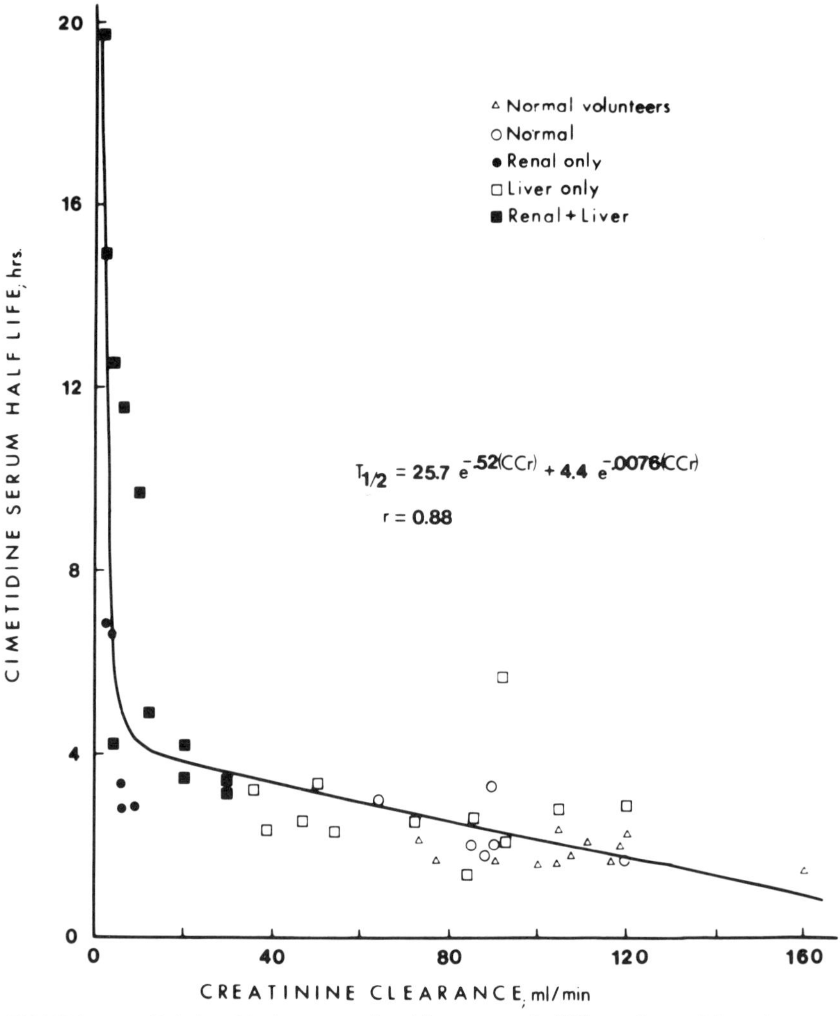

FIGURE 11-4. Relationship between cimetidine serum half-life and creatinine clearance (CCr), illustrating the primary half-life dependence on renal function and the importance of metabolic capability after creatinine clearance falls below 10 ml/min. Data were rank-ordered and fit to a biphasic equation using nonlinear least squares regression analysis (84). The equation describing the relationship between half-life and CCr is described in Figure 11-3, with strong correlation, r = 0.88. From Schentag et al. (81), with permission.

phasic and could be described by the following equation:

$$\text{Cimetidine } t - 1/2 = 25.7e^{-0 \cdot 52(\mathrm{CCr})} + 4.4e^{-0 \cdot 0076(\mathrm{CCr})} \quad \mathbf{(1)}$$

Since most of the renal excretion of cimetidine depends on tubular secretion, we evaluated this pathway by plotting the ratio of cimetidine renal clearance–CCr against creatinine clearance. Both pathways decline in parallel with the deteriorating renal function.

Effects of Age on Cimetidine Clearance

The effects of age on cimetidine total clearance were evaluated (Fig. 11-5). The data show primary dependence of creatinine clearance on disease state, but some further decline in cimetidine clearance was also possibly due to age. Multiple linear regression analysis was used to assess both effects, using total clearance as the dependent variable, and both creatinine clearance and age as independent variables. The increase in correlation due to regression with age was minimal; the correlation coefficient of Figure 11-3 rose from 0.87 to only 0.89. The regression equation describing the effects of both creatinine clearance and age on cimetidine total clearance is given as

$$Cl_B = 155 + 4.1(\mathrm{CCr}) + 0.22(\mathrm{age}) \quad (2)$$

Age had no influence on steady-state distribution volume; the slope of this regression was essentially zero. The absence of a relationship between age and steady-state volume is also clear in Table 11-1. In nine patients with liver dysfunction and 12 patients with liver and renal dysfunction who re-

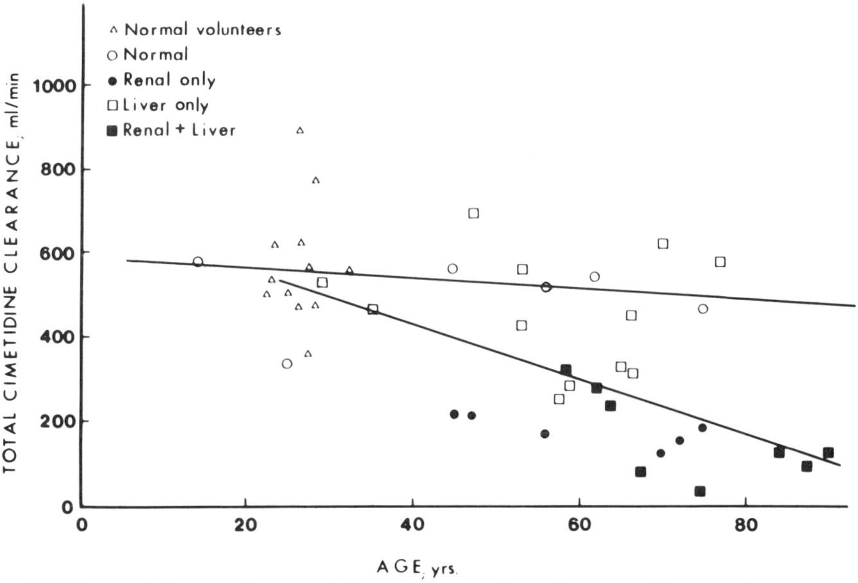

FIGURE 11-5. Influence of age and disease on cimetidine clearance. Diseases have more influence than age at each age group. The upper regression line applies to all study patients with normal renal and liver function, and the lower regression line applies to all study patients with abnormal liver and renal function. Schentag et al. (81), with permission.

ceived cimetidine, CSF samples were available for analysis. The lumbar punctures had been performed as part of the workup for mental status alteration. Although cimetidine was detected in all the CSF samples, there was little correlation between the cimetidine CSF level and the corresponding blood level. However, the liver disease patients had a higher CSF cimetidine level for a given serum concentration (e.g., 0.4 vs. 0.2 μg/ml CSF at a blood level of 0.5 μg/ml).

Results in 21 patients with CSF–serum ratios indicated an influence of disease on CNS penetration. The CSF–serum ratio was nearly twice as high in patients with liver disease as in normal patients (Fig. 11-6), and in patients with combined renal and liver disease the ratios were intermediate ($p < 0.02$).

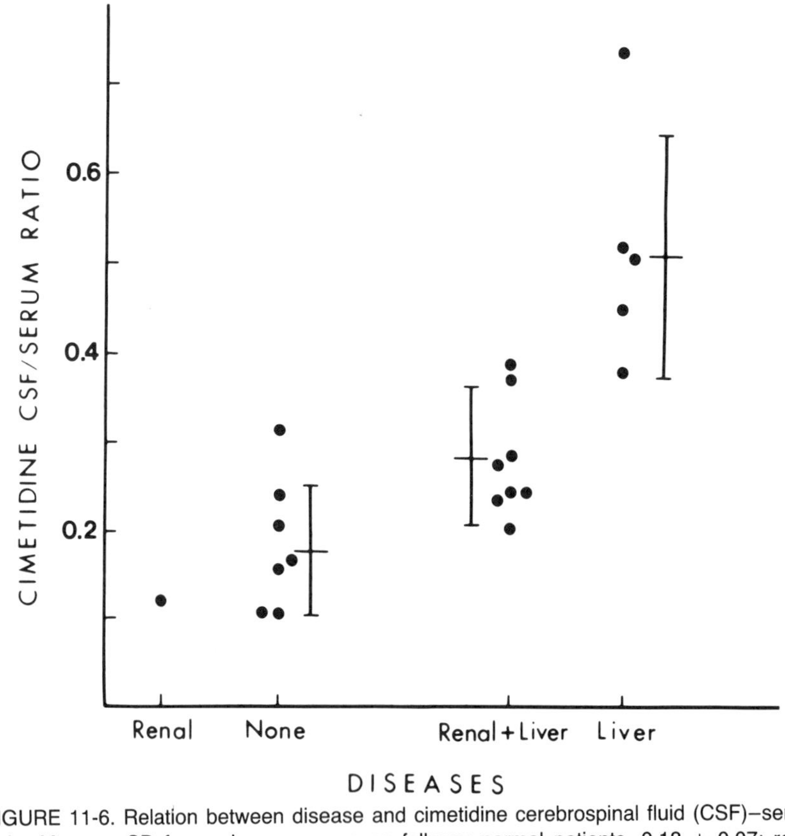

FIGURE 11-6. Relation between disease and cimetidine cerebrospinal fluid (CSF)–serum ratio. Mean ± SD for each group were as follows: normal patients, 0.18 ± 0.07; renal and liver disease patients, 0.28 ± 0.06; liver disease patients, 0.50 ± 0.14. Liver disease CSF–serum ratio was greater than that of either normal patients ($p < 0.001$) or renal and liver disease patients ($p < 0.02$). From Schentag et al. (81), with permission.

Discussion

In spite of the advanced age and critical illness of most of our patients, cimetidine kinetics were similar to that in healthy subjects provided there was no disease in eliminating organs. In contrast to the work of Somogyi and co-workers (88) and Redolfi and co-workers (89), we found no direct age influence on either steady-state distribution volume or total clearance. Even though we used larger numbers of patients and a broader age range than either of these investigators, we found no explanations for the difference in interpretation. The possibility exists that there were unrecognized age-related decreases in renal function in the patients of one or both of these studies. The effects of age on creatinine clearance are well known (90).

In our series of patients, the predominant variable influencing cimetidine clearance was disease of the eliminating organs; the kidney clearly plays a greater role in cimetidine clearance than the liver. Despite the predominant renal component, provided metabolic capacity remains intact in end-stage renal disease, serum half-life only doubles. However in patients with end-stage renal failure and concurrent liver disease, cimetidine serum half-life may be 10 times the normal value of 2.0 hr, and drastic adjustments are needed to prevent serious dose-related side effects such as mental confusion. Although there were pronounced disease effects on cimetidine clearance, we found little disease effect on either the central or the steady-state distribution volume.

We reported cimetidine CSF passage in five patients (45), and three additional cases were later reported (13). The surprising observation of our CSF penetration studies was that cimetidine CSF concentrations were influenced by disease. With 21 patients studied, a difference in CSF–serum ratio emerged that demonstrates that patients with hepatic disease accumulate cimetidine in CSF to a greater degree. For a given cimetidine serum concentration, almost twice as much cimetidine accumulates across the blood-brain barrier as in a patient with normal hepatic function. On the basis of these data, hepatic disease patients are at greatest risk for mental confusion, despite only a small reduction in cimetidine total clearance, and despite their normal trough concentrations. This is consistent with our observations in critical-care patients (Table 11-9). A two-way ANOVA confirmed the statistical significance of the disease effect on cimetidine concentrations as well as its CNS concentrations.

Patients with hepatic disease who need cimetidine should receive it with caution: Mental status changes can be anticipated with trough concentrations as low as 0.25–0.5 μg/ml (91). These values are lower than the usual toxic trough serum value we have proposed for CNS side effects of 1.25 μg/ml (45). To cope with the effects of disease on both CNS effects, and serum concentrations, we have elected to define the therapeutic and toxic concen-

Table 11-11. Therapeutic Window for Cimetidine Serum Trough Concentrations in Diseases

Group	Description	CNS Toxic Troughs (mcg/ml)
1	Normal	1.25
2	Renal disease	1.9–2.9
3	Liver disease	0.4
4	Multiple organ failure	1.0–2.5

trations of cimetidine in terms of disease. These criteria are shown in Table 11-11. These ranges should be helpful in the interpretation of measured cimetidine serum concentrations.

A DOG MODEL OF CIMETIDINE CNS PENETRATION: MECHANISMS OF TRANSPORT AND ACCUMULATION

As evident from the CNS side effects and measurable cimetidine concentrations in both brain (81,92,93) and cerebral spinal fluid (81), this drug penetrates the blood-brain barrier. Disease may alter the CSF partitioning of cimetidine, as patients with severe hepatic impairment were found to have cimetidine CSF–serum concentration ratios higher than those in normal individuals (81). Others have proposed that CNS manifestations are due to accumulation of the sulfoxide metabolite rather than to cimetidine itself (25).

Cimetidine is a weak base with pKa 7.09, with most of the drug circulating in the ionized form (96). While it is clear that this drug penetrates into SF, the CSF pharmacokinetics of cimetidine have not been comprehensively evaluated in either animals or human beings. Since there are no animal models of CNS penetration for cimetidine, we evaluated dogs for similarities to human beings in cimetidine pharmacokinetics, CSF penetration, and tissue distribution (97).

Methods

Four male mongrel dogs ranging in weight from 15 to 20 kg were studied. The animals were studied following an overnight fast but were allowed free access to water during the study procedures. The dogs were anesthetized with intravenous pentobarbital (20 mg/kg). A 21-gauge spinal needle was inserted into the cisterna magna. The head was immobilized and the needle left in place for the entire experiment. A heating pad and thermal blanket were used to maintain body temperature. A 22 mg/kg dose of cimetidine was then administered into a peripheral vein over 2 minutes. Simultaneous CSF and serum samples were obtained to assess penetration into the CSF. The animals experienced no apparent complications from the cisternal puncture, and none of the samples contained significant amounts of blood.

Assays. Quantitation of cimetidine and its metabolites was performed using an HPLC assay previously developed in our laboratories (98).

Pharmacokinetics. All serum and CSF concentrations were analyzed using either noncompartmental analysis or nonlinear least-squares regression analysis modeling the CSF as separate peripheral compartment. For both methods, pharmacokinetic parameters were calculated using standard techniques (99). Estimates of cimetidine pharmacokinetic characteristics in dogs were compared with data obtained from 12 healthy male volunteers of the average age of 26.1 years (84). Statistical differences between groups were determined using Mann-Whitney-U tests with the level of significance being $p < 0.05$. Cimetidine partitioning into dog CSF was measured and compared with predicted values.

Actual cimetidine partition ratios were determined from cimetidine CSF and serum concentrations according to the equation

$$R = C_{\mathrm{CSF}}/C_{\mathrm{serum}} \tag{3}$$

Theoretical CSF cimetidine concentrations were derived considering principles of CSF transport, pH partitioning, and protein binding. The standard partition equation for weak bases was employed to predict partition ratio (R) based on pH (100):

$$R = \frac{1 + 10\ \mathrm{pKa\text{-}pH_{CSF}}}{1 + 10\ \mathrm{pKa\text{-}pH_{serum}}} \tag{4}$$

with serum and CSF pH values being 7.4 and 7.3, respectively. The pKa of cimetidine was 7.09 (96).

Cimetidine CSF concentrations were also predicted from the free concentration of cimetidine in serum, using the equation

$$\mathrm{CSF} = fc \cdot Cp \tag{5}$$

The free fraction of cimetidine in the dog was assumed to be 0.85 (101). To estimate the relative importance of blood brain barrier (BBB) passage via passive diffusion compared to the influence on partition of bulk flow removal, active transport, or CNS metabolism, the following equation was evaluated for estimating the CSF–serum ratio (4) of cimetidine (102):

$$R = \frac{Cl_{\mathrm{IN}}}{Cl_{\mathrm{OUT}} + Cl_{\mathrm{BF}} + Cl_{\mathrm{M}} + Cl_{\mathrm{AT}}} \tag{6}$$

where Cl_{IN} is the clearance for entry across the BBB by passive diffusion, Cl_{OUT} is the clearance (equal to Cl_{IN}) for passive efflux from CSF, Cl_{BF} is the rate of bulk flow removal (equal to 3 ml/hr CSF turnover rate) (103), Cl_{M} is the clearance for cimetidine removal by brain metabolism, and Cl_{AT} is the clearance for removal of cimetidine from CSF by active transport.

Results

Serum concentrations of both cimetidine and the sulfoxide metabolite were similar to those in patients, even though the usual human dose is about 5 mg/kg. The dog demonstrates an apparent formation rate–limited excretion of cimetidine sulfoxide, similar to that of human beings. The mean elimination half-life was 2.3 hr for cimetidine sulfoxide. The hydroxymethyl metabolite of cimetidine was not detected in the serum of dogs given single doses.

The major pharmacokinetic characteristics for cimetidine in dogs were compared with those in human volunteers. There were no statistical differences in half-life total body clearance (TBC), volume of distribution at steady state (Vdss), or mean residence time (MRT).

The results of the area under the curve (AUC) determinations and AUC ratios for the dogs are shown in Table 11-12. In the dog, the sulfoxide–cimetidine area ratio of 0.173 ± 0.04 was not significantly lower than the 0.321 ± 0.15 reported in normal human beings (104).

Figure 11-7 is a representative serum and CSF time course for cimetidine in one animal. The maximum CSF concentration was 1.6 μg/ml, occurring at 0.75 hr after the dose. Cimetidine peak CSF concentrations occur at the end of the distributive phase. A CSF peak at this time is consistent with the

Table 11-12. Area Analysis After a 22 mg/kg Intravenous Dose of Cimetidine in the Dog[a]

	Serum			CSF	
Dog Number	Cimetidine (μg · hr/ml)	Sulfoxide (μg · hr/ml)	AUC_S/AUC[b]	Cimetidine (μg · hr/ml)	R_{CSF}[c]
1	33.1	4.0	0.121	3.9	0.119
2	72.0	14.8	0.206	12.4	0.172
3	54.4	10.6	0.195	5.1	0.094
4	52.7	8.9	0.168	6.0	0.114
Mean ± SD	53.1 ± 16	9.6 ± 4.5	0.173 ± 0.04	6.9 ± 3.8	0.125 ± 0.03

[a]Based on area analysis extrapolated to infinity.

[b]Ratio of sulfoxide–cimetidine serum area.

[c]Area distribution ratio determined from the ratio of cimetidine CSF–serum areas.

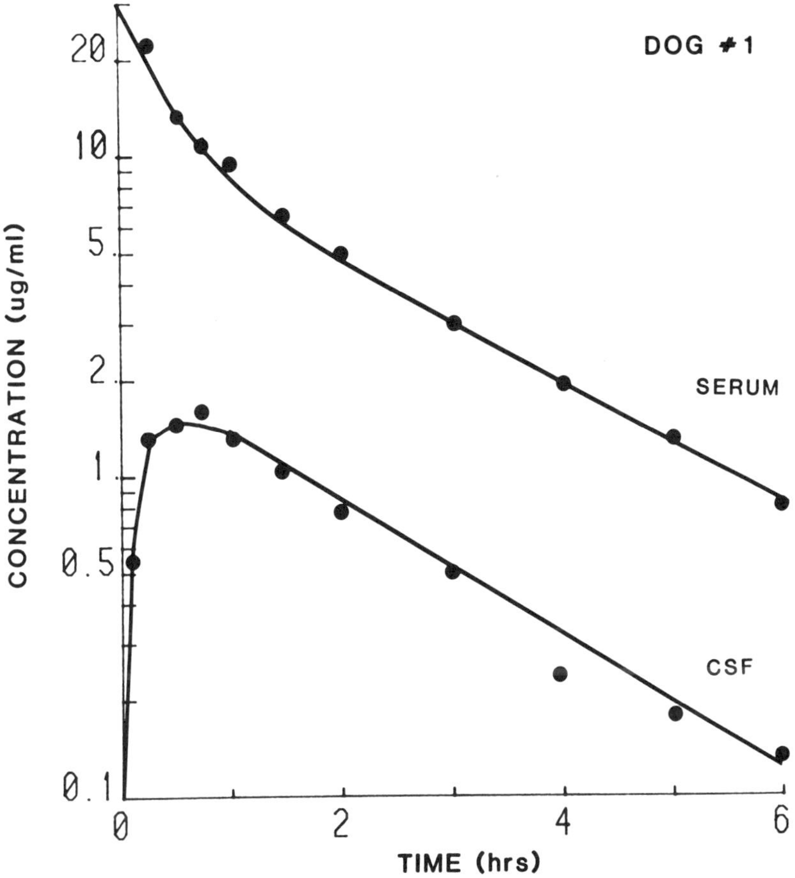

FIGURE 11-7. Cimetidine serum and CSF concentration in a dog after a 22 mg/kg intravenous dose of cimetidine. The peak CSF concentration of cimetidine was 1.6 μg/ml, and the peak occurred at 0.75 hr after the IV bolus dose. Reprinted from Ziemniak et al. (97), with permission.

CSF entry of cimetidine mediated primarily by passive diffusion. In Figure 11-8 the mean ± SD CSF time course is shown for cimetidine. The CSF half-life of 2.7 ± 1.5 hours was measured. Detectable quantities of cimetidine metabolites were not found in dog CSF. To evaluate the extent of CSF penetration, the area of distribution (R_{CSF}) was calculated from the ratio of CSF–serum AUC. In dogs, the area of distribution rates of cimetidine ranged from 0.11 to 0.17 with a mean of 0.125, as shown in Table 11-12.

The relationship between serum and CSF concentrations of cimetidine in the postdistributive phase (samples taken at least 1.5 hr after dosing) is shown in Figure 11-9. Shown for comparison are predicted relationships based on

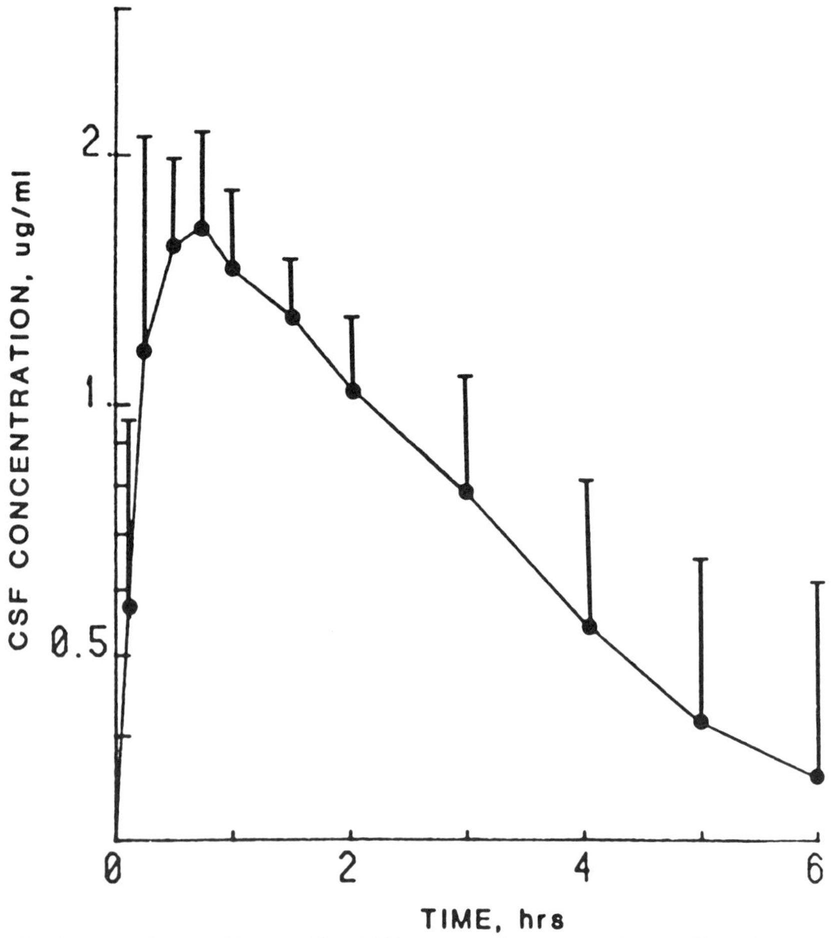

FIGURE 11-8. Mean ± SD cimetidine CSF concentrations versus time profile in four dogs after a 22 mg/kg intravenous dose. Reprinted from Ziemniak et al. (97), with permission.

pH partitioning and serum protein binding. The experimental values were clearly lower than those predicted by either pH or protein binding.

The experimental finding of a CSF–serum ratio of 0.125 was described using equation 4, assuming a rapid influx/efflux clearance of 33 ml/hr, the physiologic rate of bulk flow 3.0 ml/hr, and by the assumption of active removal with a clearance of 220 ml/hr.

Discussion

During the initial toxicologic studies, the dog was noted to metabolize cimetidine similarly to human beings (101). The present study confirms these findings and demonstrates further similarities between dogs and human beings.

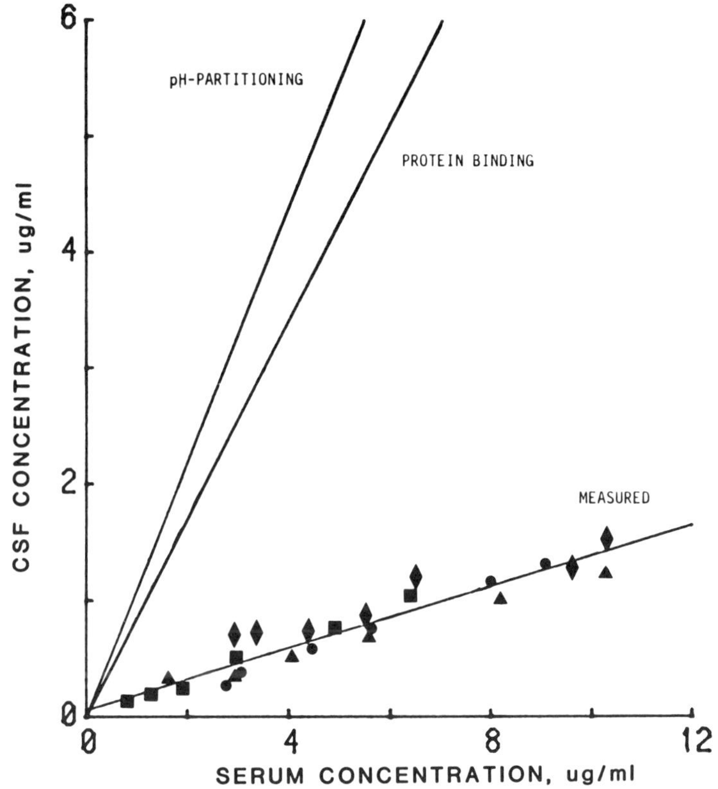

FIGURE 11-9. Measured and predicted CSF to serum relationships in four dogs. Both pH partitioning and protein binding overestimated cimetidine partitioning in dogs. Reprinted from Ziemniak et al. (97), with permission.

Cimetidine penetrates the intact blood brain barrier in both dogs and human beings. Maximum CSF concentrations in the dog are reached within 1 hour after intravenous bolus administration, a time in agreement with the time of maximum neurologic impairment observed in patients with mental confusion (45,74). The extent of cimetidine penetration in the dog, as judged by post-distributive CSF–serum concentration ratio, is also similar to that seen in normal human beings (45,81). In dogs, the rate of cimetidine elimination from the CSF parallels the decline of serum concentrations. Cimetidine sulfoxide does not appear to be formed in the CSF.

The multiple CSF sampling techniques employed in this study provide a time-averaged assessment of cimetidine CSF uptake. Therefore, a CSF penetration calculated from the ratio of CSF–serum AUC represents an apparent value. This ratio is not an actual measurement of the amount of drug entering the CSF, but it does normalize the CSF concentrations for differences in serum concentration. Provided that no dose dependence is present, it allows comparisons between individuals.

Protein binding and pH partitioning have been shown to influence the uptake of some compounds into the CSF (100,103); both overestimate the experimental data for cimetidine CSF partitioning in both dogs and human beings.

Cimetidine has minimal protein binding, is a relatively small molecule (MW 257), and is lipophilic (octanol–water, 2.5). Penetration should be excellent based on these characteristics, but, as shown in Figure 11-9, neither factor can adequately explain the experimental data.

Passive diffusion requires that the area under the unbound serum concentration time curve must equal the area under the unbound tissue concentration curve. For cimetidine, whose serum binding is minimal, the CSF–serum area ratio should approach unity if diffusion is the sole determinant of partitioning. If the ratio is significantly less than 1, factors other than passive diffusion must be involved (103).

Equation 6 incorporates the factors that may influence CSF partitioning. Any possible explanation for the lower-than-predicted cimetidine CSF concentrations must include the role of bulk flow on CSF removal, as has been demonstrated in the case of theophylline (105). A 20-kg dog has about 16 ml of CSF, and the half-life for CSF turnover is approximately 2 hr (105,106), which corresponds to a removal rate of 3.0 ml/hr. This relatively rapid CNS turnover lowers CSF cimetidine concentrations by continuous dilution. The clearance for CSF bulk flow (3.0 ml/hr) was entered into equation four, and Cl_{AT} and Cl_{M} were assumed to be negligible and the partition ratio of 0.125 was used. These values in equation 6 estimated passive clearances in or out of the CSF to be 0.43 ml/hr. A passive clearance of 0.43 ml/hr is inconsistent with the observed CSF peak at one hour and an estimated transfer constant of 2.1 hr^{-1}, and the volume of the CSF space (16 ml in dogs). If, to obtain a partition ratio of 0.125, one assumes that distribution clearance in and out of the CSF are equal, the denominator in equation 4 must be eightfold greater than the numerator, suggesting the involvement of other elimination routes. If the CSF–serum ratios are corrected for protein binding, and no binding is assumed in the CSF, a ratio of 0.15 is obtained instead of the anticipated 1.0, if the membrane is freely permeable. The two possibilities include CNS metabolism and active removal. The experimental design of our study allows only a crude discrimination between these two possible explanations, although the lack of detectable cimetidine metabolites in the CSF favors active removal as the major component.

Subsequent studies were done by Whittico and Giacomini (107). These authors injected cimetidine and insulin into the CSF of rats and measured its rate of removal. Using this technique, they estimated a cimetidine clearance that was six times greater than the rate of bulk flow plus passive diffusion out. This value closely approximates the findings in our study and is almost identical when one adjusts for serum protein binding. Thus, active removal from CSF appears to be the primary reason why CSF–serum cimetidine ratios are not unity. These findings argue strongly that the effect of hepatic disease is to depress the rate of active cimetidine removal, rather than to accelerate the rate of influx through a disruption of the blood-brain barrier.

THE EFFECTS OF DISEASE ON CIMETIDINE CNS EFFECTS

Although the disease-dependent pharmacokinetic and toxicologic profile of cimetidine is becoming clearer, the exact mechanism of the cimetidine-associated changes in mental status is still unknown. Histamine is clearly a CNS neurotransmitter depressant effect on the reticular activating system (108). Histamine receptors have been located in multiple areas of the CNS, including the hippocampus (109) and vestibular nuclei (110). The major mental status alterations observed with cimetidine are usually stimulative, consisting of tremors, apprehension, restlessness, and disorientation. It therefore seems reasonable that some of the cimetidine effect could be a primary CNS H_2-receptor blocking effect, and there is some experimental evidence to support this concept (111). Other factors, as yet undefined, must also be at play, however, since other H_2 blockers, like ranitidine and famotidine, also cross the blood-brain barrier and are even more potent inhibitors of H_2 receptors. Yet neither of these newer compounds appears to be a more potent CNS toxin than cimetidine. In view of these data, potential factors that may also be involved in mental status changes include cimetidine metabolites, a non H_2-receptor blocking effect of the drug; effects of the imidazole nucleus rather than of H_2-blockade, or disease modulation of the receptor site itself. At least part of the story appears to be a disease-related suppression of active removal from the central nervous system, as suggested by CSF accumulation in liver disease. Other endogenous amines accumulate in CSF of liver disease patients, among them glutamine (112).

The question arises whether cimetidine should be stopped when mental status changes. The answer seems to lie in clinical judgment made after considering the reason for using cimetidine, the type and degree of mental status alteration, the dose being used, and the need for cimetidine to control gastric pH. For reasons given above, a blood level determination in a critically ill patient may be of little value in determining whether a mental status alteration is related to cimetidine because of the disease-related variance affecting CNS penetration and the relationship between concentration and effect. This perspective can be corrected using the disease-dependent ranges in Table 11-11. When blood levels are interpreted in this manner, they incorporate an understanding of the subdisciplines of toxicokinetics and toxicodynamics, and apply both to improve our understanding of this interesting class of compounds.

REFERENCES

1. T. A. Grimson. Reactions to cimetidine. Lancet *1,* 858 (1977).
2. J. C. Delaney and M. Ravey. Cimetidine and mental confusion. Lancet *2,* 512 (1977).
3. T. J. Robinson and T. O. Mulligan. Cimetidine and mental confusion. Lancet *2,* 719 (1977).
4. W. Grave, J. H. S. M. Nadorp, and J. J. M. H. Rutten. Cimetidine and renal failure. Lancet *2,* 719–720 (1977).
5. N. Menzies-Gow. Cimetidine and mental confusion. Lancet *2,* 928 (1977).
6. M. A. McMillen, D. Ambis, and J. H. Siegel. Cimetidine and mental confusion. New Eng. J. Med. 298, 284–285 (1978).
7. C. W. Quap. Confusion: An adverse reaction to cimetidine therapy. Drug Intell. Clin. Pharm. *12,* 121 (1978).
8. T. R. Vickery. Cimetidine reaction. Drug Intell. Clin. Pharm. *12,* 242 (1978).
9. C. A. Wood, M. L. Isaacson, and M. S. Hibbs. Cimetidine and mental confusion. J. Am. Med. Assoc. *239*(24), 2550 (1978).
10. S. K. Agarwal. Cimetidine and visual hallucinations. J. Am. Med. Assoc. *240*(3), 214 (1978).
11. M. L. Levine. Cimetidine-induced coma in cirrhosis of the liver. J. Am. Med. Assoc. *240*(12), 1238 (1978).
12. J. B. Spears. Cimetidine and mental confusion. Am. J. Hosp. Pharm. *35,* 1035 (1978).
13. M. E. Edmonds, R. F. U. Ashford, M. K. Brenner, and A. Saunders. Cimetidine: Does neurotoxicity occur? Report of three cases. J. Royal Soc. Med. *72,* 172–175 (1979).
14. C. C. Barnhart and C. L. Bowden. Toxic psychosis with cimetidine. Am. J. Psych. *135*(5), 725–726 (1979).
15. J. R. Graham. Psychotic reaction to cimetidine, presumably an idiosyncracy. Med. J. Aust. *2,* 491–492 (197).
16. S. A. Klotz and B. F. Kay. Cimetidine and agranulocytosis. Ann. Int. Med. *88*(4), 579–580 (1978).
17. W. J. K. Cumming and J. B. Foster. Cimetidine-induced brainstem dysfunction. Lancet *1,* 1096 (1978).
18. G. A. Arneson. More on toxic psychosis and cimetidine. Am. J. Psych. *136*(10), 1348–1349 (1979).
19. S. R. Mogelnicki, J. L. Waller, and D. C. Finlayson. Physostigmine reversal of cimetidine-induced mental confusion. J. Am. Med. Assoc. *241*(8), 826–827 (1979).
20. B. J. Kimelblatt, F. Cerra, G. Calleri, M. J. Berg, M. A. McMillen, and J. J. Schentag. Dose and serum concentration relationships in cimetidine-associated mental confusion. Gastroenterol. *78,* 791–795 (1980).
21. N. J. Basavaraju, G. Wolf-Klein, F. A. Silverstone, and L. S. Libow. Cimetidine-induced mental confusion in the elderly. New York State J. Med. *20,* 1287–1288 (1980).
22. W. L. Russel and L. M. Lopez. Cimetidine-induced mental status changes: A case report and literature review. Am. J. Hosp. Pharm. *37,* 1667–1671 (1980).
23. W. W. Weddington, A. E. Muelling, H. A. Moosa, C. P. Kimball, and R. R. Rowlett. Cimetidine toxic reactions masquerading as delirium tremens. J. Am. Med. Assoc. *245*(10), 1058–1059 (1981).

24. C. Gorden. Differential diagnosis of cimetidine-induced delirium. Psychosomatics *22*(3), 251–252 (1981).
25. J. Totte, S. Schappe, R. Verkerk, H. Neels, M. VanHaeverbeek, S. Smith, and T. J. Rousea. Neurological dysfunction associated with abnormal levels of cimetidine metabolite. Lancet *1*, 1047 (1981).
26. M. Sonnenblick, A. J. Rosen, and N. Weissberg. Neurological and psychiatric side effects of cimetidine: Report of three cases with review of the literature. Grad. Med. J. *58*, 415–418 (1982).
27. B. VanSweden, and H. A. C. Kamphuisen. Cimetidine neurotoxicity: EEG and behavior aspects. Eur. Neurol. *23*, 300–305 (1984).
28. J. P. H. Barbier and J. F. Hirsch. Confusion mentale chez un malade traité par la cimetidine. Nouv. Presse Méd. *7*, 1484 (1978).
29. S. C. Yudofsky, G. Ahern, and R. Brockman. Agitation, disorientation, and hallucinations in patients on cimetidine. A report of three cases and literature review. Gen. Hosp. Psych. *3*, 233–236 (1980).
30. J. R. Pierce Jr. Case report of cimetidine-associated depression and loss of libido in a woman. Am. J. Med. Sci. *286*(3), 31–34 (1983).
31. J. W. Jefferson. Central nervous system toxicity of cimetidine: A case of depression. Am. J. Psych. *136*(3), 346 (1979).
32. M. K. Crowder and J. K. Pate. A case report of cimetidine-induced depressive syndrome. Am. J. Psych. *137*(11), 1451 (1980).
33. R. F. Billings, S. W. Tang, and V. M. Rakoff. Depression associated with cimetidine. Can. J. Psych. *26*, 260–261 (1981).
34. J. P. Petite and F. Bloch. Syndrome dépressif au cours d'un traitement par la cimetidine. Nouv. Presse Méd. *8*(15), 1260 (1979).
35. L. E. Adler, L. Sadja, and G. Wilets. Cimetidine toxicity manifested as paranoia and hallucinations. Am. J. Psych. *137*(9), 1112–1113 (1980).
36. H. G. Kinnell and A. Webb. Confusion associated with cimetidine. Br. Med. J. *2*, 1438 (1979).
37. J. P. Titus. Cimetidine-induced mania in depressed patients. J. Clin. Psych. *44*(7), 267–268 (1983).
38. J. Johnson and S. Bailey. Cimetidine and psychiatric complications. Br. J. Psych. 134, 315–316 (1979).
39. A. B. Atkinson, J. J. Brown, A. F. Lever, D. McAreavey, J. I. S. Robertson, P. O. Behan, I. D. Melville, and A. I. Weir. Neurological dysfunction in two patients receiving captopril and cimetidine. *Lancet 1*, 36–37 (1980).
40. T. J. Walls. Pearce, Venables. Motor neuropathy associated with cimetidine. Br. Med. J. 281, 974–975 (1980).
41. M. J. Kushner. Chorea and cimetidine. Ann. Int. Med. *96*(1), 126 (1982).
42. D. N. Bateman, P. Bevan, B. P. Longley, F. Mastaglia, and I. Wandless. Cimetidine-induced postural and action tremor. J. Neurol. Neurosurg. Psych. *44*, 94 (1981).
43. C. E. Handler, C. P. Besse, and A. O. Wilson. Extra pyramidal and cerebellar syndrome with encephalopathy associated with cimetidine. Post Grad. Med. J. *58*, 527–528 (1982).
44. A. M. Lam and J. A. Parkin. Cimetidine and prolonged post-operative somnolence. Can. Anaesth. Soc. J. *28*(5), 450–452 (1981).
45. J. J. Schentag, F. B. Cerra, G. Calleri, E. DeGlopper, J. Q. Rose, and H. Bernhard. Pharmacokinetic and clinical studies in patients with cimetidine-associated mental confusion. Lancet *1*, 177–181 (1979).
46. K. J. Isselbachaer, R. D. Adams, E. Braunwald, R. G. Petersdorf, and J. D. Wilson, eds. *Harrison's Principles of Internal Medicine*. 9th ed. McGraw-Hill Book Company, New York (1980).

47. D. C. Taylor, P. R. Cressell, and D. C. Barlett. The metabolism and elimination of cimetidine, a histamine H_2-receptor antagonist, in the rat, dog, and man. Drug Metab. Disp. *6,* 21–29 (1978).
48. W. L. Burland, W. A. M. Duncan, T. Hesslepo, J. G. Mills, P. C. Sharpe, S. J. Haggie, and J. H. Wyllie. Pharmacologic evaluation of cimetidine, a new histamine H_2-receptor antagonist, in healthy man. Br. J. Clin. Pharmacok. *2,* 481 (1975).
49. S. C. Mitchell, J. R. Idle, and R. L. Smith. The metabolism of ^{14}C-cimetidine in man. Xenobio. *12,* 283–292 (1982).
50. L. M. Gifford, M. E. Aeugle, R. M. Merson, and P. J. Tannenbaum. Cimetidine post-market outpatient surveillance program. Interim report on Phase I. J. Am. Med. Assoc. *243*(15), 1532–1535 (1980).
51. T. G. David, D. L. Pickett, and J. H. Schlosser. Evaluation of a worldwide spontaneous reporting system with cimetidine. J. Am. Med. Assoc. *243*(19), 1912–1914 (1980).
52. T. J. Humphries, R. M. Myerson, L. M. Gifford, M. E. Aeugle, M. E. Josie, S. L. Wood, and P. J. Tannenbaum. A unique postmarket outpatient surveillance program of cimetidine: Report of Phase II and final summary. Am. J. Gastroent. *79*(8), 593–596 (1984).
53. J. B. Porter, H. Jick, and D. R. Perera, J. T. Tlvisaker, and J. R. Hunter. Long-term follow-up study of cimetidine. Pharmacother. *4,* 381–384 (1984).
54. B. Simon, P. Muller, and H. Dammann. Safety profile of ranitidine. Pages 181–189 in: *Ranitidine*. A. J. Riley and P. R. Salmon, eds. Proceedings of an international symposium held in the context of the Seventh World Congress of Gastroenterology. Excerpta Medica, Amsterdam, Oxford-Princeton (1982).
55. Cimetidine and ranitidine. Editorial. Lancet *1,* 601 (1982).
56. A. C. Flind and D. Rowley-Jones. Cimetidine and ranitidine. Lancet *1,* 749 (1982).
57. J. D. Hughes, W. D. Reen, and C. S. Serjeant. Mental confusion associated with ranitidine. Med J. Aust. *2,* 12–13, (1983).
58. W. A. Davies. Mental confusion associated with ranitidine. Med. J. Aust. *10,* 478, 1983.
59. R. B. Mani, J. S. Spellon, J. H. Frank, and R. Laureno. H_2-receptors and mental confusion. Lancet *2,* 98, (1984).
60. P. H. Silverstone. Ranitidine and confusion. Lancet *1,* 1071 (1984).
61. C. M. Epstein. Ranitidine and confusion. Lancet *1,* 1071 (1984).
62. P. Bories, H. Michel, B. Duclos, J. J. Beraud, and J. Mirouze. Use of ranitidine without mental confusion in a patient with renal failure. Lancet *2,* 755 (1980).
63. S. Pedrazzoli, P. Petrin, C. Pasquali, C. Militello, C. Sperti, V. Fregonese, and G. Simini. Ranitidine reverses cimetidine-induced mental confusion in a patient with Zollinger-Ellison Syndrome. Arch. Surg. *118,* 256 (1983).
64. I. L. Smith, J. J. Schentag, and H. Bernhard. Ranitidine therapy of duodenal ulceration in a patient with hepatic encephalopathy intolerant to cimetidine. Unpublished case report (1988).
65. P. C. Sharpe and W. L. Burland. Mental confusion and H_2-receptor blockers. Lancet *2,* 924 (1980).
66. R. N. Illingworth and D. R. Jarvie. Absence of toxicity in cimetidine overdosage. Br. Med. J. *1,* 453–454 (1979).
67. R. Griffiths, R. M. Lee, and D. C. Taylor. Kinetics of cimetidine in man and experimental animals. In: W. L. Burland and M. A. Simkins eds. Proceedings of the Second International Symposium on Histamine H_2-Receptor Antagonists. Excerpta Medica, Amsterdam. (1977).
68. T. J. Meredith and G. N. Volans. Management of cimetidine overdose. Lancet *2,* 1367 (1979).

69. G. V. Gill. Cimetidine overdosage. Brit. Med. J. *2,* 370 (1979).
70. J. B. Wilson. Cimetidine overdosage. Brit. Med. J. *2,* 955 (1979).
71. A. W. A. M. VanRijthoven. Cimetidine intoxication. Lancet *2,* 370 (1979).
72. P. G. Nelson. Cimetidine and mental confusion. Lancet *2,* 928 (1977).
73. J. J. Schentag. Cimetidine associated mental confusion: Further studies in 36 severely ill patients. Therap. Drug Monitor *2,* 133–142 (1980).
74. F. B. Cerra, J. J. Schentag, M. McMillen, W. V. Karwande, G. C. Fitzgerald, and M. Leising. Mental status, the intensive care unit and cimetidine. Ann. Surg. *196*(5), 570 (1982).
75. A. Paazian, J. P. Capron, J. L. Dupas, and G. Boudin. Does cimetidine induce dizziness. Gastroenterology *79*(1), 179 (1980).
76. J. Brynskov, H. Thyssen, E. Jansen, and J. Munster-Swendsen. Cimetidine and Romberg's test. Lancet *1,* 1421 (1980).
77. E. C. Jansen, J. Brynskov, and H. H. Thyssen. Influence of ranitidine on postural stability. Lancet *1,* 55–56 (1982).
78. E. Szabadi, N. Theofilopuolos, and C. M. Bradshaw. Effects of ranitidine on psychomotor function: Comparison with cimetidine and thioridazine. Br. J. Clin. Pharmacol. *15,* 153 (1983).
79. E. Szabadi, C. M. Bradshaw, and P. Gaszner. The comparison of the effects of DL-308, a potential new neuroleptic agent, and thiordiazine on some psychological and physiological functions in healthy volunteers. Psychopharmacology *68,* 125–134 (1980).
80. D. A. Chiarmonte, and J. J. Schentag. A specific and sensitive high pressure liquid chromatographic procedure for cimetidine and creatinine. Ther. Drug Monit. *1,* 545–554 (1979).
81. J. J. Schentag, F. B. Cerra, M. Calleri, M. A. Leising, M. A. French, and H. Bernhard. Age, disease and cimetidine disposition in healthy subjects and chronically ill patients. Clin. Pharmacol. Ther. *29,* 737–743 (1981).
82. W. C. Randolph, W. L. Osborne, S. S. Walkenstein, J. W. Dubb, and R. M. Stote. High pressure liquid chromatographic analysis of cimetidine, a histamine H_2-receptor antagonist, in blood and urine. J. Pharm. Sci. *66,* 1148–1150 (1977).
83. C. M. Metzler. NONLIN: A computer program for parameter estimation in nonlinear situations. Technical Report No. 7292/69/7292/005. The Upjohn Company, Kalamazoo, MI, November 25, 1969.
84. M. Gibaldi and D. Perrier. Drugs and the pharmaceutical sciences. Pages 119–125 in: *Pharmacokinetics.* J. Swarbrick, ed. Marcel Dekker, Inc., New York (1975).
85. S. S. Walkenstein, J. W. Dubb, W. C. Randolph, W. J. Westlake, R. M. Stote, and A. P. Intoccia. Bioavailability of cimetidine in man. Gastroenterology *74,* 360–365 (1978).
86. E. Burgess, R. E. Cutler, and A. D. Blair. Cimetidine pharmacokinetics in hemodialysis patients and inhibition of creatinine secretion in healthy subjects. Clin. Pharmacol. Ther. *27,* 247 (1980).
87. K. W. Ma, D. C. Brown, D. S. Masler, and S. E. Silvis. Effects of renal failure on blood levels of cimetidine. Gastroenterology *74,* 473–477 (1978).
88. A. Somogyi, H. G. Rohner, and R. Gugler. Pharmacokinetics and bioavailability of cimetidine in gastric and duodenal ulcer patients. Clin. Pharmacokinet. *5,* 84–94 (1980).
89. A. Redolfi, E. Borgogelli, and E. Lodola. Eur. J. Pharmacol. *15,* 257–261 (1979).
90. K. Siersbaek-Nielsen, J. M. Hansen, J. Kampmann, and M. Kristensen. Rapid evaluation of creatinine clearance. Lancet *1,* 1133–1134 (1971).
91. B. J. Kimelblatt, F. B. Cerra, G. Calleri, M. J. Berg, M. A. McMillen, and J. J. Schentag. Dose and serum concentration relationships in cimetidine associated mental confusion. Gastroenterology *78,* 791–795 (1980).

92. W. P. Burkard. Histamine H_2-receptor binding with ^3H-cimetidine in brain. Eur. J. Pharmacol. *50,* 449–450 (1978).
93. D. A. Kendall, J. W. Ferhany, and S. J. Enna. Properties of ^3H-cimetidine binding in rat brain membrane fractions. Life Sci. *26,* 1293–1302 (1980).
94. I. R. Smith, M. T. Cleverby, C. R. Ganellin, and K. M. Melters. Binding of ^2H-cimetidine to rat brain tissues. Agents and Actions *10,* 422–426 (1980).
96. J. M. Bonati, J. Kanto, and G. Tognoni. Clinical pharmacokinetics of CSF. Clin. Pharmacokinet. *7,* 312–335 (1982).
97. J. A. Ziemniak, R. G. Shank, J. J. Schentag. The partitioning of cimetidine into canine cerebrospinal fluid. Drug. Metab. Disp. *12,* 217–221 (1984).
98. J. A. Ziemniak, D. A. Chairmonte, and J. J. Schentag. A HPLC procedure for cimetidine, its known metabolites, and creatinine in serum and urine. *Clin. Chem. 27,* 272–275 (1981).
99. W. J. Jusko. Guidelines for collection and pharmacokinetic analysis of drug disposition data. Pages 639–680 in: *Applied Pharmacokinetics*. W. E. Evans, J. J. Schentag, and W. J. Jusko, eds. Applied Therapeutics, Inc., San Francisco, CA (1980).
100. S. I. Rapoport. *Blood Brain Barrier in Physiology and Medicine*. Raven Press, New York (1976).
101. D. C. Taylor, P. R. Cresswell, and D. C. Bartlett. The metabolism and elimination of cimetidine, a histamine H_2-antagonist, in the rat, dog, and man. Drug Metab. Disp. *6,* 21–29 (1978).
102. I. J. Kopin, E. K. Gordon, D. C. Jimerson, and R. J. Polinsky. Relation between and cerebrospinal fluid levels of 3-methoxy-4-hydroxy-phenylglycol. Science *219,* 73–75, (1983).
103. M. A. Gonzalez, T. N. Tozer, and D. T. Chang. Nonlinear tissue disposition: Salicyclic acid in rat brain. J Pharm. Sci. *64,* 99–103 (1975).
104. R. Larsson, P. Erlanson, G. Bodemar, A. Walan, A. Bertler, L. Fransson, and B. Norlander. The pharmacokinetics of cimetidine and its sulfoxide metabolite in patients with normal and impaired renal function. Br. J. Clin. Pharmacol. *13,* 163–170 (1982).
105. M. D. Karol, P. Veng-Pedersen, and R. E. Brashear. Diffusion and flow transfer of theophylline across the blood-brain barrier: Pharmacokinetic analysis. J. Pharmacokinet. Biopharm. *11,* 273–287 (1983).
106. H. Davson. *Physiology of Cerebrospinal Fluid*. Churchill-Livingstone Press, London (1967).
107. M. T. Whittico and K. M. Giacomini. Cimetidine transport from cerebrospinal fluid to blood. Abstract 127. American Association of Pharmaceutical Scientists, November 2–6, 1986, Washington, DC.
108. J. C. Schwartz. Histamine as a transmitter in brain. Life Sci. *17*(4), 503–517 (1975).
109. G. Barbin, M. Garbarg, J. E. Schwartz, et al. Histamine synthesizing afferents to the hippocampal region. J. Neurochem. *26*(2), 259–263 (1976).
110. J. Satayavivad and E. B. Kirsten. Iontophoretic studies of histamine and histamine antagonists in the feline vestibular nuclei. Eur. J. Pharmacol. *41*(1), 17–26 (1977).
111. B. S. Sastry and J. W. Phillis. Depression of rat cerebral cortical neurons by H_1 and H_2 histamine receptor agonists. Eur. J. Pharmacol. *38*(2), 269–273 (1976).
112. B. T. Hourani, E. M. Hamlin, and T. B. Reynolds. CSF glutamine as a measure of hepatic encephalopathy. Arch. Intern. Med. *127,* 1033–2036, 1971.

Chapter 12

Gastrointestinal Toxicity: Dispositional Considerations

K. Rozman and M. J. Iatropoulos

Department of Pharmacology, Toxicology and Therapeutics,
University of Kansas Medical Center
and
Institut für Toxikologie der Gesellschaft für Strahlen-und
Umweltforschung München mbH, D-8042 Neuherberg,
Federal Republic of Germany
and
American Health Foundation
American Standard Testing Bureau

INTRODUCTION

Pharmacokinetics describe the time course of a compound in an organism as affected by absorption, distribution, biotransformation, and excretion, whereas pharmacodynamics examine the biochemical and physiological interactions between a compound or its metabolites with a biological system. One important goal of therapeutic intervention is specificity of the pharmacologic action of a drug at a receptor site. Often, there is a good correlation between amount (dose) or concentration of a drug in plasma and tissues and the desired pharmacologic effect, although this is not always the case.

Toxicokinetics usually do not differ from pharmacokinetics except that they are broader in scope since any compound at some dose will have a toxic effect, whereas relatively few chemicals will exert a pharmacologic effect. In contrast to pharmacodynamics, toxicodynamics—in particular those involving the gut—are more often than not unrelated or not directly related to plasma concentrations of the toxic agent. Nevertheless, in spite of the enormous complexity of the gastrointestinal (GI) tract, it is possible to describe the toxicokinetics and to understand the toxicodynamics of substances, provided that considerations are based on sound biology.

DISCUSSION

Toxic agents may cause acute or chronic injury in the GI tract by local or systemic effects (Fig. 12-1). In humans, nausea and vomiting are the most sensitive signs of GI toxicity. Both symptoms may be caused by local or systemic action of toxicants; the former involves direct action on the chemoreceptor trigger zone of the brain, and the latter is a result of vagal or sympathetic stimulation in the stomach or the small intestine (1). Similarly, diarrhea and constipation may have local (e.g., osmotic imbalance, inhibition of intestinal smooth muscle) or systemic (e.g., modification of parasympathetic or sympathetic nerve function) origin (2). Histopathologic manifestations of toxicity may also arise as a result of a combination of local and systemic toxic insult(s). Degenerative, necrotic, inflammatory, ulcerative, and proliferative lesions are the most common injuries in the GI tract (3,4).

Compared to other organs and tissues, the GI tract displays an enormous functional, morphological, and biochemical diversity. Based primarily on morphology, the gut is divided into numerous segments, as shown in Figure 12-2. Toxic agents may be chewed and swallowed with or without food acted upon by saliva. This phase of digestion is rapid, and if toxic injury occurs, it is usually acute in nature, such as burns and other forms of denudation of the mucosa. Although chronic injuries are not uncommon in the buccal cavity and the esophagus, their toxicodynamic origin is obscure. Also, absorption may occur in the mouth, but the extent of this process for most compounds is thought to be small. Ingested material entering the stomach is acted upon by digestive enzymes and the strongly acidic environment. Again, absorption of chemicals may occur in the stomach, but absorption is generally considered of little importance for most chemicals. Since contents (depending on the constituents) may remain in the stomach for several hours, this organ is one of the most frequent targets of both acute and chronic injury.

Stomach contents released through the pylorus are neutralized and mixed with digestive juices of the liver, pancreas, and duodenum at a slightly alkaline pH. While digestion continues, nutrients and many xenobiotics are rapidly absorbed in the duodenum and jejunum, even though transit through this portion of the gut is rapid ($t_{1/2} \sim 20$ min) (5,6).

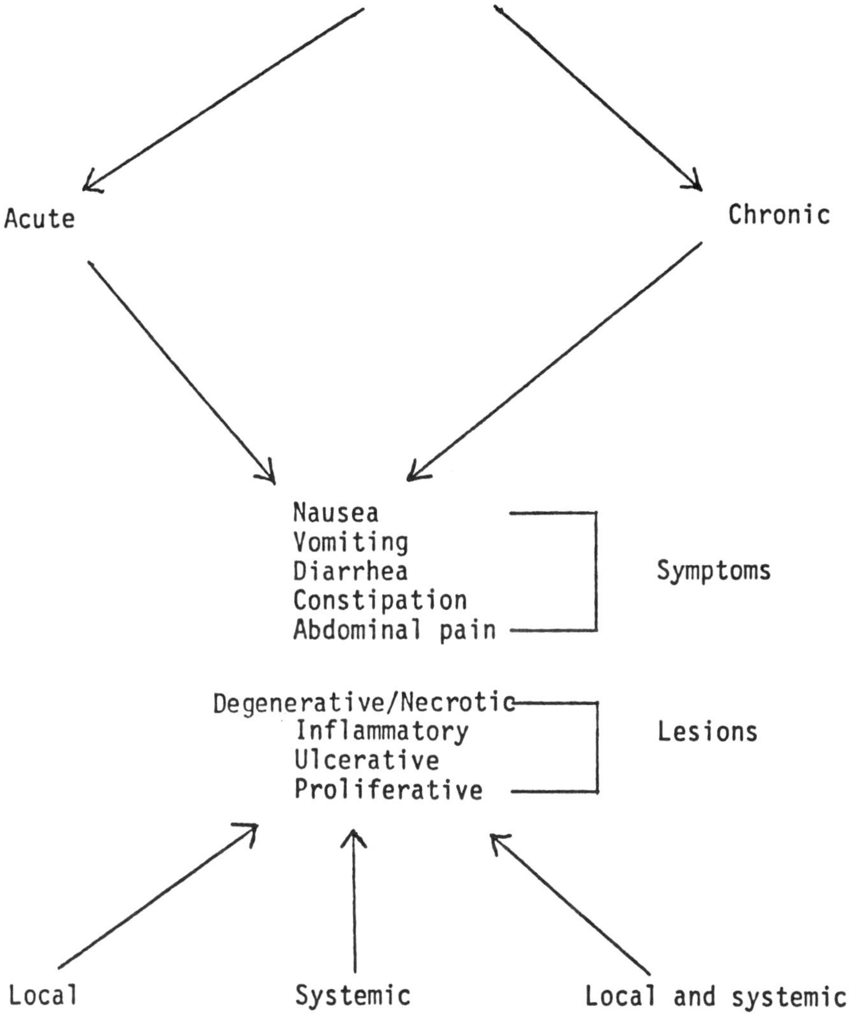

FIGURE 12-1. Gastrointestinal toxicity.

Xenobiotics absorbed in the intestine (except those absorbed from the lower part of the rectum) may or may not undergo biotransformation in the intestinal mucosa and will be either reexcreted into the lumen or transported to the liver by the portal system. In turn, the liver may biotransform these compounds to more or less toxic metabolites. Depending on the molecular weight, the liver may release the parent compound or its metabolites into the systemic circulation or into the bile (7). In either event, the bile or the arterial blood may transport the toxic substance back to the intestine.

The controversy about the relative importance of these two pathways for

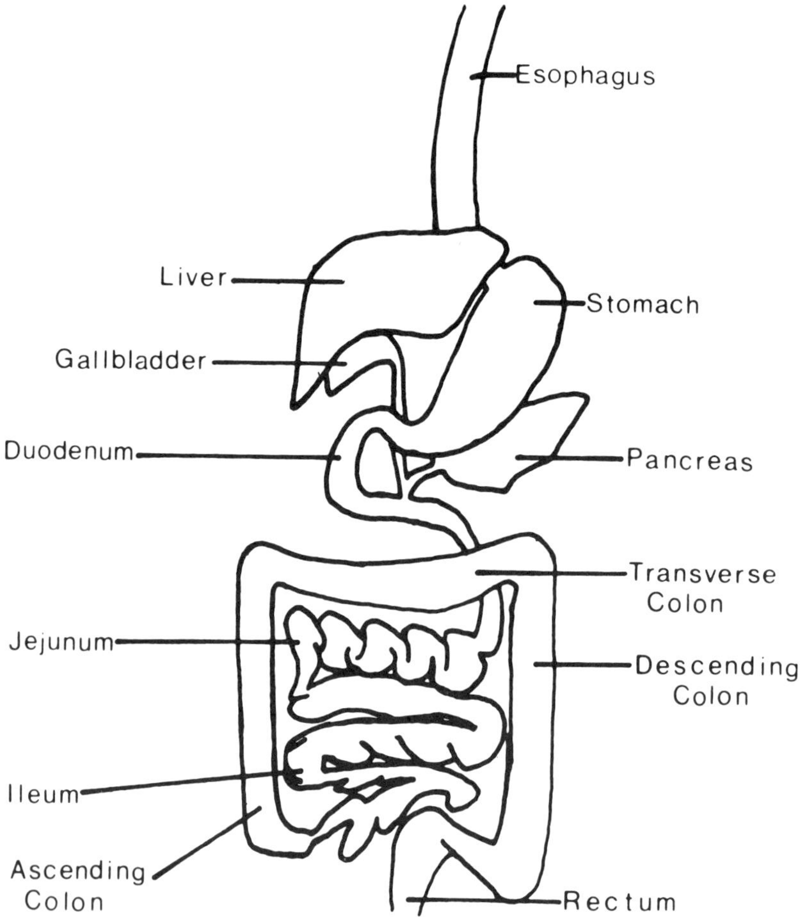

FIGURE 12-2. Schematic representation of the gastrointestinal tract.

xenobiotic toxicity in the gut has not yet been resolved (8). However, it seems that the biliary pathway may be a more frequent contributing factor to toxicity, because duodenal lesions occur often with compounds undergoing enterohepatic circulation. Furthermore, intestinal bypass surgery yields no toxicity with some xenobiotics at the site bypassed (9).

Absorption of highly lipophilic chemicals may be viewed only in the context of lipid absorption (10). This entails absorption via the lymphatics, which represents a bypassing of the liver. Another important feature of the small intestine is the extemely large surface and the rapid turnover of enterocytes (see for review 11). This may represent as much as 10 g of exfoliated cells per day in the rat (12). The desquamated cells are digested, and most of the cell constituents are reabsorbed in the lower small intestine (primarily in the ileum). These cells may also contain xenobiotics or their active metabolites, which may be absorbed and exert toxicity in the intestinal mucosa or systemically.

GI contents passing through the ileocecal valve will remain in the large intestine for 24 hr and longer, being churned and mixed by paristalsis and antiperistalsis (see for review 13). The most prominent feature of the large intestine is the large number of microorganisms (14), which may constitute 30–42 percent of fecal dry matter, although several other factors (nonabsorbed material, intestinal excretion, absorption of water) also contribute to the formation of feces (13). The intestinal flora as well as the mucosa of the large intestine are metabolically highly active biological systems, which may decisively influence the toxicity of xenobiotics (14,15,16).

In light of this multitude of interactions in the GI tract, a few examples shall demonstrate the importance of careful biological considerations for the disposition and toxicity of xenobiotics in the GI tract.

Example 1

Many compounds pass the GI tract with little or no absorption, biotransformation, or interaction with the gut flora. Nevertheless, such compounds may alter or cause intestinal and systemic toxicity, directly or indirectly. For example, xylitol, a very slowly absorbable polyol, causes a pronounced enlargement of the cecum, presumably by altering gastric emptying and, more importantly, by affecting the osmolarity of the large intestinal contents (17).

Charcoal, which is essentially nonabsorbable, does not exert any observable toxicity in the gut but significantly alters the disposition and toxicity of other compounds. Table 12-1 shows that the urinary excretion of paracetamol sulfate is significantly reduced by pretreatment with charcoal, indicating interruption of its enterophepatic circulation.

Cholestyramine is a cationic resin, which can cause toxicity in the gut as

Table 12-1. Reduced Reabsorption: Urinary Excretion of Paracetamol Sulfate in Rats[a] Treated with Activated charcoal or Cholestyramine

Treatment	Paracetamol Sulfate (% of dose in 24 hr)
Control	70.6 ± 4.0[a]
Activated charcoal	55.3 ± 3.4[b]
Cholestyramine	39.3 ± 1.5[b]

Note: Rats were dosed IV with 100 mg/kg paracetamol 2 hr after 1 g/kg charcoal or cholestyramine orally.

[a]Mean $\pm$ SE ($n = 4$).

[b]Significantly different from controls; $p < 0.05$.

well as systemic toxicity. Constipation is nearly always associated with cholestyramine treatment, and is thought to be due to altered water absorption as a result of a disturbance of electrolyte absorption (sodium and chloride) and secretion (potassium and bicarbonate). In addition, cholestyramine may trap certain acidic vitamins in the gut lumen and cause systemic toxicity in the form of various vitamin-deficiency syndromes. Moreover, this resin can significantly alter the disposition of other toxicants such as paracetamol and pentachlorophenol (Table 12-1 and 12-2). For example, cholestyramine reduces the urinary excretion of paracetamol sulfate from 70 to 40 percent of the dose, indicating prevention of intestinal reabsorption. In pentachlorophenol, a predominantly urinary excretion is changed into nearly complete fecal excretion as a result of interruption of the enterophepatic circulation. Since the bile could not entirely account for total excretion in cholestyramine-treated animals, it is possible that a nonbiliary process is also affected (Table 12-1). These considerations illustrate that numerous toxicodynamic effects in the gut are possible without measurable plasma levels of the causative agent.

Example 2

Other compounds are neither absorbed nor biotransformed to any measurable extent by the mucosa or the intestinal flora. Nevertheless, they may exert profound toxicodynamic effects locally or systemically. One such compound is pectin, which induces various enzymes of the gut flora (12-3). Induction of nitrate reductase activity results in a nearly 10-fold increase in blood methemoglobin levels after a single dose of $NaNO_3$ (19). Table 12-4 shows changes in the number of dimethylhydrazin-induced colorectal cancer

Table 12-2. Increased Excretion: Urinary, Fecal, and Biliary Excretion of Pentachlorophenol in Rhesus Monkeys Treated with Cholestyramine

Route of Excretion	Pentachlorophenol (% of dose)[b]	
	Controls	Cholestyramine
Urine	35.4 ± 5.7[c]	5.0 ± 0.7[d]
Feces	2.8 ± 0.5	54.4 ± 10.4[d]
Urine + feces	38.2 ± 6.2	59.4 ± 11.1
Bile[e]	70.4 ± 16.8	51.8 ± 9.8

[a]Monkeys were dosed with 50 mg/kg pentachlorophenol orally; cholestyramine treatment (4% of diet) was started 24 hr later.

[b]Excreted during days 2–6 after dosing.

[c]Mean ± SE (n = 3).

[d]Significantly different from controls, $p < 0.05$.

[e]Bile was collected for 24 hr and reinfused during the subsequent 24-hr period.

Table 12-3. Cecal Microbial Enzyme Activities in Rats Fed a Diet With or Without Pectin

Enzyme activity (μmol/hr/g content)	Controls	Pectin
β-Glucuronidase	14.5 ± 1.5[a]	27.1 ± 1.9[b]
Nitrate reductase	8.0 ± 1.1	47.4 ± 4.7[b]

Note: Modified from Rowland et al. (18).

The animals were fed a purified diet with (50 pectin/kg diet) or without pectin.

[a]Mean ± SE (n = 12).

[b]Significantly different from controls; $p < 0.05$.

in rats fed a basal or a pectin-containing diet. Weisburger (9) showed that dimethylhydrazin-induced colon cancer is caused by liberation of the proximate carcinogens methylazomethanol and methylazoxymethanol from the respective glucuronides by bacterial β-glucuronidase. Thus, induction of this enzyme by pectin (Table 12-3) was suggested by Bauer et al. (20) as the explanation for the significantly elevated number of large intestinal tumors (Table 12-4) in their experiment.

A related example shows in a different context the critical role of the intestinal flora in the toxicity of a xenobiotic, cycasin (methylazoxymethanol-β-glucoside). This is a poorly absorbed glucoside, which is a colon carcinogen when given orally but not when administered subcutaneously or intraperitoneally. More importantly, it does not cause tumors in gnotobiotic animals, indicating that the microflora is required for the activation of this compound. It is known that the aglycon of cycasin, methylazoxymethanol, causes duodenal tumors when administered orally. Similarly, it has been documented that β-glucosidase (the enzyme responsible for the hydrolysis of cycasin) is absent in the small intestine but abundant in the flora of the large intestine. The combination of this experimental evidence allows the

Table 12-4. Average Number of Dimethylhydrazine-induced Colorectal Tumors in Rats Fed a Basal or a Pectin-containing Diet

Diet	Number of Rats[a] with Tumors	Number of Tumors per Rat
Basal	35	2.0 ± 1.6[b]
Pectin	39	3.5 ± 2.0[c]

Note: Modified from Bauer et al. (20).

[a]Total number of rats per group is 40.

[b]Mean ± SD.

[c]Significantly different from basal diet; $p < 0.001$.

conclusion that microbial β-glucosidase is responsible for the activation of cycasin to a topically acting toxic agent.

Example 3

Loperamide and ethinylestradiol are prototypes of compounds, for which the gastrointestinal mucosa represents the key factor in their toxicodynamics.

Loperamide is an antidiarrheal drug that inhibits intestinal motility. Increasing doses result in constipation. It is known that the bioavailability of this compound is very limited. Nevertheless, most of an oral dose is excreted in feces as metabolites. The bile and the intestinal flora were excluded as potential sources of fecal metabolites, and intestinal slices indicated the possibility of mucosal biotransformation (21). Studies with the everted intestinal sack technique confirmed the hypothesis that the intestinal mucosa plays a pivotal role in the disposition of this compound. In this in vitro system, loperamide did not penetrate to the serosal side. However, both biotransformation in the tissue and excretion of metabolites back to the luminal site was extensive (Table 12-5).

Schwenk and colleagues (22) studied intestinal absorption and first-pass biotransformation of ethinylestradiol in situ. This technique is more suitable to investigate absorption of compounds, since blood flow is largely intact, allowing sampling of truly absorbed material.

Table 12-6 shows that ethinylestradiol is largely absorbed within 80 min, since only 9 percent of the initial 3H-activity was recovered at the end of this period in the luminal contents of the loop. The presence of more than 90 percent metabolites indicates extensive mucosal biotransformation and reexcretion back into the lumen of both the glucuronide and the sulfate. While the glucuronide seems to be transported to about the same extent in both directions, the sulfate is more readily reexcreted into the lumen than absorbed into the venous blood (Table 12-6).

Table 12-5. Absorption and Metabolism of ^{14}C-Loperamide Incubated in the Everted Intestinal Sack for 1 Hour

Region	Site	% of Dose	% Metabolites
Duodenum	Mucosal	62	43
	Tissue	38	21
	Serosal	0	—
Jejunum	Mucosal	56	37
	Tissue	44	34
	Serosal	0	—
Ileum	Mucosal	30	43
	Tissue	70	30
	Serosal	0	—

Note: Modified from Miyazaki et al. (21).

Table 12-6. Absorption and Biotransformation of ^{3}H-Ethinylestradiol During 80 min in In Situ Isolated Intestinal Loops

	% of Total Radioactivity	
Compound	Intestinal Loop	Venous Outflow
Ethinylestradiol	9	43
Ethinylestradiol glucuronide	40	54
Ethinylestradiol sulfate	51	3

Note: Modified from Schwenk et al. (22).

A toxicological problem with ethinylestradiol therapy is dose-dependent nausea. However, in chronic therapy the nausea subsides and the dose may be increased gradually. Since many estradiols are known to induce their own glucuronidation and sulfation (23,24), reduced nausea may be due to increased intestinal first-pass biotransformation of ethinylestradiol.

Example 4

Highly lipophilic compounds such as hexachlorobenzene (HCB), 2,3,7,8-tetrachlorodibenzo-p-dioxin (TCDD), mineral oil, and hexadecane display very different interactions in the gut from those discussed so far. These compounds when administered with the diet or in an oily vehicle, are very efficiently absorbed (via the lymphatics) from the small intestine, and are not known to affect the microflora. Moreover, without regard to the route of administration, they cause hyperplasia of the intestinal mucosa throughout the GI tract. This finding indicates that HCB and TCDD may exert their toxicity in the gut by reaching the site of action through the systemic circulation. In addition, these compounds do not require metabolic activation; rather, it is the parent compound that exerts the toxic effect.

The disposition of these chemicals is different from commonly described pathways in that biotransformation and subsequent urinary and biliary excretion represent minor routes of disposition, whereas fecal excretion of the parent compound is the predominant route of body clearance (Table 12-7). Furthermore, a simple calculation of the excretion of total biliary radioactivity shows that the bile cannot account for fecal excretion of HCB (Table 12-8), suggesting that sources other than the bile contribute substantially to the fecal excretion of this compound. Additional support for this contention is that bile duct ligation not only does not diminish fecal excretion of HCB, but increases it about threefold (Table 12-9). Interestingly, the same effect was observed by Sperry (25) regarding the nonbiliary excretion of endogenous lipids, indicating that not only the absorption but also the nonbiliary excretion of xenobiotics may be coupled to lipid transport. Conclusive evi-

Table 12-7. Dispositional Characteristics of 2,3,7,8-Tetrachlorodibenzo-*p*-Dioxin (TCDD) and Hexachlorobenzene (HCB) in Rats

	TCDD	HCB
Absorption	Not determined	Via lymphatics
Toxicity	Hyperplasia of the intestinal mucosa due to parent compound	Hyperplasia of the intestinal mucosa due to parent compound
Mulecular weight	322	282
Half-life in rats	31 d	26 d
Metabolism	<10%	<10%
Urinary excretion	Minor pathway	Minor pathway
Fecal excretion	>90%	>90%
Composition of fecal excretion	Unchanged TCDD	Unchanged HB
Biliary excretion	Very small	Very small
Composition of biliary excretion	Metabolites only	Metabolites only

dence for a nonbiliary source of fecal HB was obtained under physiological conditions, when rhesus monkeys were provided with complete biliary bypasses. Fecal excretion of HCB was not altered regardless of reinfusion of the monkeys' own or exogenous uncontaminated bile, showing that biliary excretion does not play any major role in the fecal excretion of this compound (Table 12-10).

The question then arose as to what is the source of fecal HCB. Cell exfoliation and exudation (transfer from blood across the mucosa into the luminal contents) are considered the two most important nonbiliary sources of fecal excretion of endogenous lipids (12). To distinguish between these two possibilities, fecal excretion of HCB was studied in partially jejunectomized or colectomized rats. Results in Table 12-11 demonstrate that the colon is a much more important source of fecal HCB than is the jejunum. The data also allow the indirect conclusion that exudation is a more important pathway of excretion than is cell exfoliation, since cell exfoliation is orders of magnitude greater in the small intestine than in the large intestine.

Other important questions relating to this intestinal excretion of lipophilic

Table 12-8. Comparison of Biliary and Fecal Excretion of Radioactivity in Rhesus Monkeys Dosed with ^{14}C-Hexachlorobenzene

	Volume (ml or g/kg per day)	Concentration (μg/kg)	Excretion (μg/kg per day)
Bile	39	0.06	2.3
Feces	15	0.42	6.1

Table 12-9. Effect of Bile Duct Ligation on the Fecal Excretion of Hexachlorobenzene

Day	Fecal Excretion of Hexachlorobenzene[a] (μg/kg per day)	
	Sham Operated	Bile Duct Ligated
1	73.4 ± 3.8[b]	162 ± 16.2[c]
2	62.7 ± 4.6	190 ± 28.5[c]
3	66.0 ± 6.3	179 ± 11.6[c]

[a]Rats were dosed with (^{14}C)hexachlorobenzene (100 mg/kg) 10 days prior to surgery.

[b]Mean ± SE (n = 3).

[c]Statistically different (p <0.05) from sham-operated controls.

Table 12-10. Effect of Bile Replacement on Fecal Excretion of Hexachlorobenzene (HCB) in Rhesus Monkeys

	Fecal Excretion of HCB (μg/kg per day)	
	Own Bile	Exogenous Bile
Monkey 1[a]	6.14 ± 1.08[b]	5.81 ± 1.04
Monkey 2[c]	22.3 ± 2.51	15.5 ± 2.22
Monkey 3[d]	118.0 ± 15.7	87.6 ± 4.34
Monkey 4[e]	189.0 ± 20.3	155.0 ± 9.77

[a]Dosed with single dose of HCB (100 mg/kg) in 1% methyl cellulose suspension.

[b]Mean ± SE of seven days.

[c]Dosed with five consecutive doses of HCB (20 mg/kg) in 1% methyl cellulose.

[d]Dosed with single dose of HCB (100 μg/kg) in olive oil solution.

[e]Dosed with five consecutive doses of HCB (20 mg/kg) in olive oil solution.

Table 12-11. Effect of Partial Jejunectomy or Colectomy on Fecal Excretion of Hexachlorobenzene (HCB) in Rats

	Fecal Excretion of HCB[a] (μg/day)
Sham-operated	8.3 ± 1.4[b]
Jejunectomized	7.3 ± 0.7
Sham-operated	10.0 ± 0.4
Colectomized	5.4 ± 0.3[c]

[a]Rats were dosed with 1.5 mg/kg ^{14}C-HCB Iv.

[b]Mean ± SE (n = 3).

[c]Significantly different from sham-operated; p <0.05.

xenobiotics are whether and by what mechanism this process may be altered. It has been shown that fecal excretion of many lipophilic chemicals may be enhanced by adding low levels of paraffins to the diet (13). Initially it was thought that the nonabsorbed portion of these hydrocarbons creates a more lipophilic environment in the large intestine and thus triggers a redistribution of HCB. However, the effect of mineral oil is much less pronounced when given by enema than when administered orally, suggesting that a mobili-

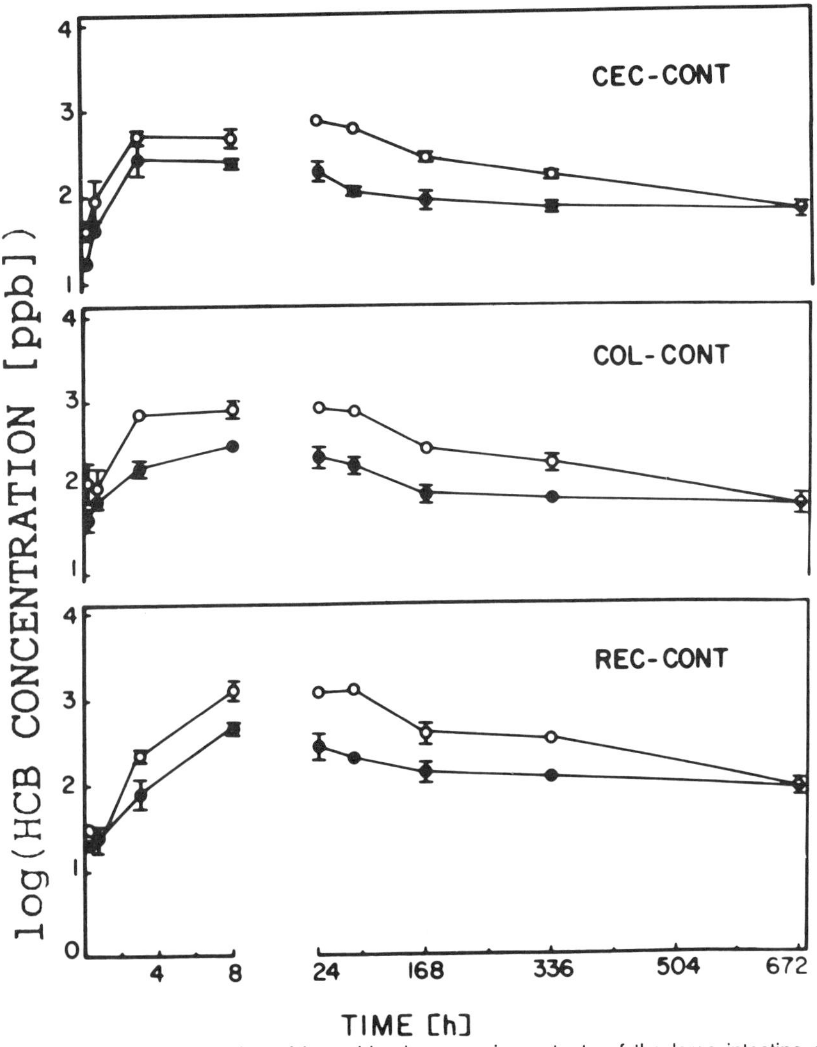

FIGURE 12-3. Concentration of hexachlorobenzene in contents of the large intestine of control (●) and hexadecane-treated (○) rats (n = 3).

zation effect from tissue stores is also involved in the enhanced nonbiliary excretion of xenobiotics (26).

Additional problems were encountered with the pharmacokinetic characterization of the intestinal excretion of xenobiotics. The usual pharmacokinetic analysis, assuming that elimination occurs from the central compartment, yielded results incompatible with the experimental data (27). However, the concentration profile of HCB in the large intestine of both untreated and paraffin-treated rats displays the characteristics of a peripheral compartment (Fig. 12-3). Since fecal excretion is the major route of HCB excretion and since the large intestine is the final site of feces formation, it is reasonable to assume that, for such compounds, elimination occurs from the peripheral rather than the central compartment (Fig. 12-4). Indeed, calculations based on this assumption according to Nagashima (28) resulted in a satisfactory description of the experimental data (26).

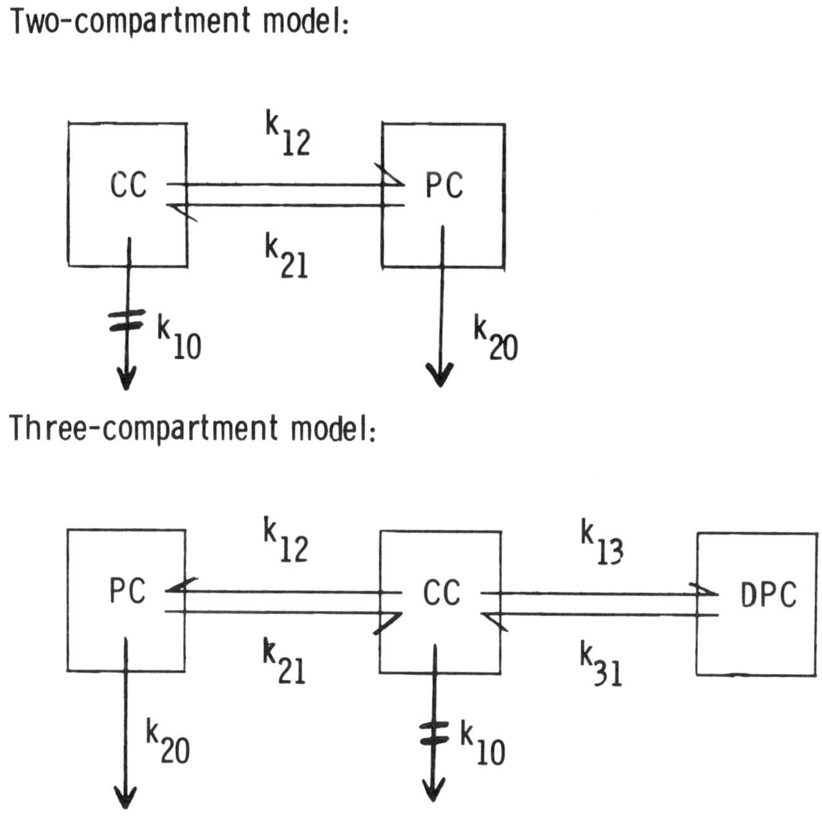

FIGURE 12-4. Two and three-compartment model for intestinal excretion of hexachlorobenzene.

CONCLUSION

This paper, using four examples, illustrates that toxicokinetic and toxicodynamic considerations in the GI tract require a careful evaluation of events in the context of the enormous complexity of this organ, which in this regard probably surpasses by far any other organ or tissue in the body. A more detailed examination of the issues raised in this report may be found in the recently published *Gastrointestinal Toxicology* (29).

REFERENCES

1. P. L. Smith. Gastrointestinal physiology. Pages 1–28 in: *Gastrointestinal Toxicology*. K. Rozman and O. Hänninen, eds. Elsevier, Amsterdam (1986).
2. V. M. K. Venho. Toxicant in the gastrointestinal tract: Drugs. Pages 363–396 in: *Gastrointestinal Toxicology*. K. Rozman and O. Hänninen, eds. Elsevier, Amsterdam (1986).
3. M. J. Iatropoulos and T. E. Davis. Ulcerative and inflammatory lesions. Pages 267–288 in: *Gastrointestinal Toxicology*. K. Rozman and O. Hänninen, eds. Elsevier, Amsterdam (1986).
4. H. J. Van Kruiningen. Proliferative lesions. Pages 289–337 in: *Gastrointestinal Toxicology*. K. Rozman and O. Hänninen, eds. Elsevier, Amsterdam (1986).
5. L. D. Scott and R. W. Summers. Correlation of contractions and transit in rat small intestine. Amer. J. Physiol. *230*, 132–137 (1976).
6. J. J. Stewart, N. W. Weibrodt, and T. F. Burks. Central and peripheral actions of morphine on intestinal transit. J. Pharmacol. Exp. Ther. *205*, 547–555 (1978).
7. P. C. Hirom, P. Millburn, and R. L. Smith. Bile and urine as complementary pathways for the excretion of foreign organic compounds. Xenobiotica *6*, 55–64 (1976).
8. E. Scheufler and K. Rozman. Industrial and environmental chemicals. Pages 397–415 in: *Gastrointestinal Toxicology*. K. Rozman and O. Hänninen, eds. Elsevier, Amsterdam (1986).
9. J. H. Weisburger. Colon carcinogens: Their metabolism and mode of action. Cancer *28*, 60–70 (1971).
10. J. S. Patton. Gastrointestinal lipid digestion. Pages 1123–1139 in: *Physiology of the Gastrointestinal Tract*. L. R. Johnson, ed. Raven Press, New York (1981).
11. M. J. Iatropoulos. Morphology of the gastrointestinal tract. Pages 246–266 in: *Gastrointestinal Toxicology*. K. Rozman and O. Hänninen, eds. Elsevier, Amsterdam (1986).
12. P. B. Cotton. Non-dietary lipid in the intestinal lumen. Gut *13*, 675–681 (1972).
13. K. Rozman. Fecal excretion of toxic substances. Pages 119–145 in: *Gastrointestinal Toxicology*. K. Rozman and O. Hänninen, eds. Elsevier, Amsterdam (1986).
14. K. Pelkonen and O. Hanninen. Interactions of xenobiotics with the gut flora. Pages 193-212 in: *Gastrointestinal Toxicology*. K. Rozman and O. Hänninen, eds. Elsevier, Amsterdam (1986).
15. R. R. Scheline. Metabolism of foreign compounds by gastrointestinal microorganisms. Pharmacol. Rev. *25*, 451–523 (1973).
16. M. Laitinen and J. B. Watkins III. Mucosal biotransformations. Pages 169–192 in: *Gastrointestinal Toxicology*. K. Rozman and O. Hänninen, eds. Elsevier, Amsterdam (1986).
17. A. Hallikainen and S. Salminen. Foods, food additives and contaminants. Pages 338–362 in: *Gastrointestinal Toxicology*. K. Rozman and O. Hänninen, eds. Elsevier, Amsterdam (1986).
18. I. R. Rowland, A. K. Mallett, and A. Wise. A comparison of five microbial enzymes

in fecal content from rats, mice and hamsters in response to dietary pectin. Toxicol. Appl. Pharmacol. *69,* 143–148 (1983).

19. A. Wise, A. K. Mallet, and I. R. Rowland. Dietary fiber, bacterial metabolism and toxicity of nitrate in the gut. Xenobiotica *12,* 111–118 (1982).
20. H. G. Bauer, N.-G. Asp, R. Oste, A. Dahlquist, and P. E. Fredlund. Effect of dietary fiber on the induction of colorectal tumors and fecal β-glucuronidase activity in the rat. Cancer Res. *39,* 3752–3756 (1979).
21. H. Miyazaki, K. Nambu, and M. Hashimoto. Loperamide in rat intestines: A unique disposition. Life Sci. *30,* 2203–2206 (1982).
22. M. Schwenk, C. Schiemenz, V. Lopez del Pinto, and H. Remmer, First pass biotransformation of ethinylestradiol in rat small intestine in situ. Naunyn-Schmiedeberg's Arch. Pharmacol. *321,* 223–225 (1982).
23. G. J. Dutton. The influence of hormones and xenobiotics on glucuronidation. Pages 135–142 in: *Glucuronidation of Drugs and Other Compounds*. G. J. Dutton, ed. CRC Press, Boca Raton, FL (1980).
24. B. W. Jakoby, R. D. Sekura, E. S. Lyon, C. L. Marcus, and J.-L. Wang, Sulfotransferases. Pages 199–228 in: *Enzymatic Basis of Detoxification*. Vol. II. W. B. Jakoby, ed. Academic Press, New York (1980).
25. W. M. Sperry. Lipid excretion IV. A study of the relationship of the bile to fecal lipids with special reference to certain problems in sterol metabolism. J. Biol. Chem. *71,* 351–378 (1926/27).
26. K. Rozman. Intestinal excretion of toxic substances. Arch. Toxicol. Suppl. 8, 87–93 (1985).
27. E. Scheufler and K. Rozman. Effect of hexadecane on the pharmacokinetics of hexachlorobenzene. Toxicol. Appl. Pharmacol. *75,* 190–197 (1984).
28. R. Nagashima, G. Levy, and R. A. O'Reilly. Comparative pharmacokinetics of coumarin anticoagulants. IV. J. Pharm. Sci. *57,* 1888–1895. (1968).
29. K. Rozman, O. Hanninen. *Gastrointestinal Toxicology* K. Rozman and O. Hänninen, eds. Elsevier, Amsterdam (1986).

Chapter 13

Renal Toxicity: Structural, Functional, Kinetic, and Dynamic Considerations

M. J. Iatropoulos

American Health Foundation
American Standard Testing Bureau

INTRODUCTION

The kidneys assume and play a central and very special role in the homeostasis of the body. They are therefore involved fundamentally in both pharmacokinetic and pharmacodynamic processes. They modulate both the definition of dosing as well as its major regulation. Maintaining the tissue integrity of the kidneys is of paramount importance. The kidneys have a very extensive cell surface comparable only to the gastrointestinal cell surface, making them vulnerable when exposed to xenobiotics.

A special dynamic interplay occurs between the structure and function of the kidneys. As organs, they are very heterogeneous. They are composed of expanding elements (extraglomerular mesangial cells), intermediate elements (intraglomerular mesangial cells), indeterminate elements (endothelial cells), and renewing elements (epithelial cells). Therefore, disuse of the kidneys can lead to atrophy, and increased functional demand to hypertrophy; nephron loss beyond a certain point can lead to continuing progression of its toxicity (1,2).

SPECIES DIFFERENCES, STRUCTURE AND FUNCTION

Lab animal species differ from humans in some major ways. In general, nephrogenesis occurs in a centrifugal pattern, with the oldest nephrons located in the juxtamedullary region and the youngest in the superficial cortex. The time at which the kidneys are fully functioning is fundamentally different in the mouse (24 days after birth), the rat (21 days), and the dog (four to five weeks) compared to the subhuman primates and human beings, in which they are fully functional at birth (3). Perhaps this developmental peculiarity is somehow connected to the urine-concentrating status of the rat and mouse (4). These two species are very good concentrators, having simple-shaped renal pelves consisting of two pyramids; human kidneys have 14. Furthermore, rats and mice possess vesicoureteral reflux, causing urine to ascend from the bladder during voiding. The long-term effects of this reflux can be substantial, both kinetically and dynamically. Young organisms of all species possess substantially more extracellular and intracellular fluid, demonstrating a more delayed mode of excretion compared to mature organisms.

To effectively conduct appropriate species extrapolation, one needs to make use of three very important common denominators that are valid across all mammals, including human beings. The first is water conservation, the second, temperature regulation, and the third, maintenance of body size (body weight plus body surface). The kidneys play a vital role in the first common denominator and an important role in maintaining body size and regulating body temperature.

Small animals usually have a faster metabolism and circulation, consume more O_2, and produce more heat than large animals. They also have a faster rate of tissue distribution (therefore a shorter tissue half-life) and cell cycles (although not as many mitoses). Gravity is directly proportional to body weight, which in turn is directly proportional to parenchymal and regulatory cell functions. Other characteristics related to body weight are as follows:

1. Weight of all organs (except brain)
2. Weight of hemoglobins/myoglobins/cytochromes
3. Blood flow of all organs
4. Rest O_2 consumption (except in brain)
5. Duration of heartbeat/breathing
6. Water intake/output
7. Nephron number/glomerular diameter
8. Renal clearance
9. Tidal volume
10. Intestinal peristalsis

11. Nitrogen/sulfur output

On the other hand, the body surface is proportional to two-thirds of the body weight. Maintenance (including metabolism) and transport functions vary directly with the body surface.

The kidney, while receiving 22 percent of the renal blood flow (Table 13-1) utilizes 7 percent of O_2, making it very vulnerable to xenobiotics causing hypoxia. From the total body water (TBW = 60%; plasma volume = 5%; extracellular volume = 20%), 66.7 percent is intracellular fluid, 25 percent is interstitial fluid, and 8.3 percent is plasma fluid. From this, only 20 percent reaches the kidney (or 5% is filtered each minute). The cortical regions receive 85 percent of the total renal blood flow, with 14 percent going to the outer medulla (5). Reduction in blood perfusion to the outer cortical regions and increased perfusion to the inner cortical regions result in a redistribution and are associated with natriuresis. It is therefore of paramount importance to keep the renal blood flow constant. That is why there are plexuses around superficial and deeper glomeruli. The medullary blood is cell poor, albumine poor, and hypertonic (enhancing the concentration of xenobiotics in the interstitium), whereas the medullary interstitium is albumin rich (5).

Utilization of nutrients is the principal determinant of solute excretion, just as the dissipation of heat is the principal determinant of water loss. Both modulate substantially the urinary water loss. The ratio of water excretion to glomerular filtration rate is similar across all species (Table 13-2), although the efficiency of water conservation is inversely related to body size (as outlined earlier), so the degree of concentration varies, inversely to the body size.

Table 13-1. Percentage of Blood Flow and O_2 Utilization in Various Organs and Tissues at Rest

Organ or Tissue	Percent Blood Flow at Rest	Percent of Utilization at Rest
Liver	27	26
Portal side	21	20
Arterial side	6	6
Kidneys	22	7
Skeletal muscle	15	18
Brain	14	19
Skin[a]	6	8
Bones	5	7
Heart	4	10
Rest	7	5

[a]At cool temperatures.

Table 13-2. Comparison Across Three Selected Species of Pertinent Body/Renal Parameters

Species	Body Weight (g)	Body Surface (cm^2)	Dose by Weight (A) (mg)	Dose by Surface (B) (mg)	Ratio = (A)/(B)	Kidney Weight (C) (g)	GFR[a] (ml/mn)	GFR/(C) (ml)/(g)	OR[b] = U^c/p^d (g)
Rat	200	325	20	14	1.43	2.56	3	1.17	8.3
Dog	12,000	5,766	1,200	248	4.82	130.00	84	0.65	5.2
Human	70,000	18,000	7,000	776	9.08	300.00	136	0.45	3.6

[a]GFR = Glomerular filtration rate.

[b]OR = Osmotic ratio.

[c]U = Urine.

[d]P = Plasma.

The cortical regions receive blood that is well oxygenated; therefore, they derive most of their energy requirements from oxidative processes. On the other hand, the energy requirements in the medulla are predominantly covered by glycolytic processes. This important difference can account for selective nephrotoxicity as well as for the correlation between activity, which is usually reversible, and toxicity, which is not (e.g., diuretic effect of ethacrynic acid vs. its direct nephrotoxicity). The major cortical substrate for metabolization is not fatty acids. The acid base state of the organism plays also an important role. In acidosis, for example, glutamine accounts for 40 percent, whereas in alkalosis, lactate contributes 50 percent of the oxidative metabolism (5,6).

Major interactions occur between the liver and kidneys. These interactions go substantially beyond the partitioning of function based on solubility or molecular size. For one, the liver, being the source of serum albumins and other proteins that bind xenobiotics, may alter their availability for renal excretion. By the same token, through xenobiotic metabolism, we may also have conversion into more polar entities, which are then excreted in the kidney. At the same time, this conversion may result in creation of new nephrotoxic entities (7,8).

Protein binding is extremely important with respect to the activity of xenobiotics and their glomerular filtration. In the serum there are simple, glyco-, lipo-, and metalloproteins. Their concentration is lower in immature organisms. In electrophoresis, the various fractions carry different component substances (Table 13-3). The glomerular segment of the kidneys is involved in regulating glomerular filtration. Molecular weight up to 7,000 can be easily filtered, although the process of glomerular filtration is not related solely to molecular size. The additional factors are the molecular charge and the charge of the filtration pores (6). These factors serve as a charge-selective filter, restricting negatively charged molecules more than neutral ones (due mainly to glycoproteins and glycosaminoglycans). On the other hand, transport of cationic molecules is facilitated. The protein-free solutes are filtered freely. The plasma-bound xenobiotics are retained as effectively as the protein itself (9).

The filtration is regulated by both hydrostatic and oncotic forces. The whole process is driven by the hydrostatic pressure. Xenobiotics that alter availability of catecholamines, dopamine, bradykinin, angiotensin II, antidiuretic hormone, or prostaglandins (especially PGE_2s) have the potential of nephrotoxicity by altering renal blood flow (10). Furthermore, they can cause contraction of intraglomerular mesangial cells, thus modulating glomerular function. The basement membrane of the renal corpuscle consists of type 4 and 5 collagens, collagenous and noncollagenous glycoproteins (negatively charged one is called podocalyxin), and proteoglycans (11,12,13).

According to the new nomenclature, the proximal tubules have been di-

Table 13-3. Carrier Components of Various Electrophoretic Fractions

Albumin	Ca^{++}
	Bilirubin
	Carrier proteins (nonspecific)
	Drugs (irrespective of whether they are acidic neutral, or basic)
	Free fatty acids
	Histamine
	Nutritional proteins
	Pathological proteins (usually denatured)
	Triiodothyronine
	Uric acid
	Vitamin C
Globulin α_1	Sialic acid
	Steroid hormones
	Thyroxine
	Vitamin B_{12}
Globulin α_2	Ceruloplasmin
	Haptoglobin
	Hemoglobin
	Hormonal transport (in general)
Globulin β_1	Transferrin
Globulin β_2	Carrier proteins (specific)
Globulin pre γ	Cryoglobulins
Globulin γ	Immunoglobulins
Globulins α_1, α_2, β_1, β_2	Coagulation factors
	Glycoproteins
	Metalloproteins
Globulins β_1, β_2	Cholesterol
	Lipoproteins
	Vitamins A, K, D, E

vided into segments because this allows for clearer correlations between structure and function. The most vulnerable part of the proximal tubules is the S_3 segment, because of its relationship with the venous blood from the inner medulla (14). In the rat and mouse, the epithelial cells of the upper descending thin limb of the long looped nephrons are joined by shallow, tight junctions. This causes paracellular shunts, resulting in transportation of solutes and water (15). Organic acids and bases are actively excreted. The maximal tubular excretion of para-aminohippurate (PAH) can be used to differentiate between a transportation (toxic) effect and one caused by reduction in renal plasma flow (12). Also important here is the existence of sulfhydryl groups on the enzymes of many tubular cells, because xenobiotics can directly inhibit such groups, thus interfering with tubular transportation (5). The collecting duct system is a major site of action for the antidiuretic hormone as well as for aldosterone (16). Figure 13-1 outlines some important endocrine relationships. Of special interest is the hormone-dependent nephrotoxicity of chloroform ($CHCl_3$) in mice (17).

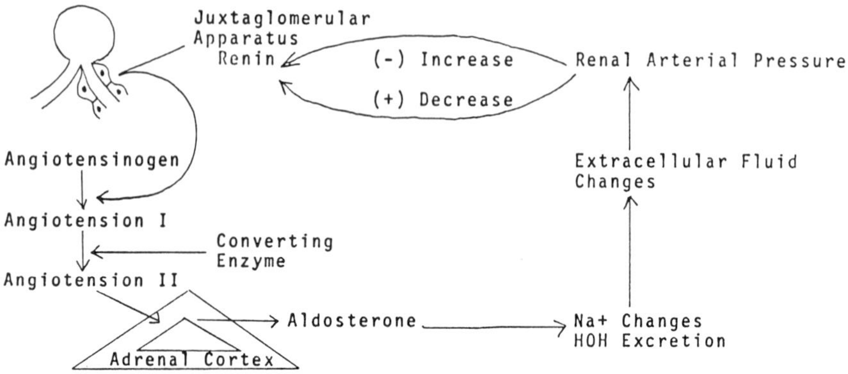

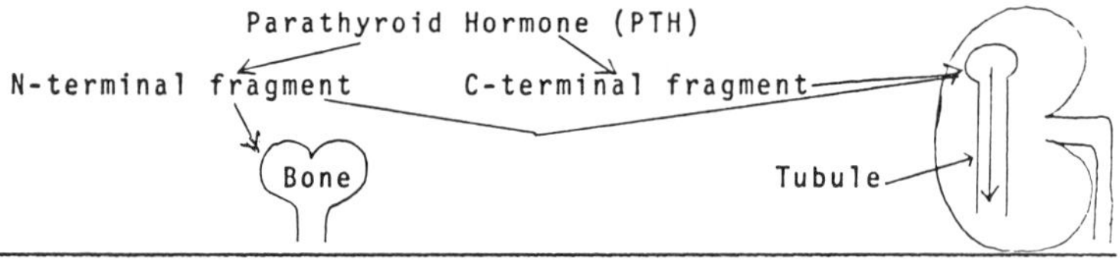

Male mouse	<27 days of age	No $CHCl_3$ renal necrosis (None)
Male mouse	>27 days of age	Necrosis (Ne)
Male mouse	<15 days of age + Testosterone	None
Male mouse	15-30 days of age + Testosterone	Ne
Male mouse	Castrated	Ne
Male mouse	Castrated + Adrenalectomized	None
Male mouse	Castrated + Testosterone	Ne
Male mouse	Castrated + Corticosteroids	Ne
Male mouse	Estrogens	Ne
Female mouse	Testerone	Ne

FIGURE 13-1.

RENAL TOXICITY

In principle, renal injury can occur from interference with circulation and the resulting hypoxia, degeneration, and necrosis, interference with the immune response pathways, and interference with growth and proliferation. The ways of response to renal toxic injury are therefore limited. For this purpose, similar morphologic derangements are repeatedly induced by different chemical substances. Even in the absence of xenobiotics, some dietary proteins, inappropriate caloric intake or utilization of nutrients, and excessive dissipation of heat can also cause renal injury (18).

In the adult kidney, the site of concentration of the xenobiotic is often the site of toxicity. Remote organs such as the liver, through manipulation of metabolic conversions into more polar or more toxic entities, or even through the fluctuations in the availability of carrier proteins, can substantially change renal toxicity (8). Remote or local endocrine or other vasoactive entities can likewise cause, directly or indirectly, renal injury by altering or redistributing renal blood flow (10). This can occur through contraction or dilation of vessels or shifts in acid base state (14). Interference with oxidative, glycolytic, metabolic, enzymatic, energy transfer, and active transport pathways can also cause renal injury. Alterations in protein binding, molecular, and filtration pore changes can likewise lead to toxicity (6,9). Even when the renal apparatus is functioning properly, prerenal as well as postrenal factors may interfere with renal function. For example, urinary obstruction causing azotemia (19) or the vesicoureteral reflux in rats can change the dynamics of xenobiotics, causing thus injury. Finally, one should always keep in mind the factor of development and aging (e.g., amyloid in human beings and in the mouse).

Some of the common pathogenic mechanisms (starting with the glomerulus/arterioles unit), including hypersensitivity (with the formation of antigen-antibody complexes), can be manifested as glomerulonephritis (which can occur also as membranoproliferative with or without crescent formation), glomerulopathies, polyarteritis nodosa, and necrotizing vasculitis. The pathogenic mechanisms of most proximal tubular lesions are direct degenerative/necrotic. In the more distal tubular segments, the underlying causes are ischemia, hypersensitivity, and direct degenerative/necrotic mechanisms. These tubular lesions are classified as interstitial nephritis and papillary necrosis.

Some basic, useful diagnostic rules are available (Table 13-4). Oliguria and polyuria are very helpful only when nonrenal factors can be excluded (3). Also serum creatinine, especially before the onset of azotemia, can be a very valuable tool. Proteinuria is likewise a very useful indicator (5). It

Table 13-4. Useful Clinical Findings Indicative of Renal Dysfunction Across Major Lab Animals and Human Beings

Site of lesion	Glomerular	Tubular
Urine volume	Anuria	Polyuria
Plasma BUN	Increased	Within normal limits (WNL)
Plasma creatinine	Increased	WNL
Plasma K	Increased	Decreased
Plasma phosphate	Increased	Decreased
Plasma urate	Increased	Decreased
Urine specific gravity	WNL	Decreased
Urine osmolality	WNL	Decreased
Urine pH	WNL	Decreased

can be practically classified by the molecular weight (MW) of occurring proteins into five types. The MW of the glomerular proteinuria (larger albumines) is 60,000–500,000. In the tubular proteinuria, the MW is 1,500–40,000 (mainly hormones, enzymes, peptides, and immunoproteins). The failure here is in the tubular reabsorption. In histuria, the MW is less than 90,000, and it is due primarily to tissue death, viral infections, and neoplasms. In secretory proteinuria, the MW is greater than 100,000 and consists of a glycoprotein (constituent of urinary casts or Tamm-Horsfall). It is localized at the thick ascending loop of Henle and comes about in response to increased concentration of electrolytes or immune complexes. The last one is the overflow proteinuria of an abnormal protein (Bence-Jones) of a molecular weight of less than 45,000, which is present at a concentration that exceeds the tubular capacity for reabsorption. In the rat, care must be taken in cases of marginal proteinurias, because this species has the tendency to demonstrate proteinuria under normal conditions (5).

RENAL XENOBIOTIC TOXICANTS

The proximal tubules, as stated earlier, are the target for most of the known nephrotoxic agents (Table 13-5). They are followed by the renal corpuscle, in particular the glomerulus. The hemodynamic/vascular site is followed by the distal interstitial sites, which in turn are followed by the distal tubular units. Many therapeutic entities involve two or three of these distinct sites, although not simultaneously. Some of their most prominent findings are depicted in Table 13-6. The pattern of involvement follows the intrarenal distribution of blood; external cortical regions are involved first and are then followed by the inner cortical, medullary, papillae, and interstitial connective tissue. Many of these chemical entities cause both acute and chronic types of injury.

One of the most important therapeutic classes is the antibiotics, which cause nephrotoxicity. These agents are further characterized by the absence of general pharmacologic activity (e.g., vasoactivity). Therefore, their dose is not limited by the general pharmacologic effect. Consequently, as a rule, high doses are administered. Of particular interest is the cephalosporin nephrotoxicity. Clinically, this nephrotoxicity is manifested in proteinuria, hematuria, and azotemia, with the damage usually reversible upon discontinuation (20). Cephaloridine seems to be the most nephrotoxic of all cephalosporins. The site is the proximal tubular brush border. There, interference with the amionic (carboxylic acid moiety function) and cationic (quaternary nitrogen of the pyridinium side chain) transport systems serves as the basis of toxicity (21). The tubular basement membrane is always preserved, explaining the reversibility of the process. The possibility of met-

Table 13-5. Target Structures of Known Nephrotoxic Agents

Arteriole/ Hemodynamic	Glomerulus	Proximal Tubules	Distal Tubules	Interstitum	Papilla
Allopurinol	Bacitracin	Aminoglycosides	Amphotericin B	Ampicillin	Aspirin
Cadmium	Bismuth tartrate	Amphotericin B	Lithium	Aspirin	Paracetamol
Carbon tetrachloride	D-Penicillamine	Bismuth	Vitamin D intoxication	Methicillin	Phenacetin
Iodides	Gold	Carbon tetrachloride		Paraacetomol	
Mercury	Heroin	Cephaloridine		Penicillin G	
Penicillin G	Hydrocarbons	Cephalothine		Phenindione	
Propylthiouracil	Hydralazine	Chromium		Rifampin	
Sulfonamide	Immunoglobulin G	Cisplatinum			
Thiazides	Kamamycin	Cyclosporine			
	Mercurial Diuretics	Ethylenidiamine tetracetic acid (EDTA)			
	Polymixin B	Gentamycin			
	Practolol	Glycols			
	Probenecid	Gold			
	Procainamide	Halothane			
	Sulfadiamine silver	Hydrocarbons[a]			
	Trimethadione	Kamamycin			
		Lead			
		Mercury			
		Merthoxyflurane			
		Neomycin			
		Polymixin B			
		Rifampin			
		Streptozotocin			
		Sulfonamides			
		Tetracyclines (degraded)			
		Tobramycin			
		Uranium			

[a]=Only in male rats and is due to an $alpha_2$ globulin.

Table 13-6. Selected Findings (Urinalysis) of Known Nephrotic Agents

Proteinuria	Hematuria
Aminoglycosides+	cpds+[a]
Bacitracin+	Acetalazolamide
Caffeine+	Anticoagulants
Carbamazepine	Capreomycin
Carbontetrachloride	Cyclophosphamide
Cephalosporins	Mefenamic acid
Clofibrate+	6-Mercaptopurine
D-Penicillamine+	Methotrexate
D-Serine	Mitotane
Glycols	Phenyclyclidine
Heavy metals+	Probenecid
Lithium	Thiazides
Merethoxylline procaine+	
Methenamine+	
Methicillin+	
Minocycline+	
Mithramycin	
Paramethadione	
Penicillin G+	
Phenylbutazones+	
Procainamide	
Rifampin+	
Salicylates+	
Theophylline+	
Tolbutamide	
Trichloroethylene	
Trimethadione	
Versenate+	

[a] cpds + = Compounds that show hematuria and proteinuria.

abolic transformation contributing to the toxicity should also be considered. This occurs through the formation of reactive epoxide from the thiophene ring (22).

SUMMARY

Renal toxicity comes about, in most cases, through a dynamic interplay of inappropriately functioning renal processes, ending with interruption of their equilibrium. Here the toxicodynamics are related to the plasma concentration of the toxic agent.

There are few important reasons why the kidney is disproportionately vulnerable to toxic injury. These reasons include the rich vascular perfusion, their enhanced concentration in the interstitium (because of medullary hypertonicity) and tubular epithelium, the great need for oxygen, the large endothelial cell surface area in the body (prone to immune complex deposition), and finally, the changes in the luminal urinary pH (prone to precipitation).

REFERENCES

1. B. M. Brenner and T. W. Meyer. Mechanisms of progression of renal disease. Pages 1233–1246 in: *Nephrology. Vol. 2. Proceedings of the Ninth International Congress of Nephrology*. R. R. Robinson, ed. Springer-Verlag, New York. (1984).
2. A P. Evan, P. Blomgren, L. C. Knopp, and G. A. Tanner. Proximal tubular morphology after single nephron obstruction in the rat kidney. Kidney Int. *27,* 231A (1985).
3. J. T. Harrington and J. J. Cohen. Measurement of urinary electrolytes, indications and limitations. New Eng. J. Med. *293,* 1241–1244 (1975).
4. W. Kriz and H. Koepsell. The structural organization of the mouse kidney. Z. Anat. Entwoicl.-Gesch. *144,* 137–163 (1974).
5. K. C. Bovee. Renal function and laboratory evaluation. Toxicol. Path. *14,* 26–44 (1986).
6. W. O. Berndt. Use of renal function test in the evaluation of nephrotoxic effects. Pages 1–29: *Toxicology of the Kidney*. J. B. Hook, ed. Raven Press, New York (1981).
7. M. R. Boyd and J. S. Dutcher. Role of renal metabolism in the pathogenesis of renal cortical necrosis produced by 4-Ipomeanol in the mouse. Toxicol. Appl. Pharmacol. *45,* 229 (1978).
8. J. B. Pritchard. Renal handling of environmental chemicals. Pages 99–116 in: *Toxicology of the Kidney*. J. B. Hook, ed. Raven Press, New York (1981).
9. E. M. Renkin and J. P. Gilmore. Glomerular filtration. Pages 185–248 in: *Handbook of Physiology*. J. Orloff and R. W. Berliner, eds. American Physiological Society, Washington, DC (1973).
10. D. M. Clive and J. S. Stoff. Renal syndromes associated with nonsteroidal anti-inflammatory drugs. New Engl. J. Med. *310,* 563–572 (1984).
11. D. A. Ansiello, J. I. Kreisberg, C. Roy, and M. J. Karnovsky. Contraction of cultured rat glomerular cells of apparent mesangial origin after stimulation with Angiotensin II and arginine vasopressin. J. Clin. Invest. *65,* 754–760 (1980).
12. E. H. Foulkes. Effects of nephrotoxins on renal clearance. Pages 57–76 in: *Toxicology of the Kidney*. J. B. Hook, ed. Raven Press, New York. (1981).
13. D. Kerjaschki, D. J. Sharkey, and M. G. Farquhar. Identification and characterization of podocalyxin. J. Cell Biol. *98,* 1591–1596 (1984).
14. W. Kriz. Structural organization of the renal medullary counterflow system. Fed. proc. *42,* 2379–2385 (1983).
15. W. Kriz, J. Schnermann, and H. J. Dietrich. Differences in the morphology of descending limbs of short and long loops of Henle in the rat kidney. Pages 140–144 in: *Recent Advanes in Renal Physiology*. W. Kriz and F. Spinelli, eds. S. Karger, Basel (1972).
16. D. Marver. Evidence of corticosteroid action along the nephron. Am. J. Physiol. *246,* F111–F123 (1984).
17. D. Culliford and H. B. Hewitt. The influence of sex hormones on susceptibility of mice to chloroform-induced necrosis of the renal tubules. J. Endocrinol. *14,* 381–393 (1957).
18. G. A. Kaysen, W. G. Kirkpatrick, and W. G. Couser. Albumin homeostasis in the nephrotic rat. Nutritional consideration. Amer. J. Physiol. *247,* F192-F202 (1984).
19. G. Levy. Some Pharmacodynamic Aspects of Toxicokinetics. Pages 97–107 in: *Toxicokinetics and New Drug Development*. A. Yacobi, J. P. Skelly, and V. K. Batra, eds. Pergamon Press, Elmsford, NY (In press).

20. K. M. McCormack, J. B. Hook, and J. E. Gibson. Developmental anomalies of the kidney. Pages 227–250 in: *Toxicology of the Kidney*. J. B. Hook, ed. Raven Press, New York (1981).
21. J. S. Wold. Cephalosporin nephrotoxicity. Pages 251–266 in: *Toxicology of the Kidney*. J. B. Hook, ed. Raven Press, New York (1981).
22. J. R. Mitchell, R. J. McMurtry, C. N. Statham, and S. D. Nelson. Molecular basis for several drug-induced nephropathies. Am. J. Med. *62*, 518–526 (1977).

Chapter 14

Selection and Evaluation of Drug Delivery Systems for Toxicology Studies—Transdermal Dosage Forms

Vijay K. Batra, Gabriela Nicolau, A. Tonelli, John A. Morrison, and Avraham Yacobi

Pharmacodynamic Research
Medical Research Division
American Cyanamid Company

ABSTRACT

To substantiate safety evaluation of a new drug, a series of drug-disposition studies including determination of concentrations in blood and tissues are essential. This is also true for transdermal dosage forms intended for acute or chronic therapy. However, selection of a practical and reliable animal model requires careful studies to assure absorption of the drug and attainment of effective blood drug concentrations in the body.

Viprostol (I), an antihypertensive prostaglandin (1), is currently being administered transdermally in clinical trials. Transdermal absorption of ^{14}C-I, investigated in several species, indicated good absorption only in relatively small animals (mouse, rat, rabbit). To support chronic toxicity studies in large species such as the dog, the absorption of ^{14}C-labeled I was investigated following topical, subcutaneous, and oral administration. Transdermal release into the systemic circulation following topical administration was very slow because of extensive and persistent skin deposition (only about 5% of a 1 mg/kg dose was absorbed by 144 hr). Because of this poor absorption, chronic transdermal safety evaluation studies could not have generated the broad range of blood drug concentrations and toxicities required for safety evaluation studies. Hence, an alternative, more viable, route of chronic drug administration was sought.

Viprostol is completely absorbed following subcutaneous (SC) administration. As in transdermal administration, the antihypertensive effect lasted significantly longer than it did following IV dosing. The prolonged activity may be due in part to the skin acting as a depot that releases the drug gradually. This is suggested by the high affinity of I for the viable layers of the skin at the injection site. SC administration was therefore considered a viable route to support chronic toxicology studies in the dog.

INTRODUCTION

The importance of disposition studies in support of drug safety evaluation has been widely discussed and accepted. These studies are essential regardless of the route of administration of the test drug, with the ultimate goal being the association of pharmacological-toxicological response with the concentrations of the drug or active metabolites in the blood. Because of this, it becomes imperative that the absorption of the drug in the animal model is verified and substantiated using the test drug administered in a test vehicle.

Advances in drug delivery systems have made possible the administration of many existing and new therapeutic agents via the percutaneous route. In drug safety evaluation, transdermal dosage forms present a somewhat different problem because of the marked variations in skin effectiveness as a barrier between species. The process of transdermal absorption is not yet completely understood. Absorption through the skin can vary significantly among and within species, depending on where and how the drug is applied. Some factors that might affect the transdermal absorption of drugs are as follows:

1. Skin conditions: Thickness of stratum corneum, surface, site of application, pigmentation, age of the skin
2. Physical-chemical characteristics of the drug: lipophilicity and partition coefficient, volatility
3. Vehicle effects: Dosage form and concentration of drug in vehicle, the presence of penetration enhancers and mode of application on the skin
4. Environmental factors: Temperature and degree of hydration of the skin due to humidity
5. Pathological state: Skin irritation, dermatitis, psoriasis, acne, etc

6. Physiological factors: Metabolism in the skin, binding to the site of application or in the skin, blood supply, absorption mechanism, and frequency of drug application on the same site.

Chronic toxicology studies are both costly and time consuming. The most suitable transdermal dosage form that will ensure the absorption of the drug from the site of application and the presence of adequate concentrations of the test compound in blood and other biological fluids must be defined. These criteria are needed to elicit the full range of pharmacological-toxicological responses in the test species. Therefore, carefully planned pharmacodynamic and pharmacokinetic studies can be instrumental in the design of safety evaluation studies.

Ideally, the safety evaluation of drugs intended for percutaneous administration should be tested by application of the transdermal delivery system on the skin of the test species. However, several limitations might preclude the possibility of safety evaluations of such dosage forms in animals. Traditionally, potent drugs, possessing a very short biological half-life, extensive first-pass metabolism when given orally, short duration of action, and relatively narrow therapeutic index have been targeted for percutaneous application. Such agents are applied on the skin for a relatively long period of time to obtain continuous absorption and exertion of pharmacological action. Since the intended dose is relatively small, quantitation of drug or metabolite concentrations in biological fluids can be difficult. In these cases, a more suitable procedure for documentation of drug absorption is often the measurement of pharmacological-toxicological action.

The transdermal mode of drug administration during a chronic or subchronic safety evaluation will be limited to those species that retain the delivery system or the dosage form on the body without undue restrain and exhibit good skin-permeation characteristics. This will require screening of various models by both pharmacokinetic and pharmacodynamic procedures. Because the transdermal application or absorption may not be feasible in some animals, alternative modes of administration for conduction of safety evaluations must be carefully examined and considered. For this purpose, thorough pharmacokinetic-pharmacodynamic input is needed to design optimal safety evaluation studies.

Viprostol (I) is a synthetic prostaglandin effective in the reduction of blood pressure after intravenous, oral, and transdermal administration (1). It is a very potent compound with a short biological half-life in animals and human beings. In the body, viprostol undergoes rapid deesterification to the corresponding free acid (II), which is equally active in lowering blood pressure in animals and human beings (Fig. 14-1). The corresponding free acid (II) also has a short biologic half-life in animals (<30 min) and is the only measurable active compound in blood and other biologic specimens (2,3). Viprostol's duration of action is significantly longer following topical

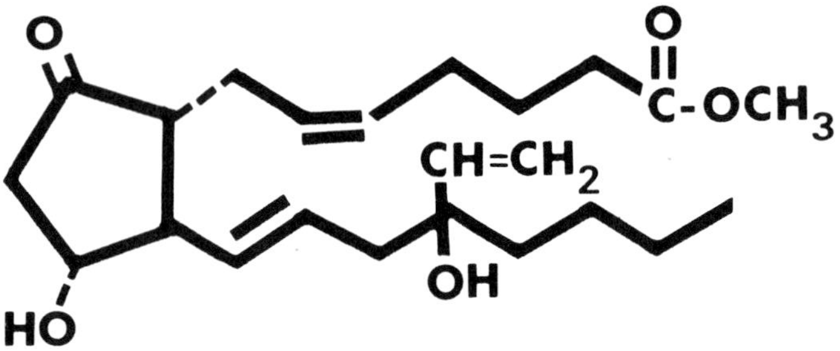

I

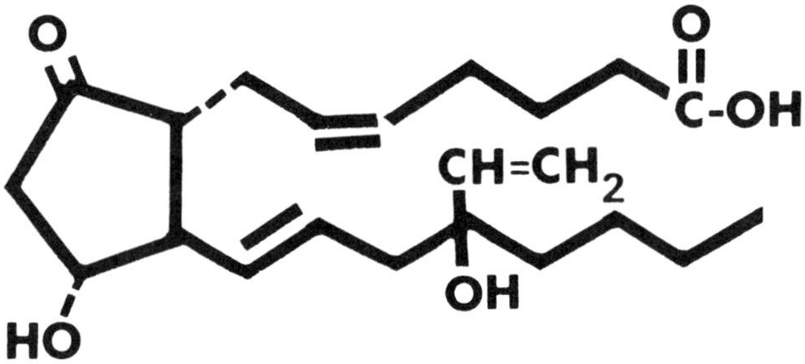

II

FIGURE 14-1. Chemical structure of viprostol (I) and the corresponding free acid (II).

administration than following oral or intravenous administration in rats. Following selection of viprostol for clinical development, drug-disposition studies to support safety evaluation were conducted in several species using carbon-14 material labeled at position C-5.[1] The results of these studies are described below.

Evaluation of Transdermal Absorption

Rat

Absorption Profile. The initial disposition studies of viprostol were conducted in the rat (2). The objectives of these studies were to compare the pharmacokinetics of drug absorption after single (1 mg/kg) topical and in-

[1]Chemical Process Research and Development, Medical Research Division, American Cyanamid Company, Pearl River, NY.

travenous ^{14}C-I administration. The drug was applied topically after removing hair from a 4 in.^{2} abdominal surface area of restrained and lightly anesthetized rats. The plasma concentration-time profiles of ^{14}C-I (total radioactivity) are shown in Figure 14-2. Transdermal absorption following topical administration was rapid, as indicated by the significant concentrations of ^{14}C-I in plasma observed within five minutes after dosing. Concentrations increased to a peak value of 200 ng/ml by one hour, plateaued at about this concentration for eight hours, and then decreased steadily. In contrast, the plasma ^{14}C-I concentration following intravenous administration declined rapidly. The data indicated that the longer duration of action observed following topical administration was probably due to rapid penetration and deposition of ^{14}C-I in the skin at the application site followed by sustained release into the systemic circulation.

Selection of Dosage Form. Two transdermal dosage forms, one as an ointment in petrolatum and the other as a viscous solution in triethylcitrate (TEC), were proposed for the safety evaluation studies. To determine which of the dosage forms had better drug delivery characteristics, a study was undertaken in the rat. Single 1 mg/kg doses of ^{14}C-I, either in petrolatum or TEC, were applied over a 4 in.^{2} abdominal surface area. The plasma concentration-time data are shown in Figure 14-3. The TEC formulation as compared to the petrolatum formulation resulted in significantly lower ^{14}C-I concentrations. Complete absorption of the drug occurred from the pet-

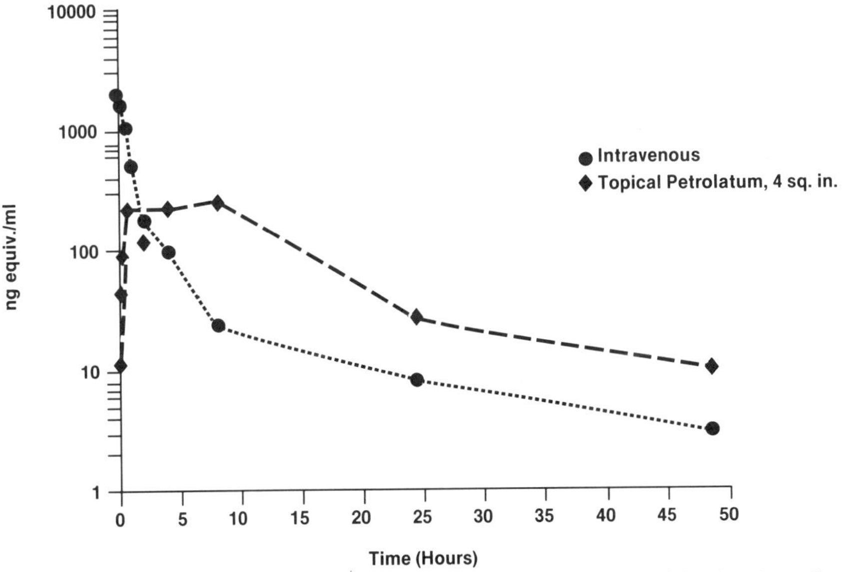

FIGURE 14-2. Plasma concentrations of total radioactivity in the rat following 2 mg/kg intravenous and topical dosing of viprostol. ● = Intravenous; ◆ = topical petrolatum, 4 in.^{2}.

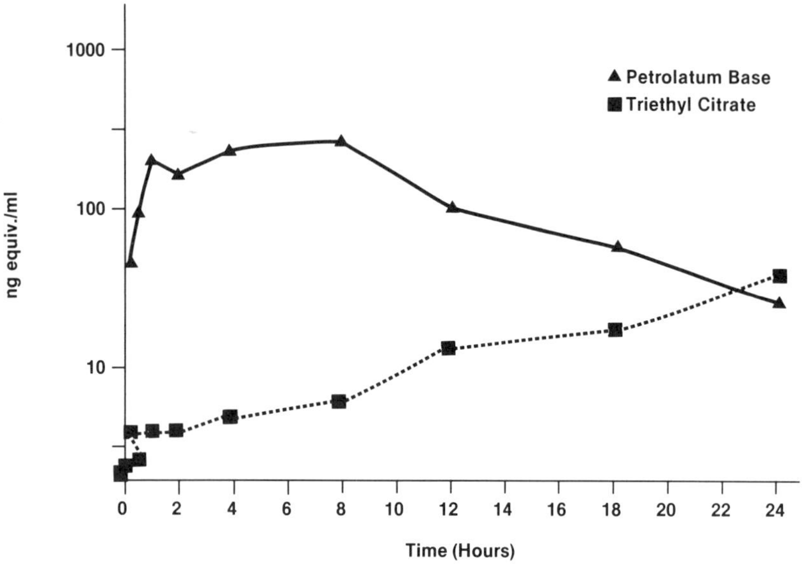

FIGURE 14-3. Rat plasma concentrations of total radioactivity following 1 mg/kg topical administration of ^{14}C-I in petrolatum base or triethylcitrate. ▲ = Petrolatum base; ■ = triethyl citrate.

rolatum base ointment by 24 hours, whereas only 36 percent of the dose was absorbed from the TEC formulation. Consequently, the TEC transdermal dosage form was not considered to be appropriate for the safety evaluation studies.

Effect of Surface Area. For drugs that have good skin-permeation characteristics, the surface area of application should have little effect on transdermal absorption. However, for drugs with poor or moderate skin-permeation characteristics, the surface area to which the drug is applied can significantly affect transdermal absorption.

A study was undertaken in the rat to determine whether the drug application surface area affected transdermal absorption ^{14}C-I. Single doses of ^{14}C-I ranging from 0.1 to 1 mg/kg were applied in 100 mg of petrolatum over abdominal surface areas of 1 to 6 in.^{2} The data obtained are listed in Table 14-1. The 0–24-hour area under the plasma concentration-time curve (AUC) following the 1 mg/kg dose increased as the surface area was increased from 1 to 2.5 in.^{2} but plateaued thereafter. The AUCs from surface areas of 2.5, 4, and 6 in.^{2} were not significantly different from each other, indicating that increasing the application on surface area beyond 2.5 in.^{2} had no effect on the transdermal absorption of ^{14}C-I. By 24 hours after dose application, the extent of absorption from the 2.5-in.^{2} application surface area and above was greater than 90 percent as compared to 70 percent from

Table 14-1. Absorption of Viprostol in Rats: Effect of Application Surface Area on Drug Absorption

Dose (mg/kg)	Route	Area (in.^{2})	Absorption[a] (% of Dose)	AUC[b] (μg.hr/ml)	C_{max}[c] (ng/ml)	T_{max}[d] (hr)
0.1	Topical	6	85	201	22	1
		4	73	172	25	1
		1	56	132	18	1
1.0	Topical	6	91	2,148	335	1
		4	91	2,153	247	1
		2.5	91	2,158	267	0.5
		2	80	1,891	244	2
		1	70	1,655	144	1
1.0	i.v.	—	—	2,364	—	—

[a]Systemic absorption $= \frac{(AUC)_{0-24}\text{ hr, topical}}{(AUC)_{0-24}\text{ hr, i.v.}}$

[b]Area under the curve, 0–24 hr (total radioactivity).

[c]Peak plasma concentration.

[d]Time of peak concentration.

[e]— = Not applicable.

the 1 in.^{2} surface area. The systemic absorption at the 0.1 mg/kg dose increased from 56 to 85 percent as the application area was increased from 1 to 4 in.^{2}. The AUC values were about one-tenth of those obtained following the 1 mg/kg dose, indicating dose-related transdermal absorption. The findings from this study indicate that the 4 in.^{2} application area chosen in most of our transdermal studies in the rat was appropriate in that the animals were well exposed to the drug.

Mouse. To investigate the performance of the petrolatum dosage form in the mouse, single doses of 1.9 mg/kg were administered topically and intravenously to two groups of mice (3). The drug was applied on the upper dorsal site of the animals and left on the skin (occluded) for various time intervals up to 24 hr. The resulting plasma ^{14}C-I concentration-time profiles of total radioactivity are shown in Figure 14-4. The data show concentration-time profiles similar to those seen in the rat, but with an earlier T_{max} and shorter duration of the plateau.

Monkey. To evaluate transdermal absorption in the monkey, single doses of ^{14}C-I were administered intravenously, topically, and orally to six monkeys in a three-way crossover design (4). The doses were 1 mg/kg for the topical and oral administration and 0.1 mg/kg for intravenous administration. For topical administration, the drug in petrolatum base was applied over a 25 cm^2 shaven area on the lower lateral back site. For the oral administration,

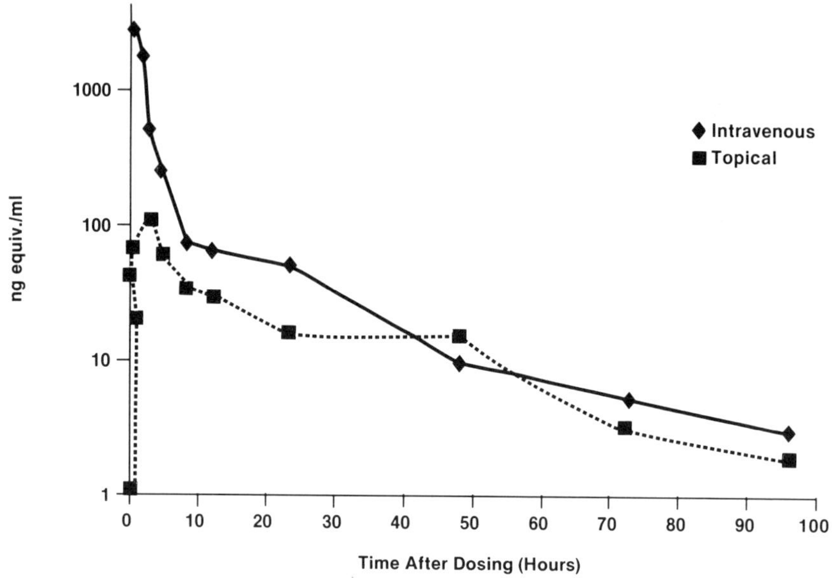

FIGURE 14-4. Serum concentrations of total radioactivity in the mouse following 1.9 mg/kg intravenous and topical administration of viprostol. ◆ = Intravenous; ■ = topical.

^{14}C-I was dissolved in Neobee and given via narogastric intubation. The plasma ^{14}C-I equivalent concentration-time profiles generated from the study are shown in Figure 14-5. The concentration values for the 1 mg/kg intravenous dose plotted in the figure are the extrapolated values (dose normalized) from the lower dose, assuming linear pharmacokinetics. Absorption (total radioactivity) following oral dosing was moderately rapid, with serum ^{14}C-I levels peaking at 2–4 hr. Significantly lower serum levels of total radioactivity were seen following topical administration, with peak times occurring very late, indicating a slow and sustained transdermal release or absorption. It is estimated that 31 percent of the dose (drug-related radioactivity) was absorbed following oral administration and only 5 percent following topical administration.

Dog. To support safety evaluation in large species, the dog was evaluated for transdermal absorption of I. Groups of three dogs each were administered single doses of ^{14}C-I intravenously (0.65 mg/kg), orally (1 mg/kg), and topically (1 mg/kg). The petrolatum ointment containing the drug was applied on the back of the dogs on a shaven 8 in.^{2} area and the application site occluded. The plasma concentrations of ^{14}C-I (total radioactivity) as a function of time for all three routes of administration are plotted in Figure 14-6. Following oral administration, the drug was absorbed rapidly, exhibiting a peak concentration of 121 ng equiv/ml in about 2 hr. In contrast,

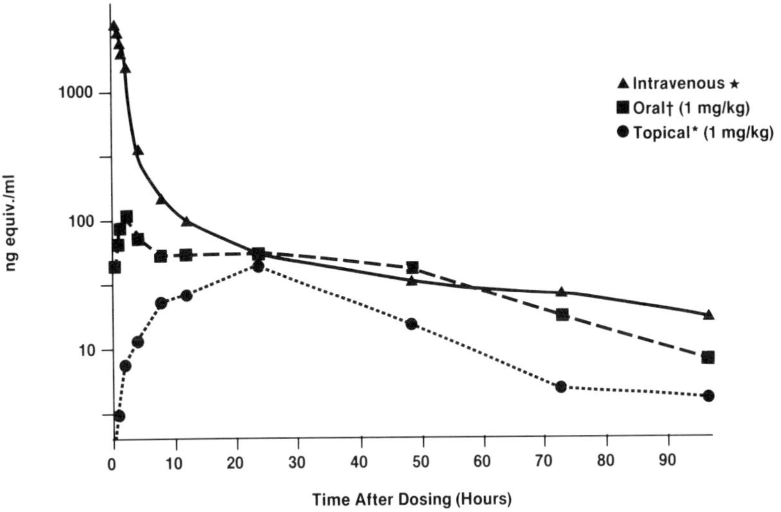

*Mean from two monkeys
†Mean from three monkeys
★ Intravenous data was extrapolated from a lower dose assuming linear pharmacokinetics

FIGURE 14-5. Serum concentrations of total radioactivity in the monkey after oral, topical, and intravenous administration of viprostol. ▲ = Intravenous (data extrapolated from a lower dose assuming linear pharmacokinetics; ■ = oral (1 mg/kg) (mean from three monkeys); ● = topical (1 mg/kg) (mean from two monkeys).

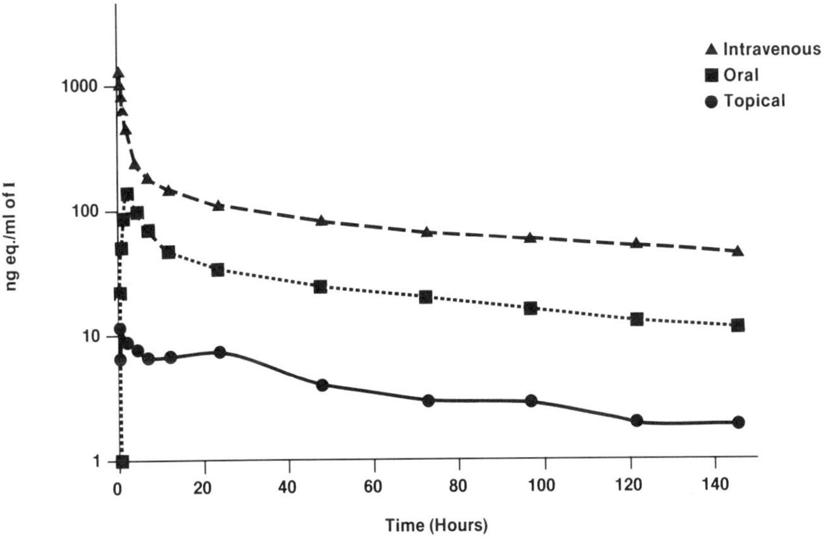

FIGURE 14-6. Plasma concentrations of total radioactivity in the dog following 1 mg/kg intravenous, oral and topical administration of viprostol. ▲ = Intravenous; ■ = oral; ● = topical.

the topically applied dose was absorbed very slowly, attaining a peak concentration of only 12 ng equiv/ml, and showing persistently low plasma ^{14}C-I levels (7–10 ng/ml) up to 24 hr after dosing. The 0–144-hour area under the plasma concentration-time curve was only 2 percent of that following intravenous dosing, indicating poor transdermal absorption. Urine was also collected in these dogs, and the urinary drug-excretion data were consistent with the plasma concentration data (Table 14-2). The mean percentages of ^{14}C-I dose recovered in urine over 10 days was 45.5 percent following intravenous administration, 25.8 percent following oral administration, and only 2.4 percent following topical administration. Based on these percentages, it is estimated that 57 percent of the oral and only 5 percent of the topical dose were absorbed.

Species Differences

Pharmacokinetic studies similar to those described above were also conducted in the guinea pig and the rabbit (3). Relevant absorption parameters comparing transdermal delivery performance among all tested species are shown in Table 14-3. In most of the transdermal studies, the excess topical dose was removed 12–24 hours after application, counted, and the resulting value subtracted from the applied dose to obtain the amount of drug that actually penetrated the skin. This penetration value, expressed as a percentage of the applied dose, varied from a value of 49 in the dog to 95 in the rat. The monkey, guinea pig, and rabbit exhibited similar skin-penetration values (76–86%). In the rat and mouse, almost all of the penetrated dose was released by skin into the systemic circulation by 24 hr after dosing. In all other species, the systemic absorption values were lower than the penetration values, indicating that not all of the penetrated dose was released for systemic absorption over the course of the study. These data, as well as data from skin deposition studies in several species (5), suggest that the skin

Table 14-2. Percent of Dose Absorbed in the Dog Based on the Urinary Excretion Data

Route	Dog No.	Excretion[a] 0–144 hr	Percent Absorption	Mean Absorption
IV	9	45.5	100	—[b]
Oral	1	33.9	75	
	2	17.2	38	56.7
	3	21.7	48	
Topical	5	3.4	7.5	5.3
	6	1.3	2.9	

[a]Expressed as percentage of applied dose.

[b]— = Not applicable.

Table 14-3. Summary of Viprostol Studies Conducted by the Transdermal Route

	Rat	Mouse	Monkey	Dog	Guinea Pig	Rabbit
Dose (mg/kg)	1	1.9	1	1	1	1
Surface area (cm^2)	25	1.5	25	50	10	37
Skin penetration (by 24 hr)	95%	56%	76%	49%	86%	84%
Systemic absorption (calculated from serum concentrations topical/IV)	>90%	46%	5%	2%	No IV data	23%
Peak serum concentration (ng equiv/ml)	200	83	43	12	18	75

Note: Values corrected for dose equivalence assuming linear pharmacokinetics.

sequesters the drug to a varying extent depending upon the species and site, and then releases it into the systemic circulation at a sustained rate. The skin thus acts as a natural reservoir or delivery system for ^{14}C-I. The ability to release the drug following penetration varied considerably among species, being relatively rapid in the rat and mouse, moderate in the rabbit, and poor in the monkey and dog. About 4.7 percent of the penetrated dose remained in the skin of the dog at the application site 20 days after dosing. The systemic availability in the guinea pig could not be calculated becuse of the absence of intravenous data.

Safety Evaluation Route in the Dog

From the above studies, it was concluded that the topical route was not appropriate for safety evaluation studies in the dog because of the poor transdermal drug-release characteristics. However, the dog was considered to be a reliable and practical animal model for toxicity testing. The subcutaneous route was considered as a possible alternative route. The suitability of the model was tested by pharmacokinetic-pharmacodynamics studies. The study was done in a two-way cross-over design with about three weeks of washout period between the two phases. In the first phase, two dogs were given ^{14}C-I intravenously and two subcutaneously. In the second phase, the dogs were switched to the other route. The dosage for this study, selected based on initial toxicology range-finding studies, was 0.15 mg/kg. Following dosing, several blood samples were withdrawn at predetermined time intervals, and arterial blood pressure measurement readings were also made at the same time. The dogs were restrained on a specially designed table during the first 2–6 hours of the study to facilitate blood pressure measurements. A representative serum concentration-time plot of total radioactivity and the mean

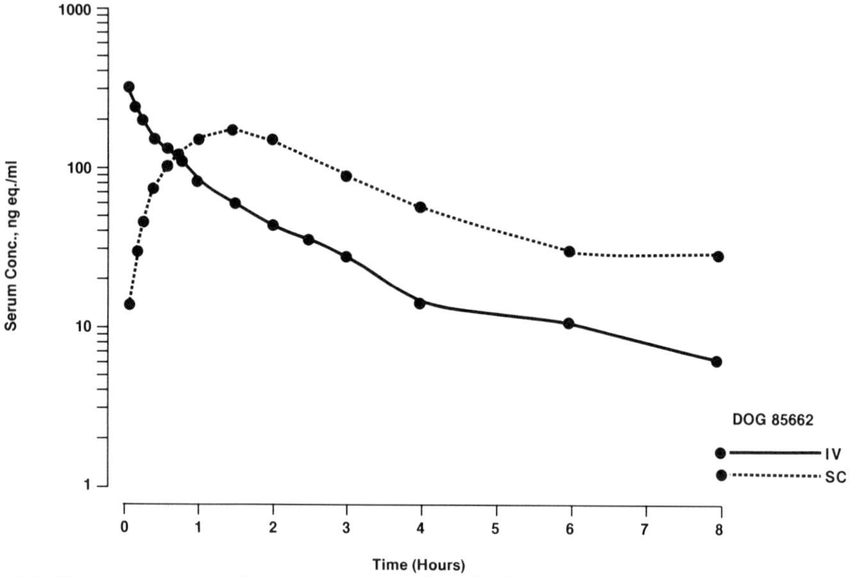

FIGURE 14-7. Serum radioactivity concentrations in dog 80716 following intravenous and subcutaneous administration of 150 μg/kg of ^{14}C-I.

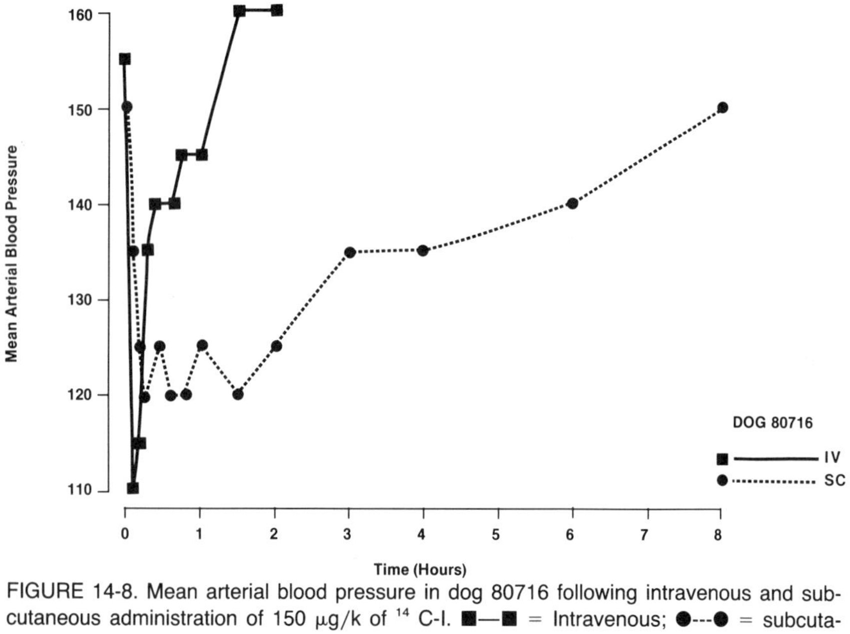

FIGURE 14-8. Mean arterial blood pressure in dog 80716 following intravenous and subcutaneous administration of 150 μg/k of ^{14} C-I. ■—■ = Intravenous; ●---● = subcutaneous.

arterial blood pressure-time plot from one of the dogs are shown in Figures 14-7 and 14-8, respectively.

The data show that absorption following subcutaneous administration was complete within 2 to 5 hours after dosing. There was a corresponding significant reduction in mean arterial blood pressure over the same period of time. The ^{14}C-I concentrations between the 0.75- and 2-hr interval were similar, giving rise to a plateau effect observed in other species following topical administration. After intravenous administration, blood pressure was reduced almost instantly, followed by a relatively shorter recovery period than that after subcutaneous administration. Thus, like the topical route in other species, the subcutaneous route in the dog provided a hypotensive response for a duration longer than that following intravenous administration. The subcutaneous route was therefore considered a viable route for evaluating chronic toxicity studies in the dog.

SUMMARY

To support the drug safety evaluations of a potent agent such as viprostol, a series of studies in various animal models were conducted. Several factors in a selection of animal model and an alternative route of administration were considered:

1. Because viprostol and the corresponding free acid are very potent, their plasma concentrations could not be measured readily by conventional procedures. ^{14}C-I enabled us to provide estimates of drug penetration into the skin and systemic absorption. The concentrations of unchanged active moieties, however, were so low that pharmacodynamics measurement provided the most reliable data.
2. Several species—mice, rats, and rabbits—showed good transdermal absorption and were useful for safety evaluation in the rodent species. The dog is the most practical animal model for large animal–second species chronic and subchronic toxicity studies, but it showed very poor transdermal absorption.
3. To develop a practical model for safety evaluation of viprostol, the subcutaneous route of administration was contemplated. Through pharmacodynamics and pharmacokinetic studies, subcutaneous administration of viprostol was verified to be a suitable route of drug delivery in dogs.

ACKNOWLEDGMENTS

The authors gratefully acknowledge the support of the scientific staff of Formulation Research, Medical Research Division, American Cyanamid, for preparing the drug formulation and the scientific and technical staff of Pharmacodynamics Research for conducting these studies.

REFERENCES

1. P. S. Chan, P. Cervoni, M. A. Rosenberg, R. C. Accomando, G. J. Quirk, P. A. Scully, and L. M. Lipchuck. Antihypertensive activity of dl-15-deoxy-16-hydroxy-16 (α/β)-vinyl prostaglandin E2 methyl ester (CL 115,347), a new orally and transdermally long-acting anti-hypertensive agent. J. Pharmacol. and Expt. Therap. *22,* 726 (1983).
2. G. Nicolau, V. K. Batra, S. Gordon, A. Tonelli, and W. McWilliams. Transdermal absorption of DHV-PGE2 prostaglandin in the rat. Abstracts, Fifth International Conference on Prostaglandins, Florence (Italy), May 18–21, (1982).
3. G. Nicolau, V. K. Batra, S. Gordon, A. Tonelli, W. McWilliams, and M. S. Pruzinski. Transdermal absorption of methyl-DHV-PGE2 prostaglandin in laboratory animals. Abstracts, Acad Pharm. Sci. *13,* 209 (1983).
4. G. Nicolau, A. P. Tonelli, D. B. Cosulich, N. A. Perkinson, A. T. DiCioccio, W. E. McWilliams, and A. Yacobi. Pre-systemic metabolism of viprostol in the monkey following oral and topical administration. Xenobiotica, *18* (7), 797–802 (1988) (In Press).
5. G. Nicolau, R. A. Baughman, A. Tonelli, W. McWilliams, J. Schiltz, and A. Yacobi. Deposition of viprostol (a synthetic PGE_2 vasodilator) in the skin following topical administration to laboratory animals. Xenobiotica *17* (9), 1113–1120 (1987).

Index